Skull Base Neuroimaging

Editor

STEVE E.J. CONNOR

NEUROIMAGING CLINICS OF NORTH AMERICA

www.neuroimaging.theclinics.com

Consulting Editor
SURESH K. MUKHERJI

November 2021 • Volume 31 • Number 4

ELSEVIER

1600 John F. Kennedy Boulevard • Suite 1800 • Philadelphia, Pennsylvania, 19103-2899

http://www.neuroimaging.theclinics.com

NEUROIMAGING CLINICS OF NORTH AMERICA Volume 31, Number 4
November 2021 ISSN 1052-5149, ISBN 13: 978-0-323-73410-3

Editor: John Vassallo (j.vassallo@elsevier.com)
Developmental Editor: Karen Solomon

Neuroimaging Clinics of North America (ISSN 1052-5149) is published quarterly by Elsevier Inc., 360 Park Avenue South, New York, NY 10010-1710. Months of issue are February, May, August, and November. Business and editorial offices: 1600 John F. Kennedy Blvd., Suite 1800, Philadelphia, PA 19103-2899. Business and editorial offices: 6277 Sea Harbor Drive, Orlando, FL 32887-4800. Periodicals postage paid at New York, NY, and additional mailing offices. Subscription prices are USD 397 per year for US individuals, USD 918 per year for US institutions, USD 100 per year for US students and residents, USD 465 per year for Canadian individuals, USD 959 per year for Canadian institutions, USD 541 per year for international individuals, USD 959 per year for international institutions, USD 100 per year for Canadian students and residents and USD 260 per year for foreign students and residents. To receive student/resident rate, orders must be accompanied by name of affiliated institution, date of term, and the *signature* of program/residency coordinator on institution letterhead. Orders will be billed at individual rate until proof of status is received. Foreign air speed delivery is included in all *Clinics* subscription prices. All prices are subject to change without notice. POSTMASTER: Send address changes to *Neuroimaging Clinics of North America*, Elsevier Health Sciences Division, Subscription **Customer Service, 3251 Riverport Lane, Maryland Heights, MO 63043. Telephone: 1-800-654-2452 (U.S. and Canada); 314-447-8871 (outside U.S. and Canada). Fax: 314-447-8029. E-mail: journalscustomerservice-usa@elsevier.com (for print support); journalsonlinesupport-usa@elsevier.com (for online support).**

Reprints. For copies of 100 or more of articles in this publication, please contact the Commercial Reprints Department, Elsevier Inc., 360 Park Avenue South, New York, NY 10010-1710. Tel.: 212-633-3874; Fax: 212-633-3820; E-mail: reprints@elsevier.com.

Neuroimaging Clinics of North America is covered by *Excerpta Medical/EMBASE,* the RSNA Index of Imaging Literature, *MEDLINE/PubMed (Index Medicus),* MEDLINE/MEDLARS, SciSearch, Research Alert, and Neuroscience Citation Index.

PROGRAM OBJECTIVE
The goal of Neuroimaging Clinics of North America is to keep practicing radiologists and radiology residents up to date with current clinical practice in radiology by providing timely articles reviewing the state of the art in patient care.

TARGET AUDIENCE
Practicing radiologists, radiology residents, and other healthcare professionals who utilize neuroimaging findings to provide patient care.

LEARNING OBJECTIVES
Upon completion of this activity, participants will be able to:
1. Review the diversity of skull base tumours and the role of imaging in their diagnosis and management.
2. Discuss the proximity of pathology to functionally important anatomical structures of the skull base.
3. Recognize how dedicated imaging protocols can be optimised for the demonstration of skull base pathologies and tailored to the particular specific tumour, region or condition.

ACCREDITATION
The Elsevier Office of Continuing Medical Education (EOCME) is accredited by the Accreditation Council for Continuing Medical Education (ACCME) to provide continuing medical education for physicians.

The EOCME designates this journal-based CME activity for a maximum of 14 *AMA PRA Category 1 Credit*(s)™. Physicians should claim only the credit commensurate with the extent of their participation in the activity.

All other healthcare professionals requesting continuing education credit for this enduring material will be issued a certificate of participation.

DISCLOSURE OF CONFLICTS OF INTEREST
The EOCME assesses conflict of interest with its instructors, faculty, planners, and other individuals who are in a position to control the content of CME activities. All relevant conflicts of interest that are identified are thoroughly vetted by EOCME for fair balance, scientific objectivity, and patient care recommendations. EOCME is committed to providing its learners with CME activities that promote improvements or quality in healthcare and not a specific proprietary business or a commercial interest.

The planning committee, staff, authors, and editors listed below have identified no financial relationships or relationships to products or devices they or their spouse/life partner have with commercial interest related to the content of this CME activity:
Ashok Adams, MBBS, BSc(Hons), EDiNR, MRCP, FRCR; Rudolf Boeddinghaus, MBChB, FCRad(D)SA, FRANZCR, FRCR; Andrea Borghesi, MD; Neeraj Chaudhary, MD, MRCS, FRCR, FACR, FAHA, FEBNI; Regina Chavous-Gibson, MSN, RN; Steve E.J. Connor, MRCP, FRCR; Davide Farina, MD; Joseph J. Gemmete, MD, FACR, FSIR, FAHA, FCIRSE; Pradeep Kuttysankaran; Leanne Lin, MD, MPHS; Ravi Kumar Lingam, MB BCh, MRCP, FRCR, EDiHNR; Davide Lombardi, MD; Roberto Maroldi, MD; Burce Ozgen Mocan, MD; Aditya S. Pandey, MD; Carlotta Pessina, MD; Gillian M. Potter, MBChB, MD, MRCP, FRCR; Marco Ravanelli, MD; Matteo Renzulli, MD; Bernhard Schuknecht, MD; Daniel J. Scoffings, MBBS, MRCP, FRCR; Jonathan Shapey, FRCS; Ata Siddiqui, MBBS, MD, DNB, FRCR; Rekha Siripurapu, MBBS, MRCP, FRCR; Federica Sozzi, MD; Ashok Srinivasan, MD; Nick W.M. Thomas, FRCS; Philip Touska, MBBS, FRCR; Sriram Vaidyanathan, MD, FRCR; Andy Whyte, BDS(Hons), MBBCh, FFDRCSI, DDMFR, FRCR, FRANZCR; Zachary M. Wilseck, MD

The planning committee, staff, authors and editors listed below have identified financial relationships or relationships to products or devices they or their spouse/life partner have with commercial interest related to the content of this CME activity:
Claudia F.E. Kirsch, MD: Consultant/advisor: Primal Pictures; Royalties: Informa

UNAPPROVED/OFF-LABEL USE DISCLOSURE
The EOCME requires CME faculty to disclose to the participants:
1. When products or procedures being discussed are off-label, unlabelled, experimental, and/or investigational (not US Food and Drug Administration [FDA] approved); and
2. Any limitations on the information presented, such as data that are preliminary or that represent ongoing research, interim analyses, and/or unsupported opinions. Faculty may discuss information about pharmaceutical agents that is outside of FDA-approved labelling. This information is intended solely for CME and is not intended to promote off-label use of these medications. If you have any questions, contact the medical affairs department of the manufacturer for the most recent prescribing information.

TO ENROLL
To enroll in the *Neuroimaging Clinics of North America* Continuing Medical Education program, call customer service at 1-800-654-2452 or sign up online at http://www.theclinics.com/home/cme. The CME program is available to subscribers for an additional annual fee of USD 265.00.

METHOD OF PARTICIPATION

In order to claim credit, participants must complete the following:
1. Complete enrolment as indicated above.
2. Read the activity.
3. Complete the CME Test and Evaluation. Participants must achieve a score of 70% on the test. All CME Tests and Evaluations must be completed online.

CME INQUIRIES/SPECIAL NEEDS

For all CME inquiries or special needs, please contact elsevierCME@elsevier.com.

NEUROIMAGING CLINICS OF NORTH AMERICA

THE CLINICS ARE AVAILABLE ONLINE!
Access your subscription at:
www.theclinics.com

Contributors

CONSULTING EDITOR

SURESH K. MUKHERJI, MD, MBA, FACR
Clinical Professor, Marian University, Director
of Head and Neck Radiology, ProScan
Imaging, Regional Medical Director, Envision
Physician Services, Carmel, Indiana, USA

EDITOR

STEVE E.J. CONNOR, MRCP, FRCR
Reader in Head and Neck Imaging, School of
Biomedical Engineering and Imaging Sciences,
King's College London, Consultant
Neuroradiologist, Department of
Neuroradiology, King's College Hospital,
Consultant Head and Neck Radiologist,
Department of Radiology, Guy's and St
Thomas' Hospital, London, United Kingdom

AUTHORS

**ASHOK ADAMS, MBBS, BSc(Hons), EDiNR,
MRCP, FRCR**
Consultant Neuroradiologist, BartsHealth NHS
Trust, Honorary Senior Clinical Lecturer, Queen
Mary University of London, Neuroradiology
Department, Royal London Hospital, London,
United Kingdom

**RUDOLF BOEDDINGHAUS, MBChB,
FCRad(D)SA, FRANZCR, FRCR**
Perth Radiological Clinic, Subiaco, Western
Australia, Australia; Department of Surgery,
University of Western Australia, Perth, Western
Australia, Australia

ANDREA BORGHESI, MD
Department of Medical and Surgical
Specialties, Radiological Sciences, and Public
Health, University of Brescia, Brescia, Italy

**NEERAJ CHAUDHARY, MD, MRCS, FRCR,
FACR, FAHA, FEBNI**
Associate Professor of Radiology,
Neurosurgery, Neurology, and Otolaryngology,
Department of Radiology, University of
Michigan, Ann Arbor, Michigan, USA

STEVE E.J. CONNOR, MRCP, FRCR
Reader in Head and Neck Imaging, School of
Biomedical Engineering and Imaging Sciences,
King's College London, Consultant
Neuroradiologist, Department of
Neuroradiology, King's College Hospital,
Consultant Head and Neck Radiologist,
Department of Radiology, Guy's and St
Thomas' Hospital, London, United Kingdom

DAVIDE FARINA, MD
Department of Medical and Surgical
Specialties, Radiological Sciences, and Public
Health, University of Brescia, Brescia, Italy

**JOSEPH J. GEMMETE, MD, FACR, FSIR,
FAHA, FCIRSE**
Professor of Radiology, Neurosurgery, and
Otolaryngology, Department of Radiology,
University of Michigan, Ann Arbor, Michigan,
USA

CLAUDIA F.E. KIRSCH, MD
Professor of Radiology and Otolaryngology,
Division Chief Neuroradiology, Northwell
Health, Donald and Barbara Zucker School of
Medicine at Hofstra/Northwell, Northshore
University Hospital, New York, New York, USA

LEANNE LIN, MD, MPHS
Neurointerventional Radiology Fellow,
Department of Radiology, University of
Michigan, Ann Arbor, Michigan, USA

**RAVI KUMAR LINGAM, MB BCh, MRCP,
FRCR, EDiHNR**
Consultant, Department of Radiology,
Northwick Park and Central Middlesex
Hospitals, London North West University
Healthcare NHS Trust, Imperial College
London, London, United Kingdom

DAVIDE LOMBARDI, MD
Department of Otorhinolaryngology–Head and
Neck Surgery, University of Brescia, Brescia,
Italy

ROBERTO MAROLDI, MD
Department of Medical and Surgical
Specialties, Radiological Sciences, and Public
Health, University of Brescia, Brescia, Italy

BURCE OZGEN MOCAN, MD
Associate Professor, Department of Radiology,
University of Illinois at Chicago, Chicago,
Illinois, USA

ADITYA S. PANDEY, MD
Professor of Neurological Surgery, Radiology
and Otolaryngology – Head and Neck Surgery,
Department of Neurosurgery, University of
Michigan, Ann Arbor, Michigan, USA

CARLOTTA PESSINA, MD
Department of Medical and Surgical
Specialties, Radiological Sciences, and Public
Health, University of Brescia, Brescia, Italy

**GILLIAN M. POTTER, MBChB, MD, MRCP,
FRCR**
Consultant Neuroradiologist, Department of
Neuroradiology, Manchester Centre for Clinical
Neurosciences, Salford NHS Foundation Trust,
Greater Manchester, England, United
Kingdom; Honorary Senior Lecturer, University
of Manchester

MARCO RAVANELLI, MD
Department of Medical and Surgical
Specialties, Radiological Sciences, and Public
Health, University of Brescia, Brescia, Italy

MATTEO RENZULLI, MD
Department of Radiology, IRCCS Azienda
Ospedaliero-Universitaria di Bologna,
Bologna, Italy

BERNHARD SCHUKNECHT, MD
Prof. Dr. med., Medical Radiological Institute,
Zürich, Switzerland

**DANIEL J. SCOFFINGS, MBBS, MRCP,
FRCR**
Department of Radiology, Cambridge
University Hospitals, NHS Foundation Trust,
Cambridge, United Kingdom

JONATHAN SHAPEY, FRCS
Department of Neurosurgery, King's College
Hospital NHS Foundation Trust, School of
Biomedical Engineering and Imaging Sciences,
King's College London, London, United
Kingdom

ATA SIDDIQUI, MBBS, MD, DNB, FRCR
Consultant Neuroradiologist, Department of
Neuroradiology, King's College Hospital,
London, United Kingdom

REKHA SIRIPURAPU, MBBS, MRCP, FRCR
Consultant Neuroradiologist, Department of
Neuroradiology, Manchester Centre for Clinical
Neurosciences, Salford NHS Foundation Trust,
Greater Manchester, England, United
Kingdom; Honorary Senior Lecturer, University
of Manchester

FEDERICA SOZZI, MD
Department of Medical and Surgical
Specialties, Radiological Sciences, and Public
Health, University of Brescia, Brescia, Italy

ASHOK SRINIVASAN, MD
Professor of Radiology, Department of
Neurosurgery, University of Michigan, Ann
Arbor, Michigan, USA

NICK W.M. THOMAS, FRCS
Department of Neurosurgery, King's College
Hospital NHS Foundation Trust, London,
United Kingdom

PHILIP TOUSKA, MBBS, FRCR
Department of Radiology, Guy's and St. Thomas' NHS Foundation Trust, London, United Kingdom

SRIRAM VAIDYANATHAN, MD, FRCR
Consultant, Department of Radiology and Nuclear Medicine, St James's University Hospital, Leeds Teaching Hospitals NHS Trust, Leeds, United Kingdom

ANDY WHYTE, BDS(Hons), MBBCh, FFDRCSI, DDMFR, FRCR, FRANZCR
Department of Medicine and Radiology, University of Melbourne, Parkville, Victoria, Australia; Department of Dentistry, University of Western Australia, Perth, Western Australia, Australia

ZACHARY M. WILSECK, MD
Neurointerventional Radiology Fellow, Department of Radiology, University of Michigan, Ann Arbor, Michigan, USA

PHILIP TOUSKA, MBBS, FRCR
Department of Radiology, Guy's and St.
Thomas' NHS Foundation Trust, London,
United Kingdom

SRIRAM VAIDYANATHAN, MD, FRCR
Consultant, Department of Radiology and
Nuclear Medicine, St James's University
Hospital, Leeds Teaching Hospitals NHS Trust,
Leeds, United Kingdom

ANDY WHYTE, BDS(Hons), MBBS,
FDSRCSI, DDMFR, FRCR, FRANZCR
Department of Medicine and Radiology,
University of Melbourne, Parkville, Victoria,
Australia; Department of Dentistry, University
of Western Australia, Perth, Western Australia,
Australia

ZACHARY M. WILSECK, MD
Neurointerventional Radiology Fellow,
Department of Radiology, University of
Michigan, Ann Arbor, Michigan, USA

Contents

Perineural extension is an increasingly recognized pathway of extension of cutaneous, mucosal, and salivary gland neoplasms associated with a severe adverse prognosis. Imaging identification is feasible by MR imaging 3-dimensional contrast-enhanced submillimetric sequences. The trigeminal nerve branches and facial nerve are the most commonly involved. PET with computed tomography may aid in the identification of the primary tumor location or recognition of recurrence, but only in conjunction with MR imaging does it achieve similar detection rates for perineural extension. Computed tomography scanning is an adjunct to MR imaging to increase specificity and for surgical treatment planning.

We review and illustrate the radiology of facial pain, emphasizing trigeminal neuralgia, relevant anatomy, current classification, concepts about etiology, and the role of imaging and its influence on the choice of treatment. We discuss glossopharyngeal neuralgia, other neuropathic causes of facial pain, postinflammatory and neoplastic causes, and nociceptive (end-organ) causes of facial pain, as well as referred otalgia. Other conditions that may present with facial pain, including trigeminal autonomic cephalgias and giant cell arteritis, are reviewed briefly. We discuss the elements of a comprehensive MR imaging protocol to enable detection of these diverse causes of facial pain.

Acquired skull base cerebrospinal fluid (CSF) leaks can result from trauma, tumors, iatrogenic causes, or may be spontaneous. Spontaneous skull base CSF leaks are likely a manifestation of underlying idiopathic intracranial hypertension. The initial assessment of rhinorrhea or otorrhea which is suspected to be due to an acquired skull base CSF leak requires integration of clinical assessment and biochemical confirmation of CSF. Imaging with high-resolution CT is performed to locate osseous defects, while high-resolution T2w MRI may detect CSF traversing the dura and bony skull base. When leaks are multiple or if samples of fluid cannot be obtained for testing, then recourse to invasive cisternography may be necessary.

The petrous apex may be affected by a range of lesions, commonly encountered as incidental and asymptomatic findings on imaging performed for other clinical reasons. Symptoms associated with petrous apex lesions commonly relate to mass effect and/or direct involvement of closely adjacent structures. Petrous apex lesions are optimally assessed using a combination of high-resolution CT and MRI of the skull base. Management of petrous apex lesions varies widely, reflecting the range of possible pathologies, with imaging playing a key role, including lesion characterization, surveillance, surgical planning, and oncological contouring.

some of the embryology, developmental anatomy, including ossification, and related abnormalities of the anterior, central and posterior skull base using illustrative cases and tables. Pathologies such as dermoids/epidermoids, cephaloceles, nasal gliomas, glioneuronal heterotopias, various notochordal remnants, persistent craniopharyngeal canal, teratomas, platybasia, basilar invagination, clival anomalies and Chiari malformations will be discussed. Developmental pearls and pitfalls will also be highlighted.

Zachary M. Wilseck, Leanne Lin, Joseph J. Gemmete, Aditya S. Pandey, Ashok Srinivasan, and Neeraj Chaudhary

Neurodiagnostic and neurointerventional radiology (NIR) play a central role in the diagnosis and treatment of skull base disorders. Noninvasive imaging modalities, including computed tomography and magnetic resonance imaging, are important in lesion localization, evaluation of lesion extent, and diagnosis, but cannot always be definitive. Image-guided skull base biopsy and percutaneous and endovascular treatment options are important tools in the diagnosis and treatment of head, neck, and skull base disorders. NIR plays an important role in the treatment of vascular disorders of the skull base. This article summarizes the imaging evaluation and interventional therapies pertinent to the skull base.

Philip Touska and Steve E.J. Connor

The skull base and cranial nerves are technically challenging to evaluate using magnetic resonance (MR) imaging, owing to a combination of anatomic complexity and artifacts. However, improvements in hardware, software and sequence development seek to address these challenges. This section will discuss cranial nerve imaging, with particular attention to the techniques, applications and limitations of MR neurography, diffusion tensor imaging and tractography. Advanced MR imaging techniques for skull base pathology will also be discussed, including diffusion-weighted imaging, perfusion and permeability imaging, with a particular focus on practical applications.

Foreword
Skull Base Neuroimaging

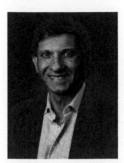

Suresh K. Mukherji, MD, MBA, FACR
Consulting Editor

The reason I decided to become a Head and Neck radiologist was because of the skull base! I still remember the neuroradiology fellow (Jane Wiseman) and my neuroradiology attending (Robert Schick) reviewing the foramen of the skull base with me on the first day of radiology residency…in 1988! I knew I wanted to be a Head and Neck radiologist by the end of my second day and have always been indebted to Drs Wiseman and Schick for taking the time to introduce me to this wonderful subspeciality.

The anatomy and pathology are very daunting, and this issue has clearly achieved its goal to demystify the challenging anatomy and complex pathology of the skull base. The issue has specific articles devoted to anatomy, neoplasms, infections, developmental anomalies, trauma, and interventional techniques. There are also articles focused on the complex subjects of perineural spread, trigeminal neuralgia, facial nerve, and cerebrospinal fluid leaks. The article authors are all recognized experts in their subject matter, and I thank them for their wonderful contributions.

I specifically would like to thank my long-time colleague and friend, Dr Steve Connor, for accepting our invitation to guest edit this issue. I have known Steve for many years, and he is an internationally renowned head and neck radiologist and one of the premier skull base radiologists in the world. Steve…thank you this wonderful issue and for our continued collaboration and friendship!

Suresh K. Mukherji, MD, MBA, FACR
Marian University
Head and Neck Radiology
ProScan Imaging
Carmel, IN, USA

E-mail address:
sureshmukherji@hotmail.com

Neuroimag Clin N Am 31 (2021) xv
https://doi.org/10.1016/j.nic.2021.08.001
1052-5149/21/© 2021 Published by Elsevier Inc.

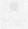

Preface
Skull Base Neuroimaging

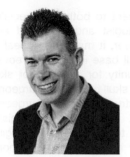

Steve E.J. Connor, MRCP, FRCR
Editor

The skull base has often been referred to as a "frontier" or an "interface" between the intracranial compartment and the extracranial head and neck. Such descriptions are pertinent, since the intricate anatomy has resulted in it becoming a "frontier" for the development of minimally invasive surgical approaches, while the skull base team now represents an "interface" between an array of different subspecialty professionals. Thus, this issue of *Neuroimaging Clinics* seeks to demystify the complex radiological skull base anatomy and demonstrate how imaging can contribute to the contemporary management of skull base disease, cementing the key role of the radiologist within skull base multidisciplinary practice.

In planning this issue, we chose to encompass the full breadth of skull base imaging subjects. The topics can be categorized according to imaging for the planning and demonstration of surgical approaches (open and endoscopic), imaging of specific tumor types and patterns of tumor spread (vestibular schwannoma and perineural spread),

imaging by clinical presentation (facial pain, cerebrospinal fluid leaks), imaging by anatomical region (petrous apex, sellar/parasellar, and seventh cranial nerve), imaging by pathological condition (infection, trauma, and developmental), and contemporary or evolving radiology of the skull base (interventional and diagnostic).

The articles feature a number of recurring themes.

First, they seek to showcase the diversity of skull base tumors and the role of imaging in their diagnosis and management. Skull base tumors may arise from the meninges, traversing neurovascular structures, the bony skull base, or the subcranial soft tissues; hence, the radiologist will encounter a wide range of neoplastic histologies with differing imaging characteristics, natural histories, patterns of spread, and management. There are few less-accessible places for the clinician to examine or biopsy, so the radiologist plays a key role in diagnosing and defining the extent of disease for the surgeon or radiation oncologist.

Neuroimag Clin N Am 31 (2021) xvii–xviii
https://doi.org/10.1016/j.nic.2021.07.001
1052-5149/21/© 2021 Published by Elsevier Inc.

Particularly important and distinctive skull base tumors and patterns of tumor spread are highlighted.

Second, another characteristic feature of the skull base is the proximity of pathologic condition to functionally important anatomical structures. After all, every neurovascular structure extending to the brain will traverse the skull base. The radiologist is integral to their evaluation in order to help customize surgical approaches and define resection margins. Each of the articles guides the reader through the relevant anatomy and how to depict these structures.

Third, since "cranial base surgery" first reached the surgical literature in the 1960s, the access and corridors to skull base pathology have evolved, and this is described in several articles. Endoscopic or open surgical approaches, from below or the side, are designed to minimize brain retraction. It is important for the radiologist to appreciate the surgical options and to understand the impact of both anatomical variants and tumor extent on surgical planning. The imaging appearances of the skull base following resection and reconstruction may be complex, and these are described.

Finally, each author highlights how dedicated imaging protocols can be optimized for the demonstration of skull base pathologic conditions and tailored to the specific tumor, region, or condition under discussion. This is further developed in an article focused on new and advanced MR imaging diagnostic imaging techniques and how they are now being applied to the cranial nerves and skull base.

This issue is of interest to both the specialist skull base neuroradiologist and the head and neck radiologist; however, it may also appeal to the more reluctant skull base imager. Moreover, it provides an opportunity for an array of skull base professionals (eg, skull base neurosurgeons, ENT surgeons, reconstructive plastic surgeons, radiation oncologists, neuroophthalmologists, and neuropathologists) to enhance their imaging knowledge. I am most indebted to the authors, who have contributed their time and expertise in order to make this issue possible. These radiologists are real authorities on skull base imaging and were invited to participate on the basis of their proven ability to communicate their knowledge. I am extremely grateful to them all.

Steve E.J. Connor, MRCP, FRCR
Department of Neuroradiology
King's College Hospital
London SE5 9RS, UK

E-mail address:
steve.connor@nhs.net

Neurosurgical Approaches to the Skull Base
A Guide for the Radiologist

Jonathan Shapey, FRCS[a,b,*], Nick W.M. Thomas, FRCS[a],
Steve E.J. Connor, MRCP, FRCR[b,c]

KEYWORDS

• Neurosurgery • Skull base surgery • Surgical approaches • Neuroradiology • Endoscopy

KEY POINTS

• Neuroimaging studies can provide the surgeon with a wealth of information to assist in the planning and execution of skull base surgery.
• CT and MRI play a complementary role in the preoperative and postoperative imaging assessment.
• For each surgical approach, key anatomical structures should be identified on preoperative imaging.

INTRODUCTION

Skull base surgery is a highly specialized area of neurosurgery. It is particularly challenging because tumors originating in this region are often intricately associated with various critical neurovascular structures. In addition to characterizing the target pathology, neuroimaging studies can provide the surgeon with a wealth of information to assist in the planning and execution of surgery. We review the key imaging anatomy relevant to neurosurgical skull base approaches and highlight the pertinent features on postoperative imaging.

APPLIED SKULL BASE BONY ANATOMY

The skull base forms the floor of the cranial cavity and comprises 5 bones: the ethmoid, sphenoid, occipital, paired frontal, and paired temporal bones. The bony anatomy is typically subdivided into 3 regions: the anterior, middle, and posterior skull base (Fig. 1). The anterior limit of the anterior skull base is the posterior wall of the frontal sinus and the interface with the middle skull base is defined by the anterior clinoid processes and the lesser wing of sphenoid. The orbits and paranasal sinuses lie below the anterior cranial fossa floor and the fronto-ethmoid suture line marks the inferior extent of the anterior cranial fossa. The clivus and petrous pyramids demarcate the posterior limit of the middle skull base. The central part of the middle fossa comprises the body of the sphenoid and the sella turcica, whereas the lateral floor is formed by the greater wing of the sphenoid and anterior petrous temporal bone. The posterior skull base is primarily formed by the occipital bone and the midline clivus and the lateral wall comprises the posterior petrous temporal bone and the lateral occipital bone.

IMAGING INDICATIONS AND TECHNIQUES

Computed tomography (CT) scans and MR imaging play a complementary role in the preoperative and postoperative imaging assessment. Preoperative CT scans provide information about the bony landmarks and variants, such as the extent of skull base pneumatization or the location and bony covering of important neurovascular structures. Meanwhile, preoperative MR imaging with

[a] Department of Neurosurgery, King's College Hospital NHS Foundation Trust, Denmark Hill, London SE5 9RS, UK; [b] School of Biomedical Engineering & Imaging Sciences, King's College London, Becket House, 9th floor, 1 Lambeth Palace Road, London SE1 7EU, UK; [c] Department of Neuroradiology, King's College Hospital NHS Foundation Trust, Denmark Hill, London SE5 9RS, UK
* Corresponding author.
E-mail address: Jonathan.shapey@kcl.ac.uk

Neuroimag Clin N Am 31 (2021) 409–431
https://doi.org/10.1016/j.nic.2021.05.004
1052-5149/21/© 2021 Elsevier Inc. All rights reserved.

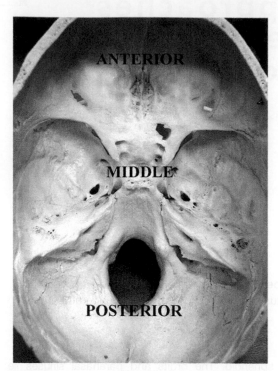

ANTERIOR

MIDDLE

POSTERIOR

Fig. 1. Bony anatomy of the skull base.

thin section T2-weighted and T1-weighted post-gadolinium MR imaging sequences provides detail on the extent of the lesion and the involvement of adjacent structures. Special 3-dimensional fast spin echo sequences (eg, SPACE and CUBE) are more resistant to a susceptibility effect at the skull base than gradient echo techniques, and the lesion conspicuity is enhanced by the addition of fat suppression or black blood techniques (eg, with motion sensitized–driven equilibrium) to T1-weighted postgadolinium imaging. Diffusion-weighted imaging may better define cellular tumors and cholesteatoma. Diffusion tensor imaging and tractography has the potential to delineate of cisternal neural structures but is yet to be widely applied. CT scan or MR imaging–based vascular imaging may be required to provide more information on variant anatomy or the involvement of vascular structures by the lesion. By using a combination of imaging modalities, key anatomic structures may be identified preoperatively and assist operative planning (Table 1). A CT scan is the key imaging modality in the postoperative period to evaluate for potential complications, in view of its accessibility and compatibility with monitoring equipment. Postoperative MR imaging is used to supplement the early imaging of postoperative infection or ischemia, assess the extent of resection at follow-up, and image for tumor surveillance.

NEUROSURGICAL APPROACHES
Frontotemporal Approaches

Pterional approach
The frontotemporal approach, popularized by Yasargil in the 1970s,[1] is among the most important and versatile approaches in neurosurgery (Fig. 2). The pterional approach was originally designed to access vascular pathology arising from the circle of Willis and for accessing lesions located in or around the subfrontal, sella, cavernous sinus, periclinoid, parasellar, and orbital regions (Table 2). The standard pterional craniotomy flap involves a frontotemporo–sphenoidal flap that is typically completed with the drilling of the sphenoid wing. For midline lesions, an approach from the nondominant side is typically preferred to prevent injury to the dominant hemisphere.

Extended frontotemporal approaches (including the frontotemporal orbitozygomatic approach)
Extending the pterional craniotomy through an isolated orbitotomy may be required to approach lesions that extend into the orbit or those that lie inside or near the cavernous sinus (Figs. 3 and 4). The medial limit of the drilling of the orbital roof is marked by the superior orbital fissure. A further surgical adjunct is the orbitozygomatic craniotomy, which increases exposure and decreases brain retraction, through the additional removal of the zygomatic arch and orbital rim and may be performed as a 1-piece[2] or 2-piece craniotomy.[3] Use of the MacCarty keyhole, located 7 mm superior and 5 mm posterior to the frontozygomatic suture,[2] enables the simultaneous exposure of the anterior cranial fossa floor. A frontotemporal craniotomy may also be extended by removal of the anterior clinoid to gain additional exposure to the adjacent internal carotid artery (ICA) or to facilitate optic nerve decompression.

Subfrontal Approaches

Supraorbital approach
The subfrontal approach may be used to access a variety of lesion originating from the anterior skull base and parasellar and suprasellar regions (see Table 2) (Fig. 5). The unilateral supraorbital craniotomy is a minimally invasive keyhole approach performed through an eyebrow incision, often with the assistance of the endoscope. A supraorbital craniotomy is commonly used to approach small to moderate sized midline or parasellar tumors. A single burr hole is made beneath the temporalis at the keyhole followed by the creation of a bone flap, which is as close to the anterior cranial fossa floor as possible.

Table 1
Key anatomic structures to be identified on preoperative imaging to assist surgical planning

	Approach	Key Anatomic Structures
Frontotemporal	1. Pterional 2. Frontotemporal orbitozygomatic	Degree of frontal sinus pneumatization Configuration of optic apparatus relative to tumor (eg, prefixed or postfixed optic chiasm) Configuration of cerebral vasculature relative to tumor (eg, relation of the ICA and associated vessels to a medial sphenoid wing meningioma)
Subfrontal	1. Supraorbital 2. Bifrontal/transbasal	Degree of frontal sinus pneumatization Configuration of optic apparatus relative to tumor Configuration of cerebral vasculature relative to tumor
Transpetrosal	1. Middle fossa transpetrosal 2. Combined petrosal 3. Translabyrinthine 4. Transcochlear	Degree of petromastoid air cell pneumatization (eg, perilabyrinthine air cells tracts) Labyrinthine anatomy (eg, arcuate eminence [MFT], greater superficial petrosal nerve [MFT], internal carotid artery variants) Venous anatomy (eg, anterolateral sigmoid sinus and high jugular bulb [TL] or inferior petrosal snus [MFT])
Lateral	1. Retrosigmoid 2. Far lateral 3. Infratemporal fossa type A 4. Petro-occipital trans-sigmoid	Degree of petro-mastoid air cell pneumatization (eg, occipital extension) Venous anatomy (eg, transverse and transverse/sigmoid sinus dominance, position of transverse-sigmoid junction and mastoid emissary veins [RS]) Vertebral artery location and dominance (FL) Bony anatomy- relationship of tumor to the occipital condyle and C1 (FL)
Endoscopic endonasal	1. Midline 2. Paramedian	Degree of paranasal sinus pneumatization Nasal cavity narrowing (septal deviation/spurs/concha bullosa) Skull base or medial orbital wall dehiscence Optic nerve and internal carotid dehiscence (in sphenoid sinus) (MEE) Anterior ethmoid artery dehiscence Intercavernous venous collaterals and medialized of cavernous carotid artery (MEE) Vidian canal (PMEE) Configuration of optic apparatus relative to tumor Configuration of cerebral vasculature relative to tumor

Abbreviations: FL, far-lateral; MEE, midline endoscopic endonasal; MFT, middle fossa transpetrosal; PMEE, paramedian endoscopic endonasal; RS, retrosigmoid; TL, translabyrinthine.

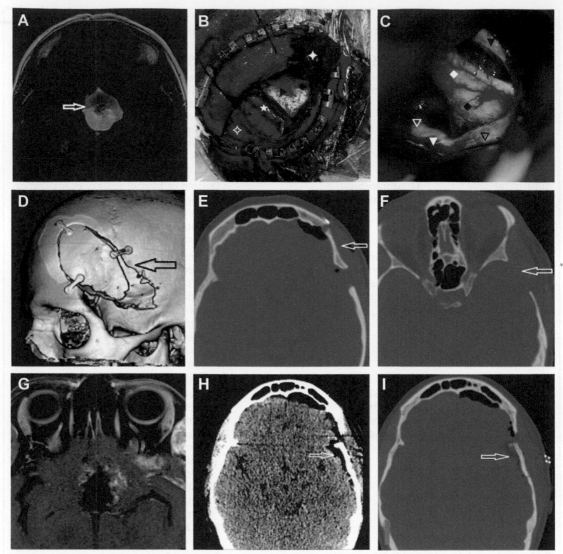

Fig. 2. Pterional craniotomy (frontotemporo-sphenoid). (*A*) T1-weighted axial postgadolinium image demonstrates a tuberculum sella meningioma. (*B*) Intraoperative photograph of a right-sided pterional approach illustrating the location of a frontotemporal and temporal burr hole before elevating the bone flap (▶). Temporalis muscle (✦) reflected inferiorly, with a cuff of muscle (★) left on the bone flap to aid closure. The pericranium (✧) is preserved on the frontal bone superior to the bone flap. (*C*) Intraoperative microscope photograph during a right-sided pterional approach to a craniopharyngioma. ▼, right internal carotid artery (ICA); ▽, right A1; ▼, ACom; ▽, left A1; ◆, right optic nerve; ◆, optic chiasm; ◇, left optic nerve; T, tumor. (*D*) Anterolateral oblique 3-dimensional rendered CT scan , (*E*) axial CT scan (superior), and (*F*) axial CT scan (inferior) demonstrates the location of the pterional craniotomy. (*G*) Axial T1-weighted postgadolinium image demonstrates the craniotomy site. There is enhancement of the temporalis muscle and parenchymal postoperative enhancement at the site of the tumor resection. T1-weighted high signal blood degradation products are present in the extraaxial space and along the surgical approach. Axial CT scan with (*H*) standard and (*I*) bone windows demonstrates low density material adjacent to the craniotomy site consistent with hemostatic material.

Bifrontal transbasal approach

For larger midline meningiomas and more extensive anterior skull base tumors (see **Table 2**), a bifrontal or extended bifrontal craniotomy is typically required (**Figs. 6** and **7**). A standard bicoronal scalp incision is turned, taking care not to incise the pericranium, which may be used as a reconstructive material at the end of the procedure. Typically, a burr hole is placed at the pterion on each side with 2 more burr holes placed on both sides of the midline just anterior to the coronal suture to protect the superior sagittal sinus. A

Table 2
Common skull base tumors encountered in each approach

	Approach	Common Tumors
Frontotemporal	1. Pterional 2. Frontotemporal orbitozygomatic	Medial sphenoid wing, parasellar, tuberculum, orbital, cavernous sinus meningioma Craniopharyngioma Pituitary adenoma Esthesioneuroblastoma
Subfrontal	1. Supraorbital 2. Bifrontal, transbasal	Olfactory groove, planum sphenoidale, parasellar, tuberculum sellae meningioma Craniopharyngioma Pituitary adenoma Esthesioneuroblastoma Sinonasal carcinoma Hemangiopericytoma Rhabdomyosarcoma
Transpetrosal	1. Middle fossa transpetrosal 2. Combined petrosal 3. TL 4. Transcochlear	Petroclival meningioma Trigeminal nerve schwannoma Facial nerve schwannoma Vestibular schwannoma (TL[a]) Cholesterol granuloma Cholesteatoma Chondrosarcoma
Lateral	1. Retrosigmoid 2. Far lateral 3. Infratemproal Fossa type A 4. Petro-occipital trans-sigmoid	Petrous, petroclival meningioma Foramen magnum meningioma (FL[a]) Vestibular schwannoma (RS[a]) Lower cranial nerve schwannoma Jugular paraganglioma (IFT-A[a], POTS[a]) Epidermoid cyst Chordoma Chondrosarcoma Cholesteatoma
Endoscopic endonasal	1. Midline 2. Paramedian	Olfactory groove, planum sphenoidale, parasellar, tuberculum sellae, cavernous sinus meningioma Craniopharyngioma Pituitary adenoma Chordoma Chondrosarcoma Esthesioneuroblastoma Sinonasal carcinoma Hemangiopericytoma Rhabdomyosarcoma Cholesterol granuloma Cholesteatoma

Abbreviations: FL, far-lateral; IFT-A, infratemporal fossa type A; POTS, petro-occipital trans-sigmoid; RS, retro-sigmoid; TL, translabyrinthine.
[a] Denotes typical approach.

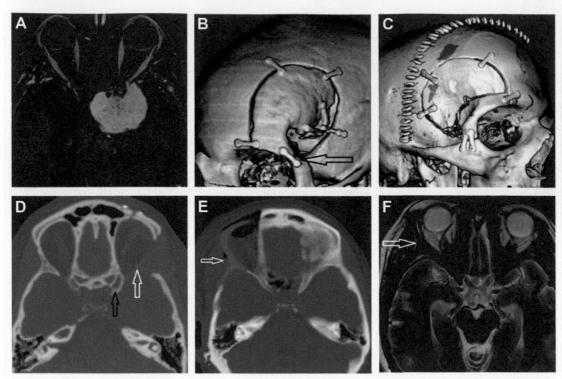

Fig. 3. Pterional craniotomy with orbitotomies. (*A*) T1-weighted fat-saturated postgadolinium axial image demonstrates a periclinoid and suprasellar meningioma. Anterolateral oblique 3-dimensional rendered CT scan for (*B*) 1-piece and (*C*) 2-piece craniotomy. *MacCarty burr hole. (*D*) Axial CT scan demonstrating extension to the orbital rim and the lateral orbitotomy extending medially to the superior orbital fissure (*white arrow*). The anterior clinoid may also be removed (*black arrow*) to decompress the optic nerve. In (*E*), the orbital defect has been replaced with a polyetheretherketone cranioplasty visible as high density on the axial CT scan (*arrow*); however, it may appear similar to cortical bone on the (*F*) axial T2-weighted MR imaging sequence (*arrow*).

standard bifrontal bone flap is then created with the anterior bone cut placed as close as possible to the frontal floor. The dura is cut in the midline, but is not reflected beyond the crista galli to avoid damaging the olfactory nerves. To prevent the development of frontal sinus mucoceles and infection, cranialization of the frontal sinus is performed by removing the posterior wall and stripping the mucosa. The bifrontal craniotomy may be extended to a transbasal approach by performing an orbital osteotomy extending from the frontozygomatic suture laterally through the roofs of the orbit in front of the crista galli and/or nasal bone. Performing this adjunct greatly decreases the extent of frontal retraction. Titanium mesh and a vascularized pericranial flap are typically used to reconstruct the floor of the anterior cranial fossa.

Transpetrosal Approaches

Middle fossa transpetrosal approach with anterior petrosectomy

The middle fossa transpetrosal approach with an anterior petrosectomy as described by Kawase[4]

is an effective approach to difficult-to-access petroclival tumors (see **Table 2**) and is often a modular component of multiple approaches such as subtemporal, transzygomatic and frontotemporal orbitozygomatic procedures to obtain the necessary extended exposure (**Fig. 8**).[5] When performed in isolation, the middle fossa transpetrosal approach is typically performed through a 4-cm wide craniotomy positioned two-thirds anterior and one-third posterior to the external auditory canal. The dura is elevated adjacent to the greater superficial petrosal nerve at the facial hiatus, whereas the arcuate eminence and the middle meningeal artery at the foramen spinosum are also identified. The goal is to create a maximal window to the clivus in the anteromedial petrous pyramid while preserving the temporal bone auditory and neurovascular structures.

Combined petrosal approach

The combined petrosal approach describes the combination of the anterior petrosal approach (extended middle fossa approach as described elsewhere in this article) with the posterior

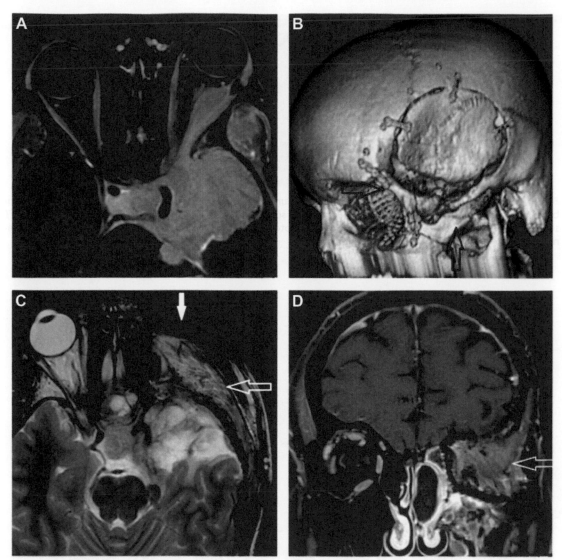

Fig. 4. Orbitozygomatic craniotomies. (*A*) S T1-weighted postgadolinium fat-saturated axial image shows a left sphenoid wing meningioma with extensive parasellar, orbital, and extracranial extension. (*B*) Anterolateral obli-que 3-dimensional rendered CT scan demonstrating orbitozygomatic craniotomies (*arrows* indicating zygomatic and orbital components). (*C*) T2-weighted axial and (*D*) T1-weighted postgadolinium coronal images demon-strate the associated orbital exenteration. The defect is filled with a rotational temporalis muscle flap, which is of increased T2-weighted signal and enhances (open *arrows* in *C* and *D*). There is an ocular prosthesis (*filled arrow*).

petrosal approach (retrolabyrinthine presigmoidal transtentorial approach) (**Fig. 9**).[6] This approach provides a wide, multidirectional corridor toward the ventral surface of the pons, the basilar trunk, and the ipsilateral cranial nerves that is, of partic-ular value when approaching large tumors of the petroclival region) (see **Table 2**). An occipitotem-poral bone flap is cut, bridging the transverse sinus and the sigmoid sinus. In addition to the anterior petrosal approach described elsewhere in this article, a total mastoidectomy and skeleto-nization of the sigmoid sinus to the jugular bulb is also performed, taking care not to open the semi-circular or facial canals. The tentorium is incised parallel to the petrous ridge where dural clips may be demonstrated. After tumor removal, the bony resection cavity may be reconstructed

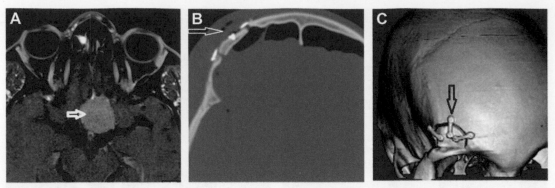

Fig. 5. Supraorbital approach. (A) T1-weighted fat-saturated postgadolinium axial image demonstrating a tuberculum sella meningioma (open *arrow*) (B) Axial CT scan and (C) oblique frontal 3-dimensional rendered CT scan indicating the site of a supraorbital key hole craniotomy (open *arrows*) close to the floor of the anterior cranial fossa for the resection of the meningioma.

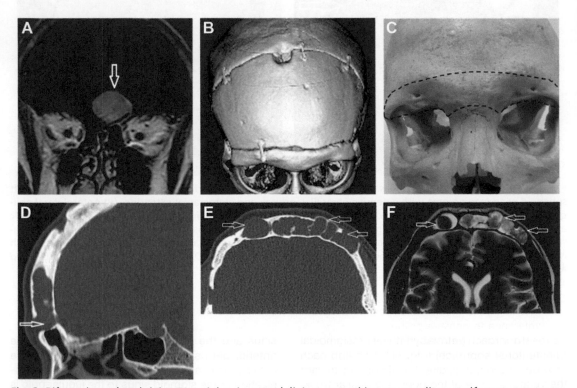

Fig. 6. Bifrontal transbasal. (A) A T1-weighted postgadolinium coronal image revealing an olfactory groove meningioma (open *arrow*). (B) A frontal 3-dimensional rendered CT scan indicating the bifrontal craniotomy. (C) Illustration of the additional osteotomies required for an extended transbasal approach. (D) A sagittal CT scan demonstrates the bifrontal craniotomies (*arrows*) involving the frontal sinuses. In this case, the frontal sinuses were not cranialized. The resulting mucoceles are demonstrated on the (E) axial CT scan (open *arrows*) and (F) axial T2-weighted MR imaging (open *arrows*).

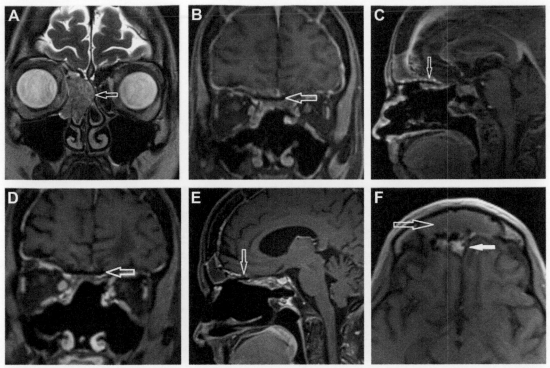

Fig. 7. Bifrontal transbasal with craniofacial resection and pericranial graft. (A) A T2-weighted coronal image of a right-sided olfactory neuroblastoma. T1-weighted postgadolinium fat-saturated (B) coronal and (C) sagittal images performed soon after bifrontal craniotomy demonstrate a low signal titanium mesh across the floor of the anterior cranial fossa (arrow) with enhancing pericranial graft both superior and inferior to the mesh. T1-weighted postgadolinium fat-saturated (D) coronal and (E) sagittal images performed 6 months later demonstrate a marked decrease in the conspicuity of the enhancing pericranial graft adjacent to the titanium mesh (arrows). (F) A T1-weighted axial image demonstrates the cranialized frontal sinus (open arrow). Some low signal foci at its periphery correspond to bone wax. There is T1-weighted hyperintense fat graft (filled arrow) related to the initial transnasal approach to the anterior skull base.

with a vascularized muscle flap or abdominal fat graft.

Translabyrinthine approach

The translabyrinthine approach is commonly used for the removal of vestibular schwannomas, particularly those with a large intrameatal component (see Table 2) (Fig. 10).[7] A mastoidectomy is performed and the sigmoid sinus is skeletonized to expose the middle fossa dura, facial nerve, and jugular bulb. After the labyrinthectomy is completed, the internal auditory canal is exposed by 270° in circumference to achieve proper dural exposure. Following tumor removal, the cavity is packed with abdominal fat graft before closing in layers.

Transotic and transcochlear approach

Although the translabyrinthine approach offers wide exposure of the cerebellopontine angle (CPA), the cochlea and petrous apex block access to the anterior aspects of the CPA and the ventral brain stem (Fig. 11). The transotic and

transcochlear approaches are most often used to access tumors medial to the porus acousticus and anterior to the brainstem (see Table 2). The transotic approach encompasses the translabyrinthine bony removal with the additional removal of the external auditory canal, middle ear contents, and the cochlea, thus permitting access to the petrous apex anterior to the internal auditory canal.[8] Closure of the external auditory canal is required and the facial nerve is skeletonized and transposed posteriorly to provide wide access to the anterior CPA. If combined with the removal of the petrous apex (transcochlear), this strategy gives wider access and is suitable for lesions with anterior extension to the prepontine cistern.

Lateral Approaches

Retrosigmoid/retromastoid suboccipital approach

The retrosigmoid/retromastoid suboccipital craniotomy is the workhorse of the infratentorial

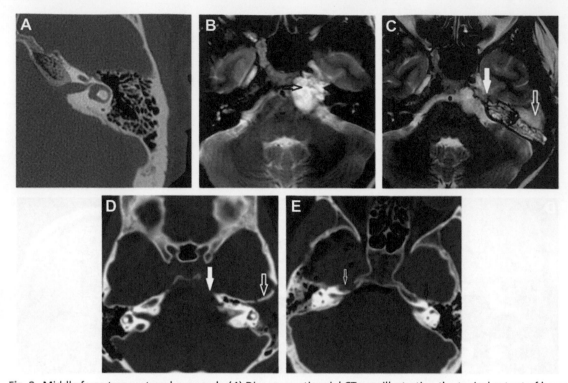

Fig. 8. Middle fossa transpetrosal approach. (*A*) Diagrammatic axial CT scan illustrating the typical extent of bony removal. (*B*) A T2-weighted axial image showing a left petrous apex chondrosarcoma. (*C*) A T2-weighted axial image and (*D*) axial CT scan demonstrates the operative corridor. There is a middle cranial fossa approach and anterior petrosectomy (*open arrows*) with fenestration of the petrous apex (*filled arrows*) to access the chondrosarcoma. (*E*) CT axial image in a patient who has undergone a right-sided middle fossa transpetrosal approach with the surgical defect seen in the right petrous apex (*white open arrow*). The landmark of the greater superior petrosal nerve is demonstrated on the left (*black open arrow*).

approaches for reaching the pathology within CPA and ventrolateral brainstem (see **Table 2**) (**Fig. 12**). Typically, a single burr hole is placed at the asterion, overlying the edge of the dural venous sinuses before completing the craniotomy. It is essential to expose the posterior edge of the sigmoid sinus; thus, additional drilling of the mastoid bone may be required after the craniotomy. In older patients and those where the dura is adherent to the bone, a full craniectomy is preferred. Bone wax is applied to the mastoid air cells to prevent cerebrospinal fluid leaks. The size of the craniotomy or craniectomy varies according to the target pathology; a smaller and more superiorly placed craniotomy is created when performing a microvascular decompression for trigeminal neuralgia whereas a larger craniotomy is required when approaching a large vestibular schwannoma. Cerebrospinal fluid is released to minimize cerebellar retraction.

Far lateral approach
The far lateral approach is used to approach lesions of the anterior/anterolateral foramen magnum and lower clivus[9] (see **Table 2**) (**Fig. 13**). During this approach, the vertebral artery (VA) is both a critical anatomic structure and a barrier that limits access as it crosses the surgical field. Detailed preoperative imaging confirming the course of the VA is required to facilitate its safe preservation and mobilization of during surgery. The suboccipital triangle is accessed, within which lies the dorsal ramus of the C1 nerve root and the horizontal segment (V3) of the VA. Removal of the C1 hemilamina allows the VA to be reflected caudally. First, a suboccipital craniotomy is performed, the size of which depends on the intracranial extent of the tumor. After this maneuver, the lateral edge of the foramen magnum is drilled, continuing laterally into the condylar fossa and condyle. Resection of the dorsal one-third of the occipital condyle improves exposure of the ventral aspect of the craniovertebral junction, minimizing brainstem retraction. Additional bone removal of the jugular tubercle and adjacent to the hypoglossal canal increases exposure of the anterior surface of the brainstem and midclivus.

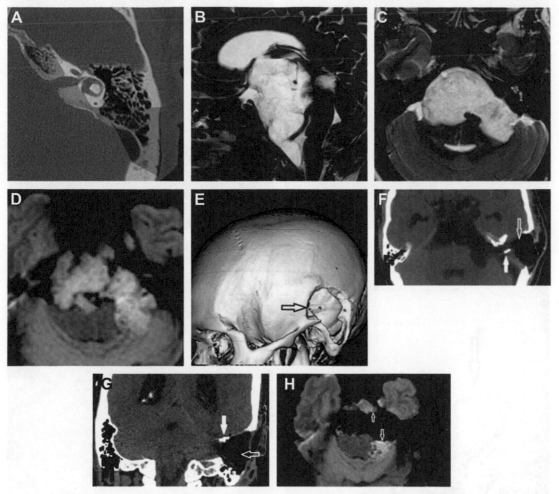

Fig. 9. Combined petrosal approach. (*A*) Diagrammatic axial CT scan illustrating the typical extent of bony removal. (*B*) Sagittal and (*C*) axial T2-weighted images together with (*D*) a diffusion-weighted axial image show an extensive epidermoid distorting the brainstem and with both supratentorial and infratentorial extension. (*E*) Lateral oblique 3-dimensional rendered CT image demonstrates a combined petrosal approach (*open arrow*) that includes a supratentorial and infratentorial craniotomy and mastoidectomy. Postoperative (*F*) axial and (*G*) coronal CT scan demonstrates the fat graft (*open arrow*) at the petrosectomy site and a dural clip (*filled arrow*) where there is sectioning of the tentorium. (*H*) A diffusion-weighted axial image shows extensive resection of the epidermoid with residual increased diffusion-weighted image signal anterior and posterior to the surgical tract (*open arrows*).

Infratemporal fossa type A approach

The infratemporal fossa type A approach as described by Fisch[10] was designed to approach tumors situated in the jugular foramen or surrounding skull base and is used primarily for the removal of jugular paragangliomas (see **Table 2**) (**Fig. 14**). Its approach is an extension of the transotic/cochlear approach and through its direct lateral exposure and medially directed surgical axis offers additional exposure of the vertical portion of the petrous ICA. Similar to the transotic/cochlear approach, the external auditory canal is transected and closed, the contents of the middle ear are removed, and the facial nerve is transposed anteriorly. However, most of the mastoidectomy, which provides access to the sigmoid sinus and petrous ICA, may be achieved through an infralabyrinthine exposure. The jugular vein is exposed in the neck and ligated, and closure of the sigmoid sinus is typically achieved by packing it with a hemostatic material such, as Surgicel. Surgicel packing may be pushed upstream as far as the transverse sigmoid junction, but care must be taken to ensure that the inferior anastomotic vein (vein of Labbé) remains patent.

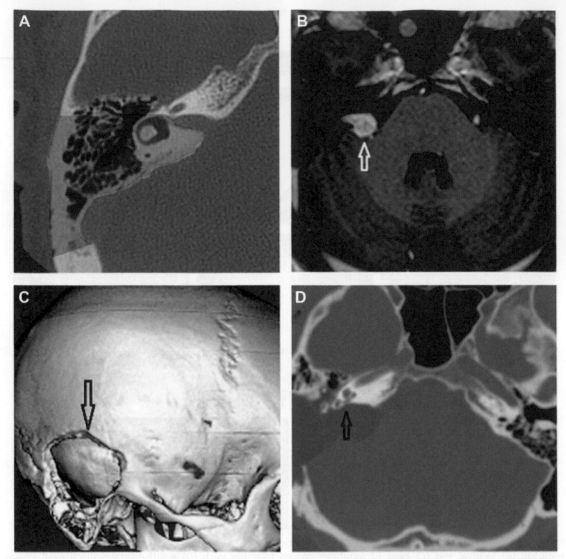

Fig. 10. Translabyrinthine approach. (*A*) Diagrammatic axial CT scan illustrating the typical extent of bony removal. (*B*) T1-weighted axial postgadolinium image demonstrating a right-sided vestibular schwannoma with a small extrameatal component. (*C*) Lateral oblique 3-dimensional rendered CT image shows the site of the presigmoid craniotomy and mastoidectomy. (*D*) Axial CT scan on bone windows demonstrates the partial labyrinthectomy, exposure of the internal acoustic meatus (open *arrow*) and the abdominal fat graft within the subtotal petrosectomy.

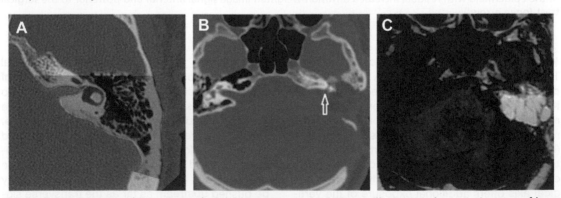

Fig. 11. Transotic/transcochlear approach. (*A*) Diagrammatic axial CT scan illustrating the typical extent of bony removal. (*B*) Axial CT and (*C*) axial T1-weighted images demonstrate a transotic resection performed for an aggressive cerebellopontine angle cistern meningioma extending medially. There is extension of the translabyrinthine approach with drilling of the cochlea in addition to the vestibule (*open arrow*) and with closure of the external acoustic meatus.

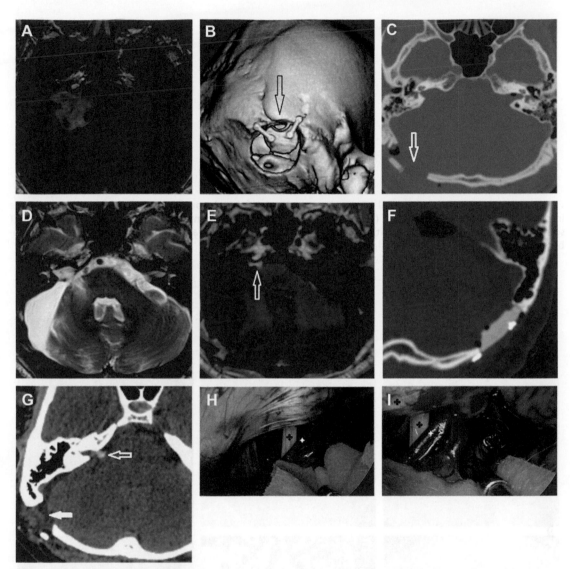

Fig. 12. Retrosigmoid/retromastoid suboccipital approach. (*A*) Postgadolinium axial T1-weighted MR imaging demonstrates a right-sided extrameatal vestibular schwannoma. (*B*) Inferolateral oblique 3-dimensional rendered CT scan and (*C*) axial CT scan illustrates a retrosigmoid craniotomy (*arrow*). (*D*) T2-weighted and (*E*) T1-weighted postgadolinium images show expected postoperative features with widening of the extra-axial spaces, some minor retraction injury, and dural enhancement. There is a thicker enhancement in the line of the facial nerve corresponding to residual tumor (*open arrow*). (*F*) In another case axial CT scan demonstrates and hydroxyapatite cement cranioplasty at the site of the retrosigmoid craniectomy. (*G*) Postoperative imaging after microvascular decompression (MVD) shows a typical small retrosigmoid craniectomy (*filled arrow*). The Teflon graft (*open arrow*) at the site of the trigeminal MVD is demonstrated. (*H*) and (*I*) Intraoperative view of the CPA from a retrosigmoid approach for MVD for hemifacial spasm: ✦, trigeminal nerve (CN V); ✣, facial-vestibulocochlear nerve complex (CN VII–VIII); ★, lower cranial nerves (CN IX–XI); ✦, anterior inferior cerebellar artery.

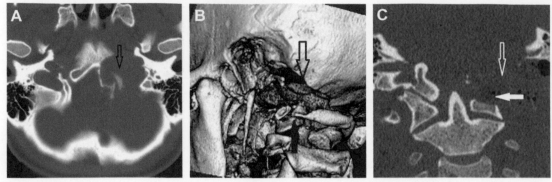

Fig. 13. Far lateral approach. (*A*) Axial CT scan demonstrates a left jugular paraganglioma extending to erode the inferior petrous apex and basiocciput (*arrow*). (*B*) Posterior oblique 3-dimensional rendered CT and (*C*) coronal CT scans demonstrate a lateral suboccipital craniotomy (*open arrows*), removal of the occipital condyle, jugular tubercle and partial resection of the atlas (*filled arrows*).

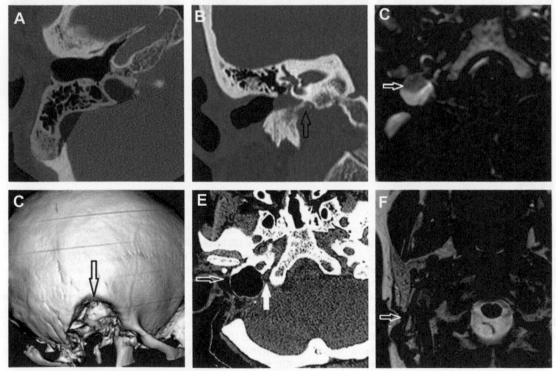

Fig. 14. Infratemporal fossa type A approach. (*A*) Diagrammatic axial CT scan illustrating typical extent of bony removal. (*B*) Coronal CT study demonstrates a jugulotympanic paraganglioma with permeative destruction of the jugular foramen (*open arrow*) (*C*) T1 postgadolinium axial image demonstrating tumor encroachment on the jugular bulb (*open arrow*). (*D*) Posterolateral oblique 3-dimensional rendered CT and (*E*) axial CT scans demonstrate the surgical corridor through the temporal bone posterior to the mandibular condyle (*open arrows* in *D*). It extends along the lowest aspect of the temporal bone to expose the jugular foramen (*filled arrow* in *E*). There is removal of the outer ear canal (*open arrow* in *E*) and anterior transposition of the facial nerve. The eustachian tube ostium was plugged with bone wax, but has recanalized with air noted in the cavity. (*F*) T2 axial image shows a retroauricular and upper neck incision (*arrow*) with exposure of the parapharyngeal region where there may also be scar tissue.

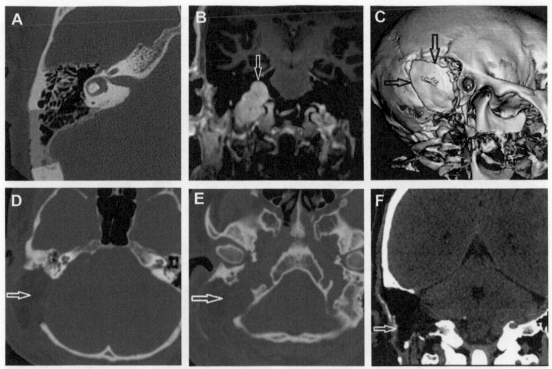

Fig. 15. Petro-occipital trans-sigmoid (POTS) approach. (*A*) Diagrammatic axial CT scan illustrating the typical extent of bony removal. (*B*) T1-weighted postgadolinium coronal image demonstrating a jugular foramen schwannoma with infracranial extension. (*C*) Inferolateral oblique 3-dimensional rendered CT scan, (*D*) superior axial CT scan, (*E*) inferior axial CT scan, and (*F*) coronal CT scan demonstrating the suboccipital craniotomy (*arrows* in *C*) with a posterolateral conservative petrosectomy with sparing of the labyrinth (*arrow* in *D*) and drilling of the inferior mastoid (*arrow* in *E*). There is an anteromedial corridor to reach the jugular fossa with the labyrinth remaining that is filled with a fat plug (*arrow* in *F*).

Petro-occipital trans-sigmoid approach

The petro-occipital trans-sigmoid approach was developed for removing tumors situated in the jugular foramen together with their local extension into adjacent parts of the skull base, CPA and parapharyngeal space[11] (see **Table 2**) (**Fig. 15**). In contrast with the infratemporal fossa type A approach, the petro-occipital trans-sigmoid approach involves a posterolateral exposure and an anteromedially directed surgical axis that preserves the external and middle ear, together with the facial nerve. The petro-occipital trans-sigmoid approach combines a retrolabyrinthine petrosectomy and retrosigmoid craniotomy. It involves removal of the inferior aspect of the mastoid and petro-occipital bones providing access to the parapharyngeal space in addition to a standard retrosigmoid craniotomy. Additional exposure may be achieved by removing the inferior aspect of the mastoid and styloid process and/or lateral mass of C1. As with the infratemporal fossa type A approach, the jugular vein is ligated and packed up to the proximal sigmoid sinus.

Endoscopic Endonasal Approaches

Median skull base approach

Endoscopic endonasal approaches to the ventral skull base include a midline corridor that extends from the from the frontal sinus to the upper cervical spine with the inferior limit roughly defined by the nasopalatine line (**Figs. 16–19**). The endoscopic endonasal approach is ideally suited for the resection of midline pathologies (see **Table 2**) and has become the preferred route of access for median ventral skull base surgery. The key points for the radiologist to analyze before endoscopic approaches are the focus of another article in this issue.

Endoscopic endonasal surgery for skull base lesions such as chordoma requires 2 surgeons using a binarial, 3- or 4-handed technique to permit dynamic endoscopy. Usually, lateralization of the middle turbinates is sufficient to provide the necessary access to the nasopharynx, but if further lateral extension is required, the middle turbinate is removed and a middle meatal

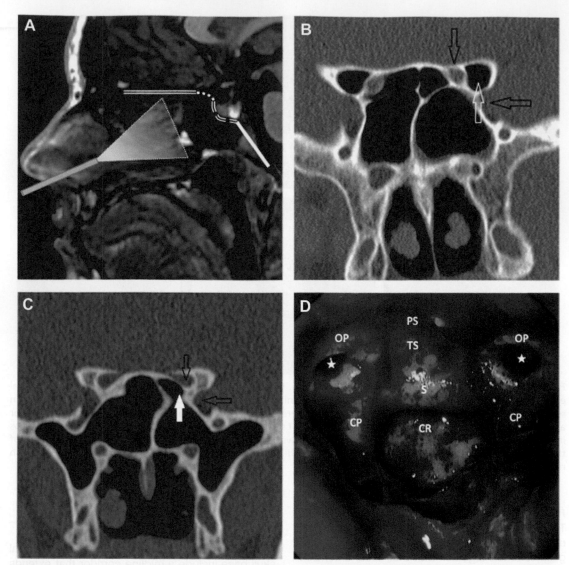

Fig. 16. Endoscopic median skull base approach-midline corridors and opticocarotid recess. (A) T1-weighted midline sagittal image illustrates the range of midline corridors to the skull base: Transcribiform (*single dashed line*), Transplanum/transtuberculum (*solid single line*), transsellar (*doubled dashed line*), and transclival (*solid double line*). (B and C) Coronal CT studies indicating the optic nerve canals (*vertical black open arrows*) and location of ICA geni (*horizontal black open arrows*). The opticocarotid recesses (OCR) are indicated (*open white arrow in B and filled white arrow in C*). There is a latero-optical OCR with extension into a pneumatized anterior clinoid in B). (D) Endoscopic view of the sphenoid sinus. CR, clival recess; OP, optic protruberence; CP, carotid pillar; PS, planum sphenoidale; S, sellar; TS, tuberculum sellae; ★, opticocarotid recess.

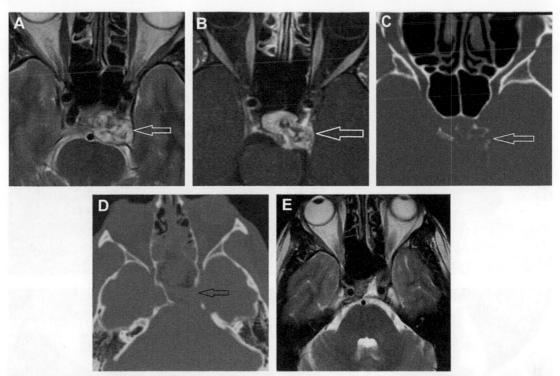

Fig. 17. Endoscopic median skull base approach—parasellar. (*A*) T2-weighted axial and (*B*) T1 postgadolinium axial images demonstrate a sella and left parasellar chondrosarcoma (*arrows*).Patchy chondroid calcification and a well pneumatized sphenoid sinus is shown on the (*C*) axial CT scan (*arrow*). (*D*) Early postoperative CT scan demonstrates the transsphenoidal surgical bony defects (*arrow*) with hemostatic and packing material in the spheno-ethmoid region. (*E*) Later postoperative T2-weighted MR imaging demonstrates the resected chondrosarcoma.

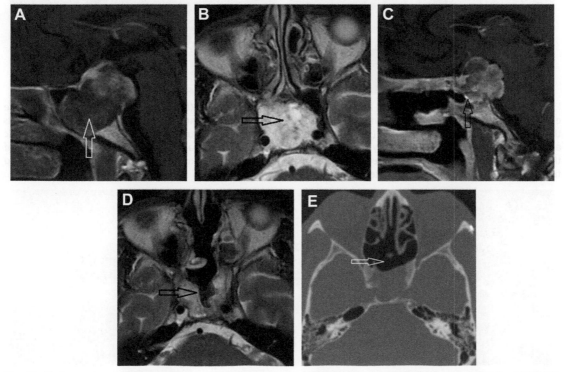

Fig. 18. Endoscopic median skull base approach-clival/basisphenoid. (*A*) T1 postgadolinium sagittal and (*B*) T2-weighted axial images demonstrate a superior clival and sellar chordoma (*arrows*). The trans-sphenoidal subtotal excision (*arrow*) is demonstrated in (*C*) T1 postgadolinium sagittal and (*D*) T2-weighted axial images. (*E*) Axial CT scan demonstrates the postsurgical defects within the nasal septum, ethmoid trabeculae and face of sphenoid (*open arrow*). The remaining tumor was removed by a transcranial approach.

426

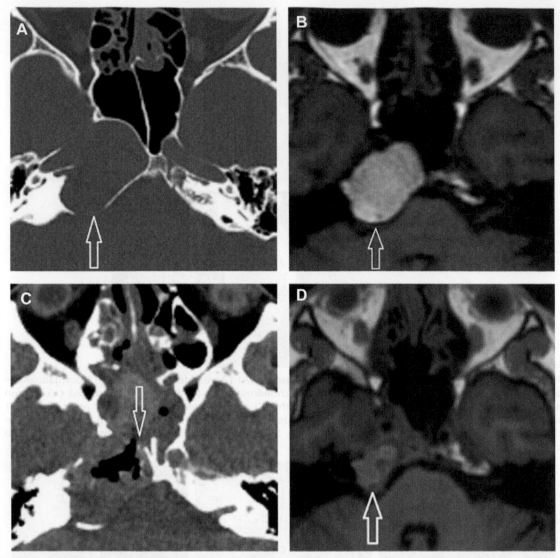

Fig. 19. Endoscopic median skull base approach—petrous apex. (*A*) CT and (*B*) T1-weighted axial images show the expansile and T1-weighted hyperintense right petrous apex cholesterol granuloma (*arrows*). It abuts and indents the dorsal wall of the sphenoid sinus. (*C*) Early postsurgical CT scan demonstrates the trans-sphenoidal endoscopic approach medial to the carotid artery with the postsurgical bony defect (*arrow*), and air seen after drainage of the cholesterol granuloma. (*D*) T1-weighted axial image at follow-up demonstrates intermediate T1-weighted fibrosis within the contracted cholesterol granuloma (*arrow*).

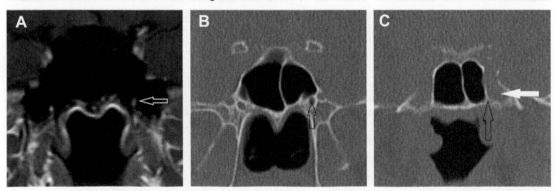

Fig. 20. Endoscopic paramedian skull base approach—vidian canal landmark for the ICA. (*A*) Postgadolinium T1-weighted coronal MR imaging indicates the location of the vidian canal (*open arrow*) in a patient with a wide inferolateral recess of the sphenoid sinus. (*B*) Coronal CT scan demonstrating the location of the vidian canal (*open arrow*). (*C*) On a coronal CT section more posteriorly, the line of the vidian canal (*open arrow*) is extrapolated to lie just inferomedial to the line of the carotid canal (*filled arrow*).

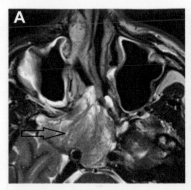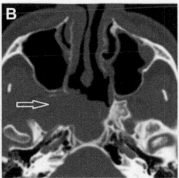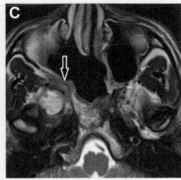

Fig. 21. Endoscopic paramedian skull base approach. (*A*) T2-weighted axial image shows a recurrent inverted papilloma (*arrow*) extending into the inferolateral recess of the right sphenoid sinus with (*B*) an axial CT image demonstrating destruction of the right pterygoid base and medial sphenoid wing (*arrow*), as well as extension to the infratemporal fossa. (*C*) Axial T2-weighted image demonstrates the endoscopic transmaxillary and transpterygoid approach used to access the lesion and the adjacent paramedian skull base with low T2 signal scar tissue at the site of resection (*arrow*) and a small remnant in the sphenoid wing.

antrostomy may be performed. The creation of a vascularized and pedicled nasoseptal flap is often required to repair the dural defect and is commonly seen on postoperative imaging.[12] Smaller free flaps fashioned from the turbinate mucosa may also be used if the nasoseptal flap is insufficient to cover the defect or if it cannot be harvested owing to tumor infiltration. To widen the working corridor and facilitate binarial access, the posterior septum is detached from the sphenoid. A wide anterior sphenoidotomy is then performed, sphenoid septations are removed and the floor of sphenoid sinus is drilled and flattened to ensure optimal placement of the nasoseptal flap at the end of the procedure. Additional

superior exposure is identical to a pituitary/sellar approach. Further inferior exposure may be achieved by exposing the medial pterygoid plates bilaterally and then resecting the nasopharyngeal mucosa and pharyngobasilar fascia from the inferior clivus.

Extended paramedian skull base approach

Expanded paramedian endonasal approaches offer a potential option for accessing lesions situated within the medial petrous apex and petroclival area, the superior and inferior cavernous sinus, and the transpterygoid/infratemporal regions[13] (see **Table 2**) (**Figs. 20** and **21**). Approaches to the medial petrous apex and petro-

Table 3
Cranioplasty material and appearance on CT scans

Cranioplasty Material	CT Imaging Appearances
Intraoperatively fashioned acrylic resins such as MMA	Intermediate density on CT scan (with foci of air owing to exothermic reaction)
Preformed acrylic resin plates	Homogenous intermediate density with predrilled holes
Hydroxyapatite cement paste	High (bone) density
Titanium mesh	Very high (metal) density and may be used as a scaffold for MMA or hydroxyapatite)
Custom made porous polyethylene	Low density on CT scan
Synthetic bone graft	Heterogeneous intermediate to high (bone) density
Autologous bone grafts (eg, split thickness calvarial bone)	High (bone) density
Customized polyetheretherketone	Low density and artifact free

Abbreviation: MMA, methyl-methacrylate.

Table 4
Graft material and imaging appearances

Type of Graft/Flap	Principle	Examples	Comments	Imaging Appearances
Neovascularized graft	Used for smaller anterior and central skull base defects however fat grafts used to seal larger petrous bone defects	Dural collagen matrix, fascia, fat, dermis, split calvarial graft, hydroxyapatite cement and titanium	With endoscopic techniques there is often a multilayer closure technique with intracranial inlay and superficial onlay components at the anterior skull base	This is variable in appearance and may be nondiscernible (eg, collagen matrix) or as much as 1 cm in thickness (eg, fascia lata). The layers often retract with decreased thickness and reduced enhancement over 2–6 mo. Fat grafts to petrosectomy defects also retract and fibrose over time.
Vascularized flap				
1. Free tissue transfer	From distal donor site and microvascular anastomosis with vessels in recipient bed (eg, temporal or facial vessels)	Fasciocutaneous, or musculocutaneous for example, radial forearm, rectus abdominis, anterolateral thigh	Particularly if previous surgery or radiotherapy or there are extensive defects	Variable MR imaging signal and enhancement (eg, owing to scar and denervation) with the visualization of striated muscle bundles and loss of volume over time.
2. Pedicled flaps	Rotated from regional location but constrained by local vascular pedicle	*Open approach:* Temporoparietal fascia/temporalis muscle, pericranial or galeal flap	Muscle used to increase bulk with larger defects (eg, if orbital exenteration)	Pericranial flap may be seen as folds with variable signal and enhancement with gradual reduction in thickness stabilizing at 6–8 wk. Temporal fossa defect or tissue expander may be seen at the site of donor temporalis muscle. Variable MR imaging signal and enhancement of the rotated muscle flap.
		Endoscopic approach: Nasoseptal flap Inferior turbinate flap		Nasoseptal flap should approximate the skull base defect and the enhancing mucosa. It may show T2 isointensity (mimicking tumor) at follow-up but it keeps the recognizable configuration

clival areas mandate isolation and mobilization of the anterior genu of the ICA. After a maxillary antrostomy, careful drilling of the medial pterygoid process posteriorly exposes the ICA. The vidian canal is a critical landmark in identifying and leading the surgeon to the anterior genu and lacerum segment of the of the ICA. For tumors extending into the infratemporal fossa, extracapsular dissection of the tumor may be pursued laterally with drilling of the lateral pterygoid plate. The cavernous sinus may be exposed fully with drilling around the foramen rotundum, exposing V2 and skeletonizing the horizontal portion of the ICA.

EXPECTED POSTOPERATIVE IMAGING APPEARANCES

Skin staples are used to close the scalp flap and will be present in the early postoperative period (see **Fig. 2**). There may be additional devices used to secure a calvarial bone flap, such as microfixation plates or clamps, but because they

are often made from titanium, they result in minimal beam hardening artifact or susceptibility effects (see **Figs. 2–6**). The bone flap margins will initially appear sharp, but become rounded with time on CT scans, whereas adjacent granulation tissue at the margins of the flap will enhance on MR imaging for up to 1 year. With the pterional approaches, there will be temporalis muscle swelling, edema, and enhancement in the early phase owing to surgical manipulation (see **Fig. 2**). Pneumocephalus usually resolves within 3 weeks of surgery (see **Figs. 2** and **5**) and is most frequently seen in the subdural space over the frontal lobes, whereas 1 to 3 mm extradural fluid collections are expected deep to the bone flap (see **Fig. 2**). MR imaging will demonstrate dural enhancement adjacent to the craniotomy from the first postoperative day; however, this may be more extensive and persist for many years. In the presence of a craniectomy, the meningogaleal complex bridging the defect may measure from 2 to 6 mm in thickness. A number of

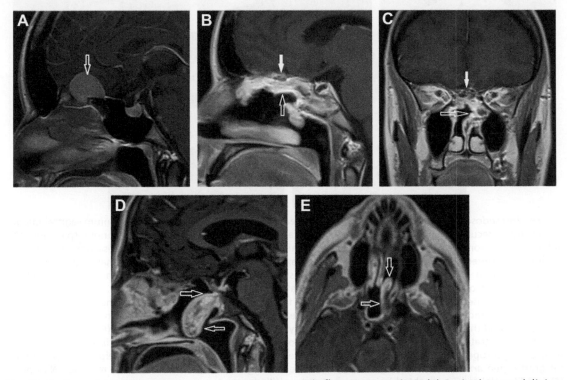

Fig. 22. Endoscopic skull base approaches with vascular pedicle flap reconstructions. (*A*) Sagittal postgadolinium T1-weighted image demonstrates an olfactory groove meningioma. A transcribriform corridor was used for endoscopic access to the anterior skull base. Postgadolinium T1-weighted (*B*) sagittal and (*C*) coronal images demonstrate the multilayered reconstruction with a vascular pedicle nasoseptal flap. Poorly enhancing inlay (collagen matrix) and onlay (fascia) graft material (*filled arrows*) is seen at the site of resection with a curvilinear enhancing nasoseptal flap underlying the surgical defect (*open arrow*). In another patient, a transplanum/transtuberculum corridor has been used to endoscopically resect a tuberculum sella meningioma. Postgadolinium T1-weighted (*D*) sagittal and (*E*) axial images demonstrate an inferior turbinate flap, which has been rotated to cover the dural defect (*arrows*).

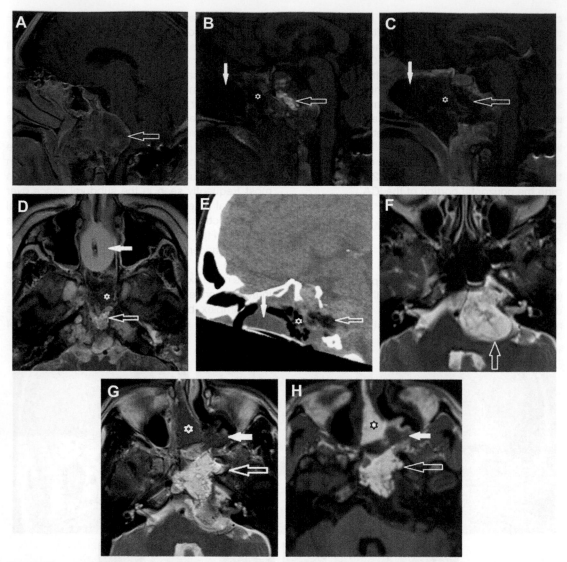

Fig. 23. Postendoscopic complex surgical imaging appearances. (*A*) T1-weighted postgadolinium sagittal images demonstrates recurrent clival chordoma (*arrow*) after a previous transoral approach and tongue split (note the enhancing oral tongue muscles) and an occipitocervical fusion. (*B*) T1-weighted and (*C*) fat-saturated postgadolinium T1-weighted sagittal images, (*D*) T2-weighted axial image and (*E*) sagittal CT reformat in the early postoperative period following endonasal endoscopic subtotal excision of the chordoma. The T1-weighted hyperintense fat graft signal is seen to null on the fat-saturated sequence (*open arrows*). A balloon catheter (*filled arrow*) is used to support the packing. Superior to some residual enhancing tumor there is also mixed intermediate and increased T1-weighted signal and decreased T2-weighted signal hemostatic material (*) between the balloon and the fat graft. This is seen as low density on the CT study. In another patient (*F*) T2-weighted axial image demonstrates a left petrous apex chondrosarcoma with exophytic extradural and interdural extension with early postoperative (*G*) T1 w and (*H*) T2-weighted axial imaging. There is T1-/T2-weighted hyperintense fat graft (open *arrow*) with T1-weighted hyperintense/T2-weighted isointense hemostatic material (Nasopore) (*) and T1-weighted/T2-weighted isointense hematoma (*filled arrow*).

absorbable topical hemostatic agents (eg, Surgicel, Surgiflo) may be intentionally left in the operative bed to control bleeding and may be deployed as sheets, sponges, or powder. This substance is resorbed over weeks to months, but may mimic a mass. They may demonstrate low density with small linear gas pockets on a CT scan (see **Fig. 2**), with intermediate to decreased T2-weighted and increased T1-weighted signals. There are ever-expanding techniques for reconstruction of surgical defects. Cranioplasty may be performed to seal bony defects with a range of materials, which display varying CT imaging appearances (**Table 3**), but are typically low signal or signal void on MR imaging (see **Figs. 3** and **12**).

Skull base defects may need to be sealed with neovascularized or vascularized tissue to separate the cranial compartment and to prevent skull base cerebrospinal fluid leaks. Neovascularized materials include dural collagen matrix, fascia, fat, dermis, split calvarial graft, hydroxyapatite cement, and titanium (see **Fig. 7**) (see **Table 3, Table 4**). Vascularized grafts (free tissue transfer or pedicled local or regional flaps) using fascia or muscle may be added to provide faster healing, support, and cosmesis for larger defects (see **Fig. 4; Fig. 22**) (see **Tables 3** and **4**). Because no sutures are possible, the postendoscopic surgical appearances of the sinonasal region are complicated by supportive nasal packing, hemostatic material and balloon catheters (**Fig. 23**).[14]

SUMMARY

Neurosurgeons rely on detailed neuroimaging studies to assist them in performing skull base surgery. This article describes the key imaging features associated with common skull base approaches, the critical anatomic and neurovascular structures to be studied when planning surgery and typical postoperative appearances.

CLINICS CARE POINTS

- CT and MRI are complementary imaging modalities.
- Key anatomical structures relevant to the tumour and the desired surgical approach should be identified on preoperative imaging.

DISCLOSURE

The authors have nothing to disclose.

REFERENCES

1. Yasargil MG. Microsurgical pterional approach to the aneurysms of the basilar bifurcation. Surg Neurol 1976;6:83–91.

2. Tubbs RS, Loukas M, Shoja MM, et al. Refined and simplified surgical landmarks for the MacCarty keyhole and orbitozygomatic craniotomy. Neurosurgery 2010;66(6 Suppl Operative):230–3.

3. Zabramski Joseph M, Talat Kiriş, Sankhla Suresh K, et al. Orbitozygomatic craniotomy. J Neurosurg 1998;89(2):336–41.

4. Kawase T, Shiobara R, Toya S. Anterior transpetrosal-transtentorial approach for sphenopetroclival meningiomas: surgical method and results in 10 patients. Neurosurgery 1991;28(6):869–76.

5. Van Gompel Jamie J, Alikhani P, Youssef AS, et al. Anterior petrosectomy: consecutive series of 46 patients with attention to approach-related complications. J Neurol Surg B Skull Base 2015;76(5):379–84.

6. Cho CW, Al-Mefty O. Combined petrosal approach to petroclival meningiomas. Neurosurgery 2002;51(3):708–18.

7. Rhoton AL Jr. The temporal bone and transtemporal approaches. Neurosurgery 2000;47(suppl_3):S211–65.

8. House William F, Hitselberger William E. The transcochlear approach to the skull base. Arch Otolaryngol 1976;102(6):334–42.

9. Rhoton AL Jr. The far-lateral approach and its transcondylar, supracondylar, and paracondylar extensions. Neurosurgery 2000;47(suppl_3):S195–209.

10. Fisch U. Infratemporal fossa approach for glomus tumors of the temporal bone. Ann Otol Rhinol Laryngol 1982;91(5):474–9.

11. Mazzoni A. The petro-occipital transsigmoid approach for lesions of the jugular foramen. Skull Base 2009;19(1):48.

12. Hadad G, Bassagasteguy L, Carrau RL, et al. A novel reconstructive technique after endoscopic expanded endonasal approaches: vascular pedicle nasoseptal flap. Laryngoscope 2006;116(10):1882–6.

13. Kassam AB, Gardner P, Snyderman C, et al. Expanded endonasal approach: fully endoscopic, completely transnasal approach to the middle third of the clivus, petrous bone, middle cranial fossa, and infratemporal fossa. Neurosurg Focus 2005;19(1):1–10.

14. Learned Kim O, Adappa ND, Lee JYK, et al. MR imaging evolution of endoscopic cranial defect reconstructions using nasoseptal flaps and their distinction from neoplasm. Am J Neuroradiol 2014;35(6):1182–9.

Anterior and Central Skull Base Tumors

Key Points for the Radiologist to Analyze Prior to Endoscopic Approaches

Davide Farina, MD[a],*, Carlotta Pessina, MD[a], Federica Sozzi, MD[a],
Davide Lombardi, MD[b], Matteo Renzulli, MD[c], Andrea Borghesi, MD[a],
Marco Ravanelli, MD[a], Roberto Maroldi, MD[a]

KEYWORDS

- Anterior skull base • Central skull base • Extended endoscopic endonasal approaches • CT
- MR imaging • CBCT • Imaging

KEY POINTS

- Surgically relevant anatomic variants should be highlighted to the endoscopic skull base surgeon on preoperative imaging.
- Computed tomography (CT)/cone-beam CT and optimized MR imaging protocols are complementary for the planning of extended endonasal approaches to the skull base.
- An understanding of the anatomic limits of endonasal approaches to the skull base helps the radiologist advise on appropriate operative corridors.
- Recognition of the expected reconstructive techniques following endoscopic resection of skull base tumors is important when interpreting follow-up imaging studies.

INTRODUCTION

Transnasal endoscopic surgery was initially developed as a minimally invasive technique to approach inflammatory conditions; however, as a result of increasing surgical expertise and technologic developments, it has progressively expanded its anatomic targets and clinical indications. This has been further enabled by more versatile and effective surgical instruments, and multidisciplinary collaboration between otolaryngologists and neurosurgeons. There are now a wide spectrum of different surgical approaches to the anterior and central skull base, referred to as EEAs. The potential targets of transnasal surgery extend from the frontal sinus anteriorly to

the atlanto-axial junction posteriorly, while laterally to include the parasellar area, the petrous apex, and the upper parapharyngeal space.[1,2] The indications for transnasal surgery have grown in parallel with the expansion of the approaches; although initially confined to chronic rhinosinusitis and pituitary surgery, experienced teams now operate on carefully selected benign lesions and malignancies.[3] The intrinsic advantage of EEA is the exploitation of a natural corridor provided by sinonasal airspaces, with no need for skin incision or osteotomy and limited soft tissue damage; moreover, fiberoptics allow a magnification of the surgical field, which was otherwise impossible with "classic" external approaches. This is generally beneficial in terms of morbidity, with a

The authors have nothing to disclose.
[a] Department of Medical and Surgical Specialties, Radiological Sciences, and Public Health, University of Brescia, Viale Europa 11, 25123 Brescia, Italy; [b] Department of Otorhinolaryngology–Head and Neck Surgery, University of Brescia, P.zzale Spedali Civili 1, 25123 Brescia, Italy; [c] Department of Radiology, IRCCS Azienda Ospedaliero-Universitaria di Bologna, Via Albertoni 15, 40138 Bologna, Italy
* Corresponding author.
E-mail address: davide.farina@unibs.it

shorter interval between surgery and adjuvant postoperative treatment and without the cosmetic consequences of facial scars or osteotomies.[4]

Schematically, EEAs for neoplastic lesions can be described as 3-step procedures: First there is creation of the most appropriate direct corridor through the sinonasal cavities to reach the lesion with the minimal morbidity, second there is the resection of the tumor, and third there is (optional) reconstruction of a barrier between the intracranial structures and the paranasal sinuses.[5]

In a multidisciplinary team, radiologists play an essential role for each of these 3 steps. Cross-sectional imaging with magnetic resonance (MR) imaging, multidetector computed tomography (MDCT), and cone-beam computed tomography (CBCT) provides the road map. This allows the evaluation of the most suitable operative corridor, the relevant variant anatomy that may jeopardize its creation, and the relationship of the lesion with adjacent neurovascular structures. In addition, postoperative scans are essential for the surveillance of complications and oncological results.

IMAGING TECHNIQUES

The cross-sectional anatomy of the skull base is demanding, because it is composed of thick and delicate bone structures as well as numerous traversing neural and vascular structures. To address these challenges, dedicated imaging techniques are applied. Axial and coronal reconstructions should be aligned to the course of the internal acoustic canal, in order to ensure symmetric representation of paired structures on the same section. Although coronal reconstructions are generally perpendicular to the hard palate, differing oblique reformats may be useful to adapt to the point of view of the surgeon during the procedure.[6]

MDCT allows acquisition with isotropic 0.5/0.7-mm voxel size (depending on the generation of the scanner). Although the spatial resolution of CBCT is superior (and may be as low as 0.1 mm), this is traded off against a lack of information on soft tissues. CBCT performed in the sitting or standing positioning may be affected by increased motion artifacts, although this is mitigated by CBCT models that allow the acquisition of images in the supine position (Table 1).

MR imaging is crucial for surgical planning and usually comprises a combination of conventional 2-dimensional sequences (turbo spin echo [TSE] T2 and TSE T1), diffusion-weighted imaging, and 3-dimensional (3D) volumetric acquisitions. A 3D gradient echo (GE) T1 with fat suppression sequence is generally obtained after the administration of contrast material (see Table 1). Although it can be reformatted in any orientation, it is generally acquired in the plane most suited to elucidate the relationships of the lesion with the key anatomic structures and surgical landmarks. A key advantage over 3D GE techniques is the marked homogeneous enhancement of vessels, which allows the depiction of nerve structures within skull base foramina and cavernous sinus,[7,8] where they are surrounded by venous plexi. Heavily T2-weighted 3D sequences depict the cisternal course of cranial nerves, by exploiting the high signal of cerebrospinal fluid (CSF) as an inherent contrast to the hypointense and filiform nerve segments. Gadolinium-enhanced 3D T2/T1 sequences also increase the conspicuity of lesional signal, which is thus contrasted against the adjacent cranial nerves (see Table 1).

RELEVANT ANATOMY AND ANATOMIC VARIANTS
Anterior Skull Base

The anterior skull base extends from the posterior wall of the frontal sinus ventrally to the planum sphenoidale dorsally. The key anatomic and surgical landmarks within the midline anterior skull base are (from medial to lateral) the cribriform plates, the lateral lamella, and the ethmoid fovea (Fig. 1, Table 2).

Midline anterior skull base

The cribriform plates are 2 horizontal laminae separated in the midline by the crista galli. These thin bony structures are perforated by multiple microscopic foramina, which offer passage to the olfactory fila. Laterally, the cribriform plates are continuous with the thicker, vertically oriented lateral lamellae. The height and obliquity of this lamina are quite variable and may be asymmetric. They define the depth of the cribriform plate, and this in turn affects the degree of surgical risk. Several anatomic classifications of this area have been formulated to define the risk of complications during endoscopic sinus surgery: the seminal paper of Keros[9] classified the depth based on the height of the lateral lamella, namely 1 to 3 mm (type I), 4 to 7 mm (type II), and >7 mm (type III). More recently, Gera and colleagues[10] measured the width of the angle between the lateral lamella and the horizontal prolongation of the cribriform plates. The risk of intracranial penetration during endoscopic surgery is increased when there is a small angle (in particular <45°), resulting from a more oblique course of the lateral lamella. The surgical relevance of the anatomic configuration of

Table 1
Summary of main imaging parameters

Computed Tomography			
Acquisition			**Reconstruction**
Voxel (mm)	MPR	Slice thickness (mm)	Orientation
0.1/0.2 CBCT	Axial	≤1	Parallel to IAC and to hard palate
0.5/0.7 MDCT	Coronal		Parallel to IAC, perpendicular to hard palate
	Sagittal		Aligned to the falx

MR Imaging								
	Voxel size (mm)		**Matrix size**		**Gap**		**TR/TE (ms)**	
	1.5T	3T	1.5T	3T	1.5T	3T	1.5T	3T
TSE T2	0.4*0.4*3	0.4*0.4*2.5	307*512	307*512	50%	10%	4750/105	5000/109
TSE T1	0.4*0.4*3	0.4*0.4*2.5	250*512	282*512	50%	10%	537/13	488/11
DWI (EPI)	1.8*1.8*3	1.0*1.0*3.0	132*132	136*136	50%	50%	4000/59	4800/64
3d GE T1	0.6*0.6*0.6	0.5*0.5*0.5	308*448	294*448	-		7.68/3.01	8.19/3.19
3d T2/T1	0.5*0.5*0.5	0.5*0.5*0.5	312*384	323*448	-		5.95/2.67	8.53/3.97

Abbreviations: CBCT, cone-beam computed tomography; DWI, diffusion-weighted imaging; GE, gradient echo; MDCT, multidetector computed tomography; MPR, multiplanar reconstruction; IAC, internal acoustic canal; DWI, diffusion-weighted imaging; EPI, echo-planar imaging; GE, gradient echo; TE, echo time; TR, repetition time; TSE, turbo spin echo.

the ethmoid roof is highlighted by a third classification[11] that defines the risk by assessing the distance between the orbital floor and both the cribriform plate and ethmoid roof. The advantage of this classification is that provides a practical measurement that can be adopted for risk stratification on pretreatment CT images and is quite easily applied to endonasal surgery.

Lateral anterior skull base

The lateral part of the anterior skull base is composed of the thicker frontal bone, which extends from the ethmoid fovea to the roof of the orbits. Three anatomic areas require accurate preoperative evaluation due to the potential for complications during endoscopic surgery.

First, the vertical lamella of the middle turbinate inserts on the skull base at the junction between the thin cribriform plate and lateral lamella. Surgical maneuvers leveraging on the middle turbinate may cause a mechanical stress on this delicate structure, thus resulting in fracture and possible CSF leakage.

Second, the ophthalmic artery provides 2 paired ethmoidal branches, namely anterior and posterior, which course into bony canals parallel to the ethmoid roof. The anterior ethmoidal artery pierces the medial orbital wall in its anterior third and then runs in a canal located close to the fronto-ethmoid suture. This canal is generally easily detected on coronal CT scans as a focal notch in the superomedial orbital wall. The position of the canal relative to the skull base is variable: it can be

enclosed in the skull base or it can float in anterior ethmoid cells, at variable distance from the skull base. In addition, the bone coverage of the canal may be focally dehiscent. The thinner posterior ethmoid artery perforates the posterior third of the medial orbital wall: due to its filiform caliber and oblique orientation, it is best seen on thin axial thick sections. Iatrogenic damage of these vessels may result in significant hemorrhage, if the artery is pulled and transected at level of the orbit medial wall. This is particularly difficult to manage because there is a tendency for the vascular stump to retract into the orbit, and for this reason, such vessels are often preventively ligated during endoscopic procedures.

Central Skull Base

Body of sphenoid and sphenoid sinus

The body of the sphenoid bone is the key element in the anatomy of the central skull base (see **Table 2**). The extent and patterns of its pneumatization are variable. This may be classified in terms of anteroposterior extent (based on the relationships between sphenoid sinuses and sella) and the lateral extent (based on the pneumatization of the greater and lesser wings). The vertical extent also becomes relevant when the sinuses extend beyond the posterior wall of the sella (post-sellar sinus).[12] Such complex analysis of the patterns of pneumatization accounts for the number of neurovascular structures that may be at risk during EEA.

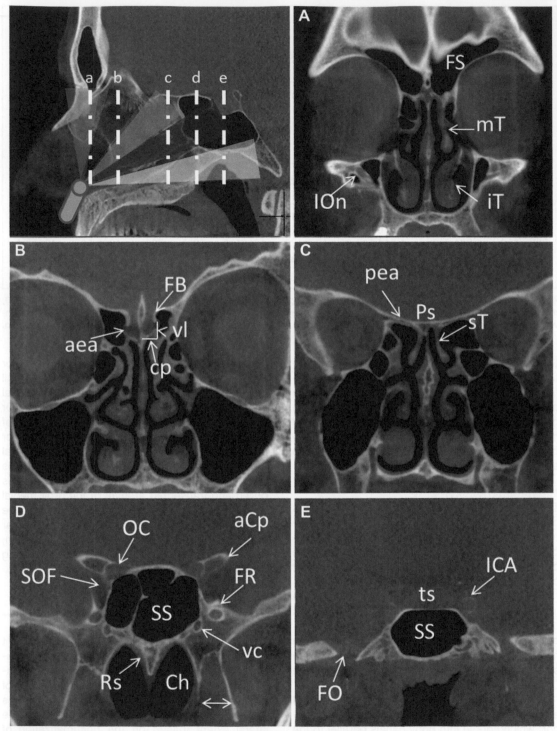

Fig. 1. Sagittal EEA: the sagittal CT scan highlights the target area for each approach; the relevant anatomic landmarks are analyzed on a coronal CT image. (*A*) Transfrontal: frontal sinus (FS), middle turbinate (mT), inferior turbinate (iT), infraorbital nerve (IOn). (*B*) Transcribriform: vertical lamella (vl), cribriform plate (cp), frontal bone (FB), anterior ethmoid artery (aea). (*C*) Transplanum/transtuberculum: posterior ethmoid artery (pea), superior turbinate (St), planum sphenoidalis (Ps). (*D*) Transsellar: superior orbital fissure (SOF), optic canal (OC), anterior clinoid process (aCp), sphenoid sinus (SS), foramen rotundum (FR), choana (Ch), sphenoid rostrum (Rs), vidian canal (vc). (*E*) Transclival: tuberculum sellae (ts), sphenoid sinus (SS), internal carotid artery (ICA), foramen ovale (FO).

Table 2
Key anatomic landmarks

Anterior Skull Base		
Bone	**Nerves**	**Vessels**
Crista galli Cribriform plate Vertical lamella Orbital roof	Olfactory fila (I)	Anterior ethmoid artery Posterior ethmoid artery

Central Skull Base			
Bone	**Nerves**	**Vessels**	**Pneumatization**
Anterior clinoid process Optic strut Pterygoid root Pterygoid laminae Greater sphenoid wing	Optic (II) Ophthalmic (III) Trochlear (IV) Ophthalmic (V1) Maxillary (V2) Mandibular (V3) Abducens (VI) Vidian Palatine nerves	Internal carotid artery Cavernous sinus Sphenopalatine artery Middle meningeal artery	Sellar region Anterior clinoid process Pterygoid root Onodi cell

The maxillary nerve (V2) traverses the foramen rotundum to course intracranially along the inferolateral sphenoid sinus wall. It is surrounded by a bony canal that may be incomplete on the intracranial aspect. The vidian nerve canal courses inferomedial to the maxillary nerve, into the spongiotic bone of the pterygoid root. When sphenoid pneumatization extends laterally to the pterygoid root and lesser wing, the 2 nerves may protrude into the sphenoid sinus cavity, protected by only thin layers of bone, and they are potentially dehiscent. The cavernous segment of the internal carotid artery may protrude into the sphenoid sinus when there is a post-sellar type of pneumatization. This results in increased surgical risk, particularly when the canal is focally dehiscent or when sphenoid sinus septum inserts on it.[13] The anterior clinoid process is the posteromedial border of the lesser wing of sphenoid and it forms an attachment for the tentorium cerebelli. Medially, the anterior clinoid process is related to the pre-chiasmatic segment of the optic nerve, whereas infero-medially it is adjacent to the roof of the superior orbital fissure, through which the oculomotor and ophthalmic nerves course. A bone spur termed the optic strut connects the anterior clinoid process to the sphenoid body, separating the optic canal from the superior orbital fissure. In the sphenoid sinus cavity, this strut corresponds to the lateral opticocarotid recess, which lies between the indentations created by the carotid protuberance and optic nerve.[14] Finally, the bone spur connecting the anterior and middle clinoid process creates a carotico-clinoid foramen, which is crossed by the internal carotid artery (**Fig. 2**). These crucial anatomic structures are potentially at risk during surgery, particularly when the lesser wings of the sphenoid bone are pneumatized (**Figs. 3 and 4**).

Finally, the surgical risk is increased by the anatomic variant of the Onodi cell. This posterior ethmoid cell expands supero-lateral to the sphenoid sinus, and in some cases extends into a pneumatized anterior clinoid process. Hence, there is the potential for surgical injury to the optic nerve and internal carotid artery, if this is overlooked.

Cavernous sinus

The cavernous sinus lies along the lateral walls of sphenoid sinuses, posterior to the superior orbital fissure. This is the crossroads for several cranial nerves and it contains the carotid siphon. Three-dimensional gadolinium-enhanced MR imaging sequences may depict the nerves along the lateral surface of the sinus (oculomotor, trochlear, ophthalmic, and maxillary nerves) or embedded in the high signal of the blood-filled venous spaces (abducens). This depiction is most consistent for the thicker oculomotor and maxillary nerves. The cavernous sinus is related to the Meckel cave (which envelops the Gasserian ganglion) posteriorly and the foramen lacerum inferiorly. The foramen lacerum is a virtual foramen, closed by a thin layer of cartilage that can be found at the petroclival junction: the intracranial aspect is related to the vidian nerve anteriorly, whereas the extracranial aspect of the foramen is related to the lateral recess of the nasopharynx. The anatomy

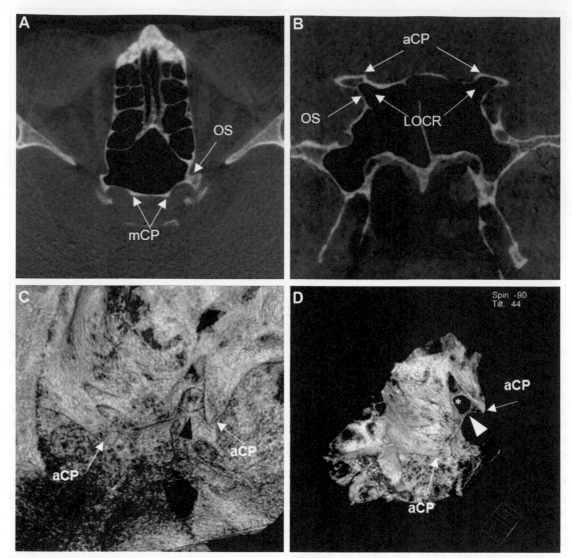

Fig. 2. CBCT scan, MPR on axial (*A*) and coronal (*B*) plane, volume rendering (*C, D*). The lateral opticocarotid recess (LOCR) is a key endoscopic landmark of the course of the optic nerve and carotid artery. On CT images it corresponds to the pneumatization of the optic strut (OS). The caroticoclinoid ligament connects the anterior (aCP) and medial clinoid process (mCP)of the sphenoid: when ossified (*arrowheads*), it contributes to delineate the caroticoclinoid foramen (*asterisks*).

of the abducens nerve is relevant to the planning of some endoscopic approaches. Before reaching the cavernous sinus, this nerve emerges at the pontomedullary junction and courses cranially and laterally in the prepontine cistern, along the dorsal surface of the clivus. At the petrous apex, it pierces the dura at the level of the Dorello canal and finally reaches the cavernous sinus.

Lateral central skull base and pterygopalatine fossa

At the lateral aspect of the central skull base, the greater sphenoid wing separates the infratemporal fossa and masticator space from the middle cranial fossa. The foramen ovale principally provides passage for the mandibular nerve whereas the more posterolateral foramen spinosum contains the middle meningeal artery.

At the inferolateral part of the sphenoid bone, the pterygoid roots and laminae contribute to the posterior border of the pterygopalatine fossa. This vertical slit can easily be found on axial CT or MR imaging scans behind the posteromedial maxillary sinus wall. The palatine nerves course vertically to its inferior aspect. The mid-pterygopalatine fossa contains the sphenopalatine ganglion and its multiple communications, which include the vidian nerve. The maxillary nerve

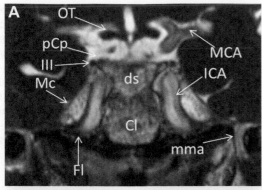

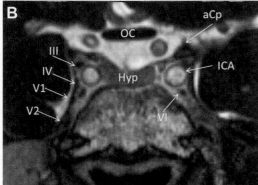

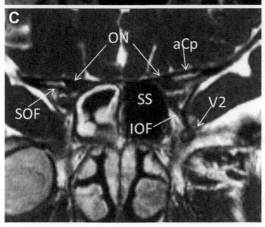

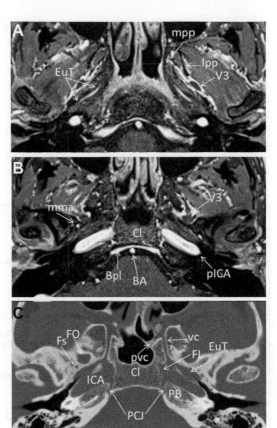

Fig. 4. Anatomy of the central skull base on the axial plane; 3D GE T1 with contrast (*A,B*) and CT (*C*). Clivus (Cl), petrous bone (PB), petro-clival junction (PCJ), foramen lacerum (FL), vidian canal (vc), palatovaginal canal (pvc). Foramen ovale (FO) and foramen spinosum (FS) are crossed, respectively, by the mandibular nerve (V3) and middle meningeal artery (mma). Petrous internal carotid artery (pICA), basilar artery (BA), basilar plexus (Bpl), Eustachian tube (EuT), medial (mpp) and lateral (lpp) pterygoid plate.

Fig. 3. MR imaging anatomy of the parasellar region (*A*), cavernous sinus (*B*) and superior orbital fissure (*C*) on coronal T2/T1 3D sequence after contrast administration. Optic nerve (ON), tract (OT), and chiasm (OC). Internal carotid (ICA), middle cerebral (MCA), and middle meningeal (mma) artery. Anterior (aCp) and posterior clinoid process (pCp), dorsum sellae (ds) clivus (Cl), foramen lacerum (Fl), sphenoid sinus (SS), superior (SOF) and inferior (IOF) orbital fissure. Oculomotor nerve (III), trochlear nerve (IV), ophthalmic nerve (V1), maxillary nerve (V2), abducens nerve (VI), Meckel cave (Mc), hypophysis (Hyp).

crosses horizontally to end in the infraorbital nerve within the more superior pterygopalatine fossa. The most superior (and wider) part of the pterygo-palatine fossa communicates with the superior

orbital fissure, thereby creating an intricate network of anatomic connections and neural pathways between the middle cranial fossa, orbit, and face.

ENDOSCOPIC APPROACHES TO THE ANTERIOR AND CENTRAL SKULL BASE

As a rule of thumb, the resectability of skull base lesions is defined by 2 main concepts: the location of the lesion and its relationships with crucial anatomic structures.

Lines can be traced on CT/MR images to define the endoscopic resectability of lesions: these are the Kassam (nasopalatine) line, which extends antero-posteriorly, from the apex of nasal bone to posterior edge of the hard palate, and the paired midorbital lines, vertically oriented and passing through the midpoint of orbital roof.[15] Lesions located above the Kassam line or in-between mid-orbital lines are amenable to an endoscopic approach. A general rule can be applied to the relationships with the adjacent neurovascular structures: if the lesion is located posteriorly or laterally, then the risk of iatrogenic damage is higher and so endoscopic resection may be contraindicated.

The site of the lesion also influences the selection of the specific procedure. Endoscopic approaches are classically subdivided in 2 classes. Sagittal approaches allow the endoscopic approach to access midline lesions; these include the transfrontal, transcribriform, transtuberculum/transplanum, transsellar, transclival, and transodontoid approaches. On the other hand, coronal approaches allow access to the paramedian part of the skull base; these include the transorbital approach anteriorly, and the transpterygoid, infratemporal fossa, transpetrous, and transcavernous approaches posteriorly[5] (Table 3).

Table 3
Endonasal endoscopic approaches to skull base pathologies: boundaries and indications

Approach	Boundaries	Indications
Transfrontal	*Anterior*: nasal bones *Posterior*: cribriform plate *Lateral*: superior orbital walls	Nasofrontal dysembryogenic and neoplastic lesions Complications of rhinosinusitis CSF leaks
Transcribriform	*Anterior*: posterior frontal sinus wall *Posterior*: planum sphenoidale *Lateral*: lamina papyracea	Nasoethmoid tumors Meningiomas Meningoceles
Transplanum/transtuberculum	*Anterior*: posterior ethmoid arteries *Posterior*: sella turcica *Lateral*: optic canals, paraclinoid ICA, opticocarotid recesses	Pituitary adenomas Meningiomas Craniopharyngiomas
Transsellar	*Anterior*: anterior intercavernous sinus *Posterior*: posterior intercavernous sinus *Lateral*: cavernous sinus	Pituitary adenomas, Rathke Cleft cysts, craniopharyngiomas, arachnoid cysts
Transclival	*Lateral*: cavernous sinus, paraclival ICA, hypoglossal canal *Superior*: orbital roof *Inferior*: orbital floor	Meningiomas, chordomas, chondrosarcomas, aneurysms
Transodontoid	*Lateral*: occipital condyles, lateral masses of the atlas *Superior*: suprasellar area *Inferior*: foramen magnum	Pannus (rheumatoid arthritis), chordomas, meningiomas, Nasopharyngeal carcinomas
Transorbital	*Anterior*: lacrimal pathway, eyeball *Posterior*: orbital apex *Superior*: orbital roof *Inferior*: orbital floor	Meningiomas, hemangiomas, schwannomas
Transpterygoid/infratemporal	*Lateral*: greater sphenoid wing, lateral pterygoid muscle *Medial*: sphenoid floor, nasopharynx *Superior*: superior orbital fissure *Inferior*: pterygomaxillary junction	Juvenile angiofibromas, schwannomas
Transcavernous	*Lateral*: dura of middle cranial fossa *Medial*: sella turcica *Superior*: anterior and posterior clinoid processes, roof of cavernous sinus *Inferior*: petroclival junction	Meningiomas, invasive pituitary adenomas, schwannomas
Transpetrous	*Anterior (lateral)*: paraclival ICA *Medial*: midclivus *Superior*: abducens nerve *Inferior*: petroclival junction	Meningiomas, chordomas, chondrosarcomas, cholesterol granuloma

Abbreviations: CSF, cerebrospinal fluid; ICA, internal carotid artery.

Transfrontal Approach

This approach may be used to treat congenital midline lesions of the anterior skull base (eg, meningo-encephaloceles, nasal gliomas, dermoid cyst and sinuses) and inflammatory lesions (eg, chronic rhinosinusitis, mucocele), as well as benign frontal sinus tumors (eg, osteomas, inverted papillomas) that do not involve the frontal sinus anterior wall or extend laterally. Boundaries of this approach are the nasal bones and anterior wall of frontal sinus anteriorly, the cribriform plate posteriorly, and orbital cavities laterally. Two main concepts guide the use of the transfrontal approach. First, the creation of a surgical corridor mandates resection of the frontal sinus floor between the nasal septum and lamina papyracea, through an anterior septectomy on both sides (Draf III procedure).[16] Second, this procedure is precluded by involvement of the anterior wall of the frontal sinus and by lateral extent of the lesion beyond the midorbital line. The vertical and oblique orientation of the corridor, the narrow channel, and the risk of iatrogenic damage of the anterior skull base also increase the technical challenge.

Transcribriform Approach

This is the mainstay for endoscopic resection of some benign (eg, meningiomas, schwannomas) and selected malignant tumors of the naso-ethmoid complex that invade the anterior skull base (**Fig. 5**). Boundaries of this approach are the bony angle between frontal sinus and anterior skull base anteriorly, the orbital cavity laterally (on one or both sides) and the spheno-ethmoidal junction posteriorly. In this procedure, resection of the anterior part of the nasal septum allows bi-nostril control of the surgical access.[1] In some cases, particularly when the septum is not invaded and the olfaction is not already compromised, a unilateral approach may be used to preserve the olfactory epithelium on the opposite side. The resection generally extends to the whole roof of the ethmoid with the wide transcranial corridor exposing a large tract of the dura mater and thus permitting intradural dissection of the tumor.[1] In the reconstructive phase, a multilayered technique (with fascial grafts or, when available, vascularized mucosal flaps) ensures complete adequate sealing of the anterior skull base.

Transplanum/Transtuberculum Approach

This approach is best suited for tumors located along the sphenoid planum and tuberculum sellae (eg, meningiomas, pituitary adenomas with extrasellar extension) (**Fig. 6**). The boundaries of this approach are the cribriform plate and planum anteriorly, the anterosuperior aspect of the sellar cavity posteriorly. The medial limit is the orbital wall, medial aspect of cavernous sinus, and

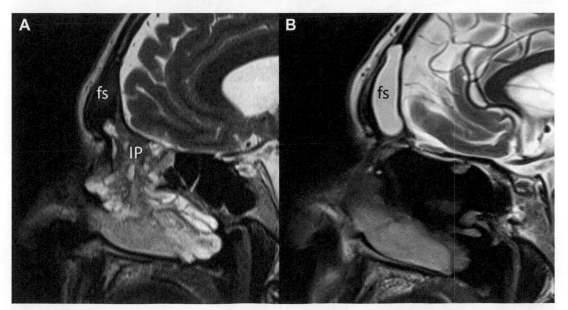

Fig. 5. Sagittal TSE T2, pretreatment (*A*) and follow-up scan (*B*). (*A*) Fronto-ethmoidal inverted papilloma widely in contact with the anterior skull base, near the midline. (*B*) After ethmoidectomy obtained through an endoscopic transcribriform approach, a smooth and regular interface separates the anterior cranial fossa from the residual cavity. The hyperintense line on the nasal side represents a free mucosal flap. The frontal sinus (fs) is blocked and filled by retained secretions.

opticocarotid recess. The transplanum/transtuberculum approach does not affect the olfactory function because the rostral insertion of the nasal septum is not resected and the craniectomy does not extend anterior to the posterior ethmoid arteries and canals.[1]

Transsellar Approach

This represents the most established and most frequently used endonasal approach, originally designed for the resection of pituitary adenomas but now used to treat other sellar lesions. This approach also allows access to the medial part of the cavernous sinus.[17] A combination with transplanum/transtuberculum or transclival approaches may be required to address superior or inferior extensions. The transsellar approach requires posterior septectomy and sphenoidotomy; however, the width of the sphenoidotomy may be tailored to the local extension of the lesion to minimize morbidity.

Transclival Approach

Resection of a wide variety of lesions (eg, chordoma, ecchordosis physaliphora, chondrosarcomas) can be achieved via this approach, which provides access to the prepontine cistern in-between the sellar and sphenoid sinus floors (midclival approach) (**Fig. 7**). Depending on the caudal extent of the lesion, bone resection can be extended inferiorly (below the level of foramen lacerum to reach the foramen magnum) or superiorly to the upper third of the clivus, above the Dorello canal. The lower rates of gross tumor resection in this settings reflects the more challenging relationships with neurovascular structures at the craniocervical junction and the cavernous sinus.

Transodontoid Approach

The resection of tumors (eg, chordoma and selected recurrent nasopharyngeal carcinoma) and treatment of non-neoplastic conditions of the

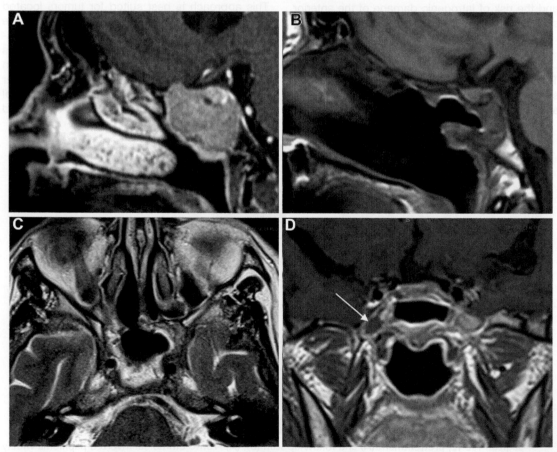

Fig. 6. (*A*) Sagittal gadolinium-enhanced 3D GE T1 shows a homogeneous solid mass filling and expanding the sphenoid sinus. Biopsy proved invasive pituitary adenoma. (*B–D*) Follow-up scan after transplanum EEA shows inflammatory thickening of the mucosa of the sphenoid sinus and retained secretions in the blocked right lateral recess (*arrow*).

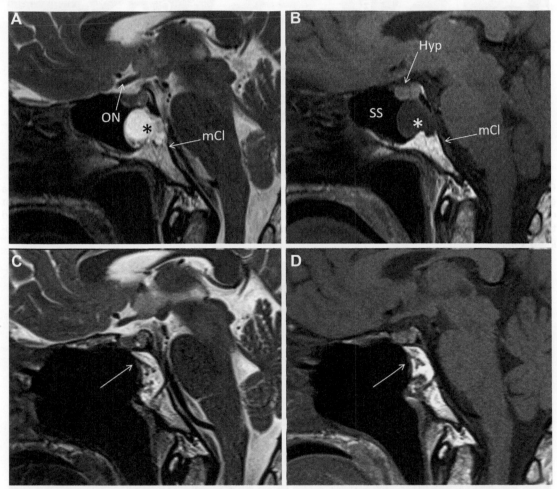

Fig. 7. Sagittal TSE T2 and SE T1; pretreatment (*A, B*) and follow-up scan (*C, D*). (*A, B*) A T2 hyperintense and T1 hypointense lesion (*asterisk*) alters the posteromedial aspect of the mid-clivus (mCl), thinning its intracranial cortical and focally invading the spongiotic; there is protrusion in the sphenoid sinus (*S*) cavity that shows post-sellar pattern of pneumatization. (*C, D*) After endoscopic resection with a transclival approach, a fat pad (*arrows*) separates the sinus cavity from the middle cranial fossa content.

craniocervical junction (eg, pannus in rheumatoid arthritis) may benefit from this approach. The boundaries are limited by the sphenoid sinus floor superiorly, hard and soft palate inferiorly, and Eustachian tube and the parapharyngeal internal carotid arteries laterally. The main constraint for the trans-odontoid approach is the Kassam (naso-palatine) line. This line defines the anatomic constraints of bone resection at the cranio-cervical junction, therefore tumors extending caudal to it should be managed with alternative or multiportal approaches.[18]

Transorbital Approach

This coronal approach to the anterior skull base entails resection of the medial orbital wall to reach lesions of the orbital roof or intraconal orbital tumors[18] (**Fig. 8**). Lesions located above

and lateral to the optic nerve and ophthalmic artery are not amenable to a transorbital endoscopic approach.[5] In some cases, this procedure provides a lateral enlargement for a trans-cribriform or transplanum approach, allowing treatment of sinonasal tumors that contact the lamina papyracea and with no sign of macroscopic orbital invasion at preoperative imaging. Besides the optic nerve and ophthalmic artery, the medial and inferior recti muscles (which may offer a corridor to reach the intraconal space) and the ethmoid arteries (which need to be ligated to expose the medial part of the orbital roof) are essential landmarks.

Transpterygoid/Infratemporal Approach

This approach requires a wide antrostomy, which may be further enlarged to an inferior medial

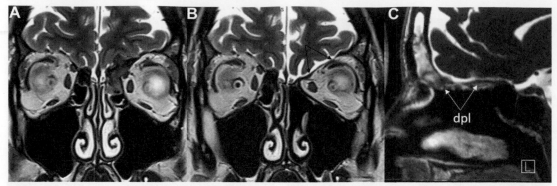

Fig. 8. (*A*) Pretreatment coronal TSE T2 shows a frontoethmoid lesion on the left, contacting the ethmoid fovea and remodeling both the roof and floor of the frontal sinus. Biopsy proved osteoblastoma. (*B, C*) Posttreatment coronal TSE T2 and sagittal gadolinium-enhanced T2/T1, obtained after combined approach (ie, craniectomy and transcribriform/transorbital EEA) shows the bone gap in the orbital roof (*arrows*) and the thin and regular duraplasty (dpl).

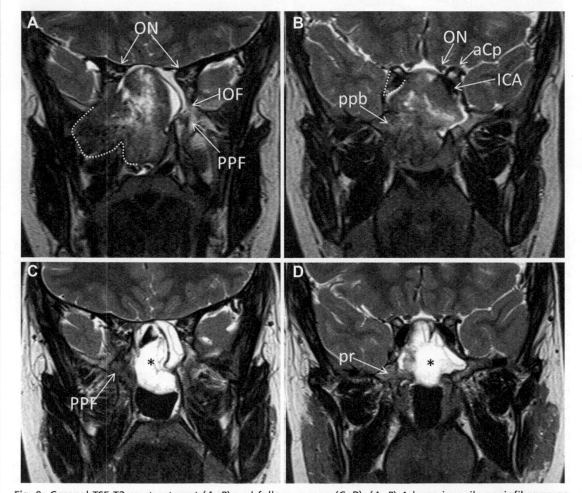

Fig. 9. Coronal TSE T2, pretreatment (*A, B*) and follow-up scan (*C, D*). (*A, B*) A large juvenile angiofibroma occupies the pterygopalatine fossa (PPF on the contralateral side for comparison), the infratemporal fossa (*dotted line* in *A*), the sphenoid sinus, and the nasopharynx. There is permeative growth in the spongiosa of the pterygoid root (ppb) and invasion of the inferior orbital fissure (IOF on the contralateral side for comparison). The lesion is in contact with both internal carotid arteries (ICA), anterior clinoid processes (aCp), and optic struts (*dotted line* in *B*), no involvement of optic nerves is seen (ON). Follow-up scan (*C,D*) shows scarring of the pterygopalatine fossa and pterygoid root and inflammatory ballooning of the mucosa of the sphenoid sinus (*asterisks*).

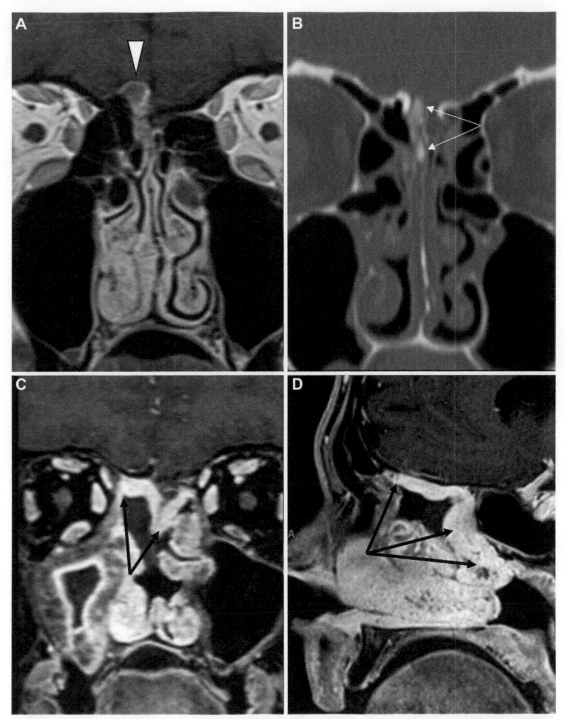

Fig. 10. (*A, B*) Gadolinium (Gd)-enhanced SE T1 and MDCT on coronal plane show a partially calcified and enhancing lesion growing across the right cribriform plate (*white arrows*). The adjacent dura is slightly thickened but continuous (*arrowhead*). (*C, D*) Gd-enhanced 3D GE T1 after EEA with transcribriform approach depicts the curvilinear pedicled flap of septal mucosa (Hadad flap) (*black arrows*) used to reconstruct the anterior skull base.

maxillectomy. The transpterygoid approach then offers a route to treat lesions that reach the pterygopalatine fossa, including lesions extending posteriorly from the maxillary sinus or laterally from the nasopharynx. More rarely, the target may be a lesion arising in the pterygopalatine fossa itself or the pterygoid root (eg, juvenile angiofibroma). The infratemporal approach allows treatment of lesions involving this space primarily or secondarily (eg, from the maxillary sinus or the skull base).[19] Access to the infratemporal fossa is also gained via the posterior maxillary sinus wall. The combination of medial maxillectomy with anteromedial maxillotomy (Denker approach) or contralateral transseptal approach provides a progressively wider angle of exposure of the infratemporal fossa, thus allowing wider control (**Fig. 9**). An important landmark is the internal carotid artery and its relationship to the tumor.

Transcavernous Approach

The cavernous sinus may be reached endoscopically following 2 distinct roots, both targeted at its anterior wall. The medial transcavernous approach reaches the medial compartment of

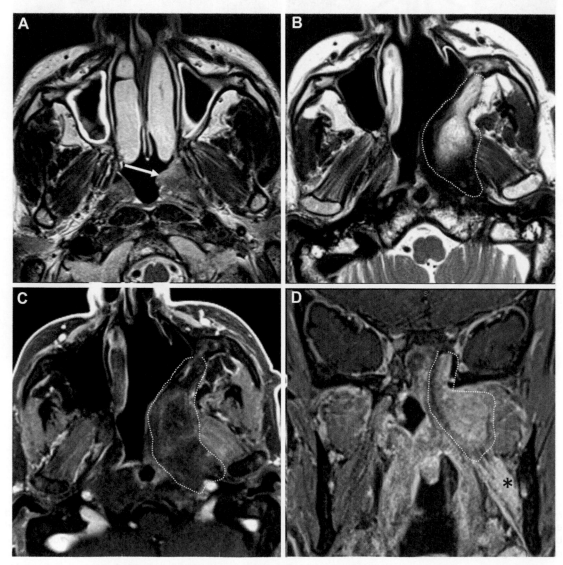

Fig. 11. (*A*) In a patient previously treated with chemoradiation for nasopharyngeal carcinoma, a nodular mass is seen thickening and obstructing the left torus tubarius (*arrow*). Biopsy proved recurrence. (*B–D*) Follow-up scan after nasopharyngeal endoscopic resection obtained with transpterygoid and infratemporal access with Denker procedure. A large fronto-parietal flap was harvested to cover the surgical bed (*dotted lines*); reactive enhancement of the internal pterygoid muscle (*asterisk*).

the sinus, between the lateral wall of the sphenoid sinus and intracavernous carotid. Such an approach is best suited for the inferior part of the sinus, rather than its posterior or superior tract. Initially designed to achieve the resection of the intracavernous extension of hypophyseal lesions, its indications are now expanded to other tumors and tumorlike conditions. The lateral transcavernous approach targets tumors involving the lateral part of the sinus beyond the internal carotid artery (eg, meningiomas, neurogenic tumors, or pituitary lesion with parasellar extension).

Transpetrous Approach

Three distinct subtypes are included under the same classification, all representing a lateral extension of the mid-lower transclival approach. The suprapetrous approach is also referred to as the Meckel cave approach, highlighting its main target. Although naturally suited for the treatment of neurogenic tumors, it also can be a route to access lesions reaching the borderland between the cavernous sinus and Meckel cave (eg, sinonasal tumors or nasopharyngeal tumors with perineural

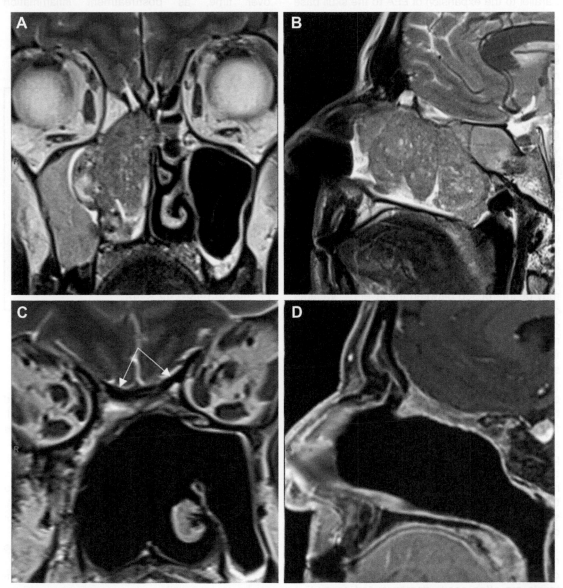

Fig. 12. (*A, B*) Pretreatment coronal and sagittal TSE T2 show a solid ethmoid mass attached to the anterior skull base with no intracranial extension. Biopsy proved adenocarcinoma. (*C, D*) Posttreatment coronal TSE T2 and sagittal gadolinium-enhanced GE T1, obtained after combined approach (ie, craniectomy and transfrontal/transcribriform/transplanum EEA). The multilayered duraplasty shows hypointense T2 signal on the intracranial side (*arrows*) and homogeneous enhancement.

spread). The medial petrous approach encompasses the petrous apex superior and anteroinferior to the carotid artery and allows resection of petroclival lesions (eg, cholesterol granulomas, chondrosarcomas, chordomas).[20] Finally, the infrapetrous approach generally combines a transpterygoid approach to open a corridor to the anteroinferior part of the petrous apex and anterior foramen lacerum, medial to the foramen ovale.

SKULL BASE DEFECT RECONSTRUCTION

Parallel to the expansion of EEA to the skull base and the widening of the surgical indications, numerous reconstructive techniques have been developed with the main aim to restore watertight separation between the neurocranium and sinonasal cavities and to avoid CSF leakage. This same technique may be adapted to provide cover for vital anatomic structures, such as the internal carotid artery, when tumor resection exposes these structures or they become friable due to previous irradiation. This can be accomplished using synthetic materials, free grafts, or pedicled flaps, either alone or in combination.

The multilayer technique is principally applied to anterior skull base reconstruction and consists of the juxtaposition of 3 layers of autologous material (eg, iliotibial tract of fascia lata), 2 of which are intracranial (intradural and extradural, respectively) whereas one is extracranial. The layers are fixed with fibrin glue, and some adipose tissue may be interposed between the layers.[21] Variants of this scheme may include the use of synthetic dural material, intracranially,[22] or apply free mucosal grafts harvested from the nasal fossa floor or the inferior turbinate on the extracranial side.

Pedicled flaps are favored for the reconstruction of surgical defects in the central skull base due to the higher pressure of CSF leaks, the irregular profile of the skull, and the need to protect critical structures (eg, internal carotid artery).Traditionally, pedicled flaps are harvested from the posterior third of the nasal septum (Hadad flap)[23] (Fig. 10); however, alternative sites may be chosen when this is not possible (principally due to previous septal resection), such as the temporoparietal fascia flap or the pericranial flap[24] (Fig. 11).

Awareness of the reconstruction technique is required for the interpretation of the normal postoperative imaging appearances. Autologous materials are often poorly demonstrated on routine 2D MR imaging sequences. When visualized, they generally display low signal intensity on all MR imaging sequences due to the lack of water content and they are nonenhancing due to the

absence of vascularization (Fig. 12). Fat pads are easily recognized by combining standard and fat-suppressed MR imaging sequences. Free flaps demonstrate enhancement on later postoperative imaging when they are integrated and there is reepithelization of the surgical cavity. In contrast, pedicled flaps display physiologic enhancement on immediate postoperative monitoring scans, and also appear significantly thicker.[25,26] Although the interface between anterior/middle cranial fossa and sinonasal cavities is expected to be sharp and regular, progressive thinning may occur over time, as posttreatment inflammation regresses.

CLINICS CARE POINTS

- Symmetric representation of paired structures on cross-sectional scans is obtained using the internal acoustic canals as a reference for acquisition and reconstruction.
- The high spatial resolution of CBCT scans may be exploited to depict the finest bone details of skull base anatomy.
- Each surgical corridor has specific boundaries and anatomic structures at risk, which require meticulous preoperative assessment.
- Details about the reconstructive technique adopted are pre-requisite for the interpretation of follow up scans.

REFERENCES

1. Kassam A, Snyderman CH, Mintz A, et al. Expanded endonasal approach: the rostrocaudal axis. Part I. Crista galli to the sella turcica. Neurosurg Focus 2005;19(1):E3.
2. Kassam AB, Gardner P, Snyderman C, et al. Expanded endonasal approach: fully endoscopic, completely transnasal approach to the middle third of the clivus, petrous bone, middle cranial fossa, and infratemporal fossa. Neurosurg Focus 2005; 19(1):E6.
3. Bossi P, Farina D, Gatta G, et al. Paranasal sinus cancer. Crit Rev Oncol Hematol 2016;98:45–61.
4. Kasemsiri P, Carrau RL, Ditzel Filho LF, et al. Advantages and limitations of endoscopic endonasal approaches to the skull base. World Neurosurg 2014; 82(6 Suppl):S12–21.
5. Roxbury CR, Ishii M, Blitz AM, et al. Expanded endonasal endoscopic approaches to the skull base for

the radiologist. Radiol Clin North Am 2017;55(1): 1–16.

6. Yano S, Shinojima N, Kitajima M, et al. Usefulness of oblique coronal computed tomography and magnetic resonance imaging in the endoscopic endonasal approach to treat skull base lesions. World Neurosurg 2018;113:e10–9.

7. Maroldi R, Farina D, Borghesi A, et al. Perineural tumor spread. Neuroimaging Clin N Am 2008;18(2): 413–29, xi.

8. Hayashi M, Chernov MF, Tamura N, et al. Usefulness of the advanced neuroimaging protocol based on plain and gadolinium-enhanced constructive interference in steady state images for gamma knife radiosurgery and planning microsurgical procedures for skull base tumors. Acta Neurochir Suppl 2013; 116:167–78.

9. Keros P. On the practical value of differences in the level of the lamina cribrosa of the ethmoid. Z Laryngol Rhinol Otol Ihre Grenzgeb 1962;41: 808–13.

10. Gera R, Mozzanica F, Karligkiotis A, et al. Lateral lamella of the cribriform plate, a keystone landmark: proposal for a novel classification system. Rhinology 2018;56:65–72.

11. Abdullah B, Chew SC, Aziz ME, et al. A new radiological classification for the risk assessment of anterior skull base injury in endoscopic sinus surgery. Sci Rep 2020;10(1):4600.

12. Bilgir E, Bayrakdar İŞ. A new classification proposal for sphenoid sinus pneumatization: a retrospective radio-anatomic study. Oral Radiol 2020. https://doi.org/10.1007/s11282-020-00467-6. Epub ahead of print.

13. Farina D, Lombardi D, Bertuletti M, et al. An additional challenge for head and neck radiologists: anatomic variants posing a surgical risk - a pictorial review. Insights Imaging 2019;10(1):112.

14. Sandu K, Monnier P, Pasche P. Anatomical landmarks for transnasal endoscopic skull base surgery. Eur Arch Otorhinolaryngol 2012;269(1):171–8.

15. Schmalfuss IM. Imaging of endoscopic approaches to the anterior and central skull base. Clin Radiol 2018;73(1):94–105.

16. Selleck AM, Desai D, Thorp BD, et al. Management of frontal sinus tumors. Otolaryngol Clin North Am 2016;49(4):1051–65.

17. Raithatha R, McCoul ED, Woodworth GF, et al. Endoscopic endonasal approaches to the cavernous sinus. Int Forum Allergy Rhinol 2012;2(1):9–15.

18. Snyderman CH, Pant H, Carrau RL, et al. What are the limits of endoscopic sinus surgery? The expanded endonasal approach to the skull base. Keio J Med 2009;58(3):152–60.

19. Prosser JD, Figueroa R, Carrau RI, et al. Quantitative analysis of endoscopic endonasal approaches to the infratemporal fossa. Laryngoscope 2011; 121(8):1601–5.

20. Mason E, Rompaey JV, Solares CA, et al. Subtemporal retrolabyrinthine (posterior petrosal) versus endoscopic endonasal approach to the petroclival region: an anatomical and computed tomography study. J Neurol Surg B Skull Base 2016;77(3): 231–7.

21. Villaret AB, Yakirevitch A, Bizzoni A, et al. Endoscopic transnasal craniectomy in the management of selected sinonasal malignancies. Am J Rhinol 2010;24:60–5.

22. Eloy JA, Shukla PA, Choudhry OJ, et al. Challenges and surgical nuances in reconstruction of large planum sphenoidale tuberculum sellae defects after endoscopic endonasal resection of parasellar skull base tumors. Laryngoscope 2013;123(6):1353–60.

23. Hadad G, Bassagatseguy L, Carrau RL, et al. A novel reconstructive technique after endoscopic expanded endonasal approaches: vascular pedicle nasoseptal flap. Laryngoscope 2006;116:1882–6.

24. Bolzoni Villaret A, Nicolai P, Schreiber A, et al. The temporo-parietal fascial flap in extended transnasal endoscopic procedures: cadaver dissection and personal clinical experience. Eur Arch Otorhinolaryngol 2013;270(4):1473–9.

25. Farina D, Zorza I, Golemi S, et al. Posttreatment imaging surveillance. Adv Otorhinolaryngol 2020;84: 218–30.

26. Kim CS, Patel U, Pastena G, et al. The magnetic resonance imaging appearance of endoscopic endonasal skull base defect reconstruction using free mucosal graft. World Neurosurg 2019;126: e165–72.

Imaging of the Vestibular Schwannoma
Diagnosis, Monitoring, and Treatment Planning

Steve E.J. Connor, MRCP, FRCR[a,b,*]

KEYWORDS

- Neoplasms • Skull base schwannoma • Vestibular computed tomography
- Magnetic resonance imaging • Cerebellopontine angle tumor • Residual tumor • Neurosurgery
- Hearing disorders

KEY POINTS

- Whilst vestibular schwannomas are the commonest tumour of the cerebello-pontine angle cistern and internal auditory meatus, imaging features suggesting an alternative diagnosis should be identified.
- 3D T2w sequences are a cost effective means to detecting vestibular schwannomas, however gadolinium enhanced imaging is required in particular settings and for equivocal findings.
- Understanding the natural history, optimal measurement and definition of tumour growth helps evaluate for the failure of conservative management and requirement for therapeutic intervention.
- MRI helps decide whether surgery or radiotherapy is the appropriate therapeutic intervention, provides important information for surgical planning and monitors tumours following treatment.

Vestibular schwannomas (VSs) account for 6% to 8% of intracranial tumors and comprise the vast majority of cerebellopontine angle (CPA) cistern and internal auditory meatus (IAM) lesions. Imaging plays a key role in the detection, characterization, and management of these tumors.

IMAGING STRATEGIES

MRI is the standard of care for the detection and follow-up of VSs. Heavily T2-weighted (T2w) 3D acquisitions provide high-spatial-resolution isotropic depiction of the CPA and IAM with a cisternographic effect. These may be based on 3D T2w gradient echo (GRE) or 3D fast spin echo (FSE) techniques (**Table 1**). They are used for the initial detection of VSs and are increasingly used

for the monitoring of tumors. The 3D T2w GRE approach uses steady-state free precession sequences which provide high signal to noise. While banding artifact may result from phase shift errors due to magnetic field inhomogeneities, these are mitigated by acquiring at least two off resonance volumes (eg, fast imaging using steady-state acquisition [FIESTA], constructive interference in steady state [CISS]). The 3D T2w FSE sequences are less affected by such susceptibility artifact; however, they have been prone to blurring in view of the long echo train lengths required. These deficiencies have been addressed by contemporary 3D T2w FSE techniques such as volume, isotropic turbo spin echo acquisition (VISTA), CUBE, and sampling, perfection with application optimized contrasts using different flip angle

a School of Biomedical Engineering & Imaging Sciences, King's College London, London, UK;
b Neuroradiology Department, King's College Hospital NHS Foundation Trust, Denmark Hill, London SE5 9RS, UK
* Neuroradiology Department, King's College Hospital NHS Foundation Trust, Denmark Hill, London SE5 9RS, UK.
E-mail address: steve.connor@kcl.ac.uk

Neuroimag Clin N Am 31 (2021) 451–471
https://doi.org/10.1016/j.nic.2021.05.006

| Table 1 | | | |
| Imaging sequences | | | |
Sequence Type	GE	Siemens	Philips
3D T2w GRE	3D FIESTA-C	3D CISS	3D -SSFP
Optimised 3D FSE (T1w and T2w)[a]	CUBE	SPACE	VISTA

Abbreviations: FIESTA, fast imaging using steady-state acquisition; SPACE, sampling perfection with application optimized contrasts using different flip angle evolution; SSFP, steady state free precession; VISTA, volume isotropic turbo spin echo acquisition.
[a] Variations in factors such as the effective echo time and flip angle are used to influence tissue contrast.

evolution (SPACE). These 3D T2w FSE techniques are characterized by significantly shortened echo spacing, and variable flip angles for the refocusing radio-frequency pulses, so suppressing blurring while reducing flow and chemical shift artifacts.

Thin section pre- and post-gadolinium-enhanced T1-weighted imaging is used to characterize lesions and may be used for the posttreatment follow-up of tumors. Fat-saturated T1w imaging may be a useful adjunct in the setting of a postoperative fat graft. While 2- to 3-mm-thin-section spin echo T1w sequences have traditionally been used to image the posterior fossa, 3D T1w sequences are now considered optimal. In particular, 3D T1w FSE sequences benefit from reduced vascular enhancement and susceptibility effects compared with 3D T1w GRE sequences (see **Table 1**).

Innovative MRI techniques such as "Slice Encoding for Metal Artifact Correction (SEMAC)" may also be applied in the setting of patients with MRI conditional auditory implants to improve visualization of the CPA and IAM. CT plays a role in patients with contraindications to MRI and may occasionally be used for presurgical planning.

IMAGING APPEARANCES AND DIFFERENTIAL DIAGNOSIS OF THE CPA CISTERN VESTIBULAR SCHWANNOMA

A CPA cistern VS usually extends from the IAM through the porus acusticus before expanding into the CPA with an "ice cream cone" configuration. MRI reveals a T1w isointense and T2w hyperintense lesion. While smaller schwannomas usually show homogenous enhancement, up to 40% are seen to enhance heterogeneously with 5% to 15% demonstrating cystic change (**Fig. 1**).[1] The presence of tumoral cysts is important to document because they predispose to rapid growth, increase surgical morbidity, and reduce the efficacy of radiotherapy. While macroscopic hemorrhage is relatively rare (<1%), microhemorrhagic change is present on haem-sensitive sequences in most cases.[2] A subgroup of hypervascular CPA schwannomas in younger patients are characterized by prominent vascular flow voids.[3] Additional imaging features include dural enhancement (25%) and adjacent parenchymal edema (40%). Although hydrocephalus most frequently relates to fourth ventricular obstruction, there may also be a communicating hydrocephalus due to the schwannoma secreting protein into the cerebrospinal fluid. A focal T2w hyperintensity in the dorsal brain stem is very occasionally observed and is likely related to degeneration of the vestibular nucleus (**Fig. 2**).[4]

Bilateral VSs are present in 5% of patients and are emblematic of neurofibromatosis type 2 (NF2). NF2 is an autosomal dominant tumor predisposition condition with birth incidence of 1 in 25 to 33,000. Patients with mosaic NF2 may present with unilateral VS, but there will usually be clinical features or a family history of NF2. NF2 VSs are characterized by a younger age at presentation, more rapid growth, and intracochlear extension. NF2 is also associated with other cranial nerve schwannomas and meningiomas with the potential for collision tumors in the posterior fossa. Whole neuro-axis imaging is appropriate as 75% of patients will also develop schwannomas and ependymomas within the spine (**Fig. 3**).

VSs comprise 60% to 70% of CPA tumors in major surgical series. The other most frequent primary extra-axial tumors of the CPA are meningiomas (10%–15%) and epidermoids (5%).[5] The distinguishing imaging features of these lesions are demonstrated in **Table 2** (**Figs. 4–6**). CPA meningiomas are important to distinguish from VSs preoperatively because they demonstrate a different relationship to neurovascular structures, variable histology, and potential invasiveness, which therefore influences the surgical approach. Non-VSs in the CPA may be derived from V, VII, IX, X, XI, and XII nerves and may mimic VS both radiologically and clinically. Other primary lesions of the CPA include arachnoid cysts, metastases, developmental lesions (eg, lipoma, dermoid), and vascular lesions (eg, hemangiomas, arteriovenous

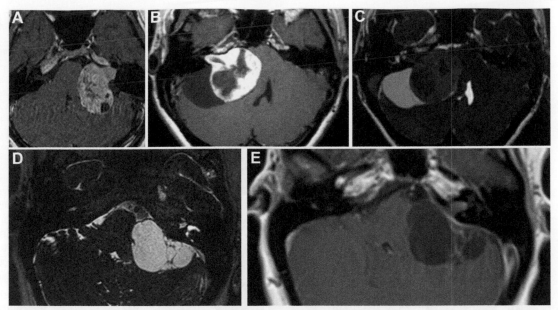

Fig. 1. Appearances of the CPA cystic schwannomas. (*A*) Post-gadolinium T1w axial image demonstrating intra-tumoral cysts while (*B*) and (*C*) post-gadolinium T1w axial and CISS axial images demonstrate a peritumoral cyst. Thin-walled cysts as shown in (*D*) CISS axial and (*E*) post-gadolinium T1w images are associated with increased risk of operative neurovascular injury.

malformations, aneurysms) (**Box 1, Table 3**). Secondary leptomeningeal involvement by metastases (eg, lung, breast, melanoma, lymphoma) and inflammatory lesions (eg, sarcoid, tuberculosis) should also be considered and will require correlation with clinical history and cerebro-spinal fluid (CSF) analysis to aid the diagnosis. It should be noted that less than 1% of patients with VS present with facial nerve dysfunction, so such a clinical presentation should raise the possibility of an alternative diagnosis such as VII nerve schwannoma, vascular lesion, or aggressive leptomeningeal disease. It should also be remembered that bilateral lesions are rare in the absence of an NF2 diagnosis, so such a finding should prompt the radiologist to consider other causes such as leptomeningeal disease.

When analyzing a CPA mass, it should be ensured that it is not arising from adjacent structures. Exophytic intra-axial lesions extending from the brain stem and cerebellum (eg, medulloblastoma in children and metastasis or hemangioblastoma in adults) or from the fourth ventricle (eg, ependymoma, choroid plexus tumor) may present as a CPA mass lesion. It should be noted that primary CPA tumors are rare in young patients, and so an exophytic intra-axial lesion should always be considered in this setting. Similarly, masses arising from the petrous apex (eg, metastasis or chondrosarcoma) or the jugular foramen (eg,

paraganglioma) may be mistaken for a CPA VS unless traced to their point of origin.

IMAGING APPEARANCES AND DIFFERENTIAL DIAGNOSIS OF THE INTERNAL AUDITORY MEATUS VESTIBULAR SCHWANNOMA

The origin of VSs is controversial, and they have been described as either arising from both the nerve sheath near the Obersteiner-Redlich zone (at the transition from central glial to Schwann cells) and from Scarpa's ganglion. The most distal part of the VIII transition zone extends over 4-5 mm which may explain the variable location of small IAM VSs. IAM schwannomas are usually hypointense to CSF on 3D FSE or GRE sequences and are described as having a nodular or fusiform morphology. Approximately 85% of VSs arise from the inferior vestibular nerve with a smaller proportion arising from the superior vestibular nerve (9%) or the cochlear nerve (6%).[6] Dumbbell-shaped schwannomas may extend from the IAM into the cochlea (trans-modiolar), vestibule (trans-macular), or middle ear (trans-otic) (**Fig. 7**).

The differential diagnosis of IAM VSs is similar to that of those centered in the CPA (see **Box 1, Table 3**) although there are differences in the frequency of each pathology (**Fig. 8**). First, an IAM lesion is statistically even more likely to represent a VS, with schwannomas comprising over 90% of

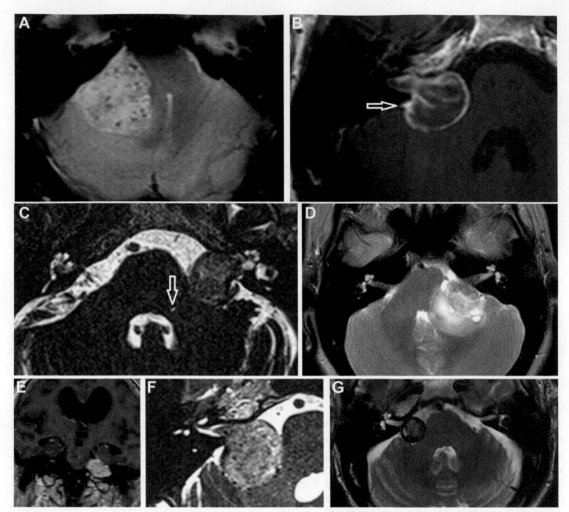

Fig. 2. Variant appearances of the CPA vestibular schwannoma. (*A*) T2* axial image demonstrates VS microhemorrhage. (*B*) Post-gadolinium T1w axial image demonstrates a cystic VS with a dural tail (*arrow*). (*C*) T2 CISS image reveals a focus of T2 high signal in the region of the vestibular nucleus (*arrow*). (*D*) T2w axial image depicts a VS with adjacent edema while associated hydrocephalus is shown on an (*E*) coronal post-gadolinium T1w imaging. Hypervascularity as shown on an (*F*) T2 CISS image and macrohemorrhage illustrated on a (*G*) T2w image are further variant imaging features.

all IAM tumors. A recent study of IAM lesions which were felt to be clinically and radiologically consistent with VS, demonstrated that alternative pathology was discovered at surgery in only 2.5% of cases.[7] Second, inflammatory and neoplastic leptomeningeal disease rather more frequently presents as an IAM lesion than is the case with CPA masses. When considering inflammatory and malignant disease of the IAM, it is always important to search for an origin in the lateral petrous bone, either from inflammatory middle ear disease or from facial nerve perineural spread.

The radiologist should be particularly alert to the possibility of alternative pathologies when there is a clinical history of systemic malignancy or immunosuppression, when symptoms are rapidly progressing, and when they include facial nerve palsy. Imaging features suggestive of another diagnosis include a linear pattern of gadolinium enhancement, bilateral lesions, and extension of disease laterally to the facial nerve or middle ear. Note that physiologic vascular gadolinium enhancement at the fundus of the IAM, normal expansion of Scarpa's ganglion, or an intrameatal vascular loop may all mimic a small VS.

CLINICAL PRESENTATION OF VESTIBULAR SCHWANNOMA AND INDICATIONS FOR DIAGNOSTIC IMAGING

Audiological symptoms are present in almost all patients with VSs. Sensorineural hearing loss is

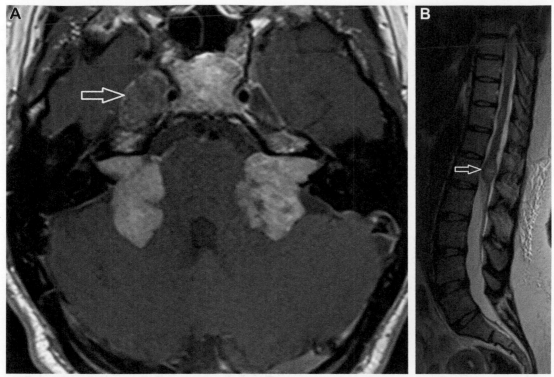

Fig. 3. Vestibular schwannomas in the context of NF2. (*A*) Post-gadolinium T1w illustrates bilateral vestibular schwannomas with a right trigeminal schwannoma (*arrow*) while a (*B*) T2w sagittal image demonstrates associated spinal cord ependymomas (largest indicated by *arrow*).

the most common symptom leading to diagnosis (95%), and this is of sudden onset in 5% of cases. Most patients also experience asymmetric tinnitus, although it is rare (<1%) for it to be an isolated presenting symptom.[8] Larger tumors will be more likely to present with symptoms related to compression of posterior fossa structures, with the possibility of unsteadiness, true vertigo, facial pain, and numbness. Incidental diagnosis after MRI for unrelated clinical presentations may now represent up to 10% of the VSs detected.

Diagnostic imaging is required to detect VSs in patients with unilateral or asymmetric audiological symptoms or other relevant localizing symptoms and signs. In addition, MRI is indicated in the setting of asymmetric hearing loss on pure tone audiometry. There are no standardized criteria as to the required interaural audiometric threshold asymmetry to prompt imaging. The optimal choice of audiometric criteria will depend on whether the aim is to achieve maximum sensitivity (with increased numbers of MRI studies) or maximum positive predictive value. The recent National Institute of Clinical Excellence guidelines state that patients with ≥15 dB interaural difference in thresholds at more than two adjacent frequencies should undergo MRI; however, the audiometric

criteria remain controversial,[9] and there are no prospective studies available. The most comprehensive criteria for imaging would be weighted for multiple factors (eg, age, history of noise exposure, other audio vestibular symptoms) and are likely to be clarified with machine learning algorithms.[10]

IMAGING PROTOCOLS FOR THE DETECTION OF VESTIBULAR SCHWANNOMA AND DIAGNOSTIC YIELD

Three-dimensional T2w FSE or GRE sequences have proven to be more cost-effective than gadolinium-enhanced T1w imaging[11] for the detection of VSs. However, there is potential for <2-mm IAM lesions, labyrinthine lesions, and leptomeningeal disease to go undetected with this approach, so there should be a low threshold to perform gadolinium-enhanced T1w imaging for equivocal cases and, in particular, clinical settings such as immunocompromised or malignancy. It should also be remembered that alternative causes for audiological symptoms (eg, inner ear pathologies) should be sought because they are detected on MRI with a similar frequency to that of VSs.[12]

Table 2
Differential diagnosis: imaging features of the three principle CPA masses

Tumour	Origin	Morphology/Location	CT Features	T1w/T2w Intensity	Enhancement	Other Sequences	Lateral to IAM Fundus
Vestibular schwannoma	Schwann cells of nerve sheath and usually inferior vestibular nerve	Centered on an expanded porus acusticus. Spherical with acute angle to dorsal petrous bone.	Variable density but principally isodense. Calcification rare.	T1 iso-intense/T2 hyper-intense	Moderate and heterogeneous with cystic non-enhancement in larger lesions	Microhemorrhage on heme-sensitive sequences. Myoinositol peak on spectroscopy	May be intral-abyrinthine extension and note any extension along facial nerve canal to suggest facial schwannoma mimic.
Meningioma	Arachnoid mening-oepithelial cells of CPA (or rarely IAM)	Centered on posterior petrous bone with hemispheric broad base, asymmetric to porus acusticus. Rugged medial contour.	Usually (70%) hyperdense with possible hyperostosis and calcification (20%). No enlargement of porus acusticus	Variable signal but maybe T1 iso-intense/T2 iso-intense to cortex	Moderate homogenous enhancement with dural tail	Decreased ADC compared to VS but overlapping. Increased CBV compared to VS. Alanine peak on spectroscopy	Perilymphatic signal is preserved on CISS sequences when IAM extension
Epidermoid	Inclusions of ectodermal cell rests	Insinuating within the basal cisterns, with a fine irregular surface. Extending to contralateral CPA and superior to tentorium.	Usually CSF density with occasional peripheral calcification and molding of petrous bone	Usually iso-intense to CSF signal with rare T1 hyper-intense, T2 hypo-intense "white epidermoids"	Non-enhancing	Increased DWI, FLAIR signal relative to CSF distinguishes from arachnoid cyst. Well defined with 3D T2w sequences. Lactate peak on spectroscopy	

Abbreviations: ADC, apparent diffusion co-efficient; DWI, diffusion weighted imaging; FLAIR, fluid-attenuated inversion recovery.

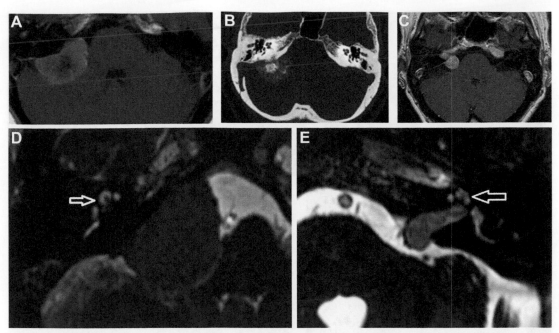

Fig. 4. CPA meningioma imaging differential diagnosis. (*A*) Post-gadolinium T1w axial image of a meningioma reveals the broad base along the posterior petrous pyramid and its location eccentric to the IAM with (*B*) calcification on CT. (*C*) Post-gadolinium T1w axial images showing meningioma with intracanalicular extension. Note how perilymphatic signal is preserved on CISS sequences when there is IAM extension from a (*D*) meningioma, whereas it may be reduced with an (*E*) VS (*arrows*).

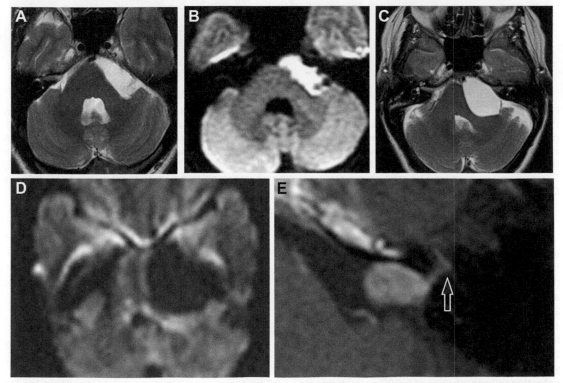

Fig. 5. Imaging differential diagnosis of CPA mass. (*A*) T2w axial and (*B*) DWI depict a CPA epidermoid and characterized by increased DWI as compared to (*C*) T2w axial and (*D*) DWI images of a CPA arachnoid cyst. (*E*) Post-gadolinium T1w axial image identifies a facial schwannoma by its tail of enhancement in the line of the nerve (*arrow*).

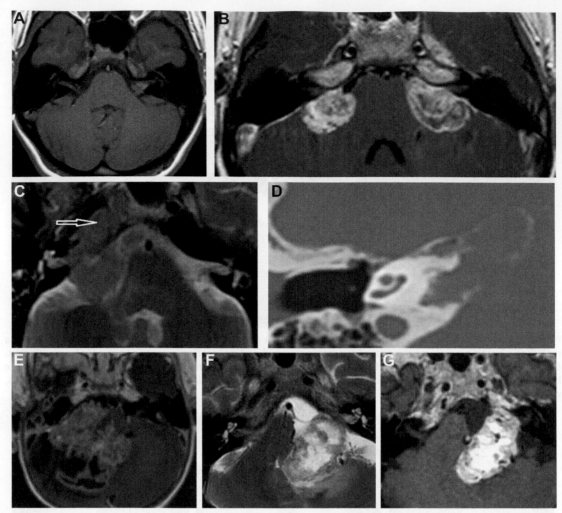

Fig. 6. Pitfalls in the characterization of a CPA mass. (*A*) T1w axial image with patchy T1 high signal due to a low flow venous malformation. (*B*) Post-gadolinium T1w axial image with bilateral CPA lesions and additional meningeal enhancement secondary to leptomeningeal atypical rhabdoid teratoid tumor. (*C*) T2w axial image with CPA exophytic extension from a petrous apex (*arrow*) metastasis with the bony changes confirmed in the (*D*) CT study. (*E*) Post-gadolinium T1w axial image demonstrates CPA exophytic extension from an intra-axial GBM. (*F*) and (*G*) T2w and post-gadolinium T1w axial images demonstrating a hemangioblastoma extending exophytically into the CPA from a pial attachment to the lateral pons.

As audio-vestibular symptoms are common, and audiometric selection criteria are now more liberally applied, the imaging for detection of VSs now represents a significant burden for many imaging departments. It has been estimated that 20% of patients referred to ear, nose, and throat secondary care will satisfy audiometric criteria for MRI.[12] As MRI has become more available, there has been a trend toward lower diagnostic yield for the detection of VS. Although varying in selection criteria, studies of (>300 patient) populations with asymmetric symptoms or audiometry over the past 20 years have demonstrated schwannomas in 1.4%-9.2% of cases.[12–14] The increasing use of MRI has also contributed to the rising incidence of VS, which has been documented on several national databases. This is associated with a reduction in mean tumor size at detection from 26 mm to 7 mm.[15]

DIFFERENT MANAGEMENT OPTIONS FOR VESTIBULAR SCHWANNOMA AND THE ROLE OF IMAGING

The three principle approaches available for the management of VSs are a "wait and scan" conservative approach, surgery, and radiotherapy. Less frequently, medical therapy may be considered;

Box 1

Radiological differential diagnosis of a CPA or IAM lesion

Vestibular schwannoma

Meningioma

Non-vestibular schwannoma

Developmental: epidermoid/lipoma/hamartoma

Vascular: aneurysm/arteriovenous malformation/venous malformation

Leptomeningeal disease: infection/inflammation/neoplasia (lymphoma or metastasis)

however, this is principally in the setting of NF2. The therapeutic decision-making is multifactorial with clinical (eg, age and symptoms) as well as imaging findings (size and growth) being considered. In addition to its influence on the choice of management option, imaging plays a key role in the planning of interventions and posttreatment monitoring.

Conservative Wait and Scan

As most VSs are small and slow growing, "wait and scan" protocols are playing an increasing role, particularly in older patients. Measurement techniques, appropriate timing of imaging, optimal imaging protocols, and definition of tumor growth will be discussed.

Tumor Measurements

Consistent measurement techniques and reliable measurements of tumor size are important to assess the tumor size and growth rate. There is considerable variation in how measurements are performed, in both clinical practice and the research setting (**Fig. 9**).[16] Standardized methods of tumor measurement have been promoted by organizations, although none have been uniformly adopted.[17] The largest extrameatal dimension was deemed the key measurement at a recent consensus meeting, and it forms the basis for most tumor staging classifications (**Table 4**). Although these single linear measurements have been widely adopted, it is known that they are prone to measurement error and that the reliability

Table 3
Pearls and pitfalls in the imaging assessment of a CPA or IAM lesion

Imaging Review Area	Why?
Evidence of cysts	Propensity for tumors to grow rapidly and impacts on effectiveness and morbidity of surgery/radiotherapy
Extension of enhancement to other cranial nerve foramina and canals	Consider a nonvestibular schwannoma which influences surgical approach
Interface with petrous apex, jugular foramen and brain	Ensure it is a primary CPA lesion rather than an exophytic extension from adjacent structures
Look for contiguity with disease in the lateral petrous bone	Acute and chronic inflammatory middle ear disease and facial nerve perineural spread can demonstrate IAM extension
Review pre-gadolinium T1w sequence	Do not misinterpret T1w hyperintensity (eg, lipoma) as gadolinium enhancement
Note if extrameatal component of the mass is eccentric to IAM and forming an obtuse angle with petrous bone	Consider a meningioma with intracanalicular component which effects surgical approach
Look for excessive flow voids and vascularity	Highlight hypervascular VS variant to surgeon or consider alternative vascular pathology
Reformat volumetric sequence to standard plane	Ensures consistent measurement technique for assessment of tumor growth
Identify other leptomeningeal lesions or bilateral lesions in absence of NF2 diagnosis	Suggest alternative diagnosis of inflammatory/infective/neoplastic leptomeningeal disease

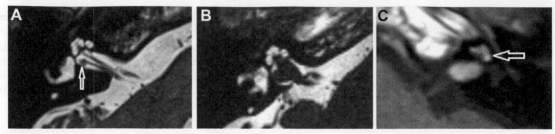

Fig. 7. IAM vestibular schwannoma appearances. CISS axial images revealing an (A) small nodular inferior vestibular nerve schwannoma (*arrow*) and a (*B*) fusiform schwannoma extending along the inferior vestibular and cochlear nerves. (C) Post-gadolinium T1w image reveals transmodiolar extension (*arrow*).

and agreement can be improved by combining multiple linear dimensions or evaluating area dimensions.[18]

Further precision may be achieved by applying volumetric analysis, which is recognized to have the optimum ability to define growth between serial scans when accounting for measurement error. Although algorithms are rapidly evolving, there are currently challenges to the routine use of volume analysis in clinical practice. Completely automatic segmentation is generally not possible, particularly in view of the difficulties posed by adjacent dural and venous enhancement, necrosis, and collisions tumors.[19] The ability to accurately segment the tumor is also dependent on the imaging acquisition, with the contrast relative to adjacent tissues being suboptimal when T2w

sequences are used, and the measurement error increasing to greater than 10% when less than five sections pass through the tumor.[20] With the exception of the monitoring of medical therapy, linear dimensions currently remain adequate for most clinical decision-making and are able to predict volumetric progression with 70% to 90% accuracy.[21,22] Artificial intelligence methods have been applied to fully automated segmentation and volumetric assessment so may have a future role in VS surveillance.

Natural history of VSs as a guide to optimizing "wait and scan" imaging follow-up interval and duration

In order to guide follow-up imaging protocols for the conservative management of VSs, it is

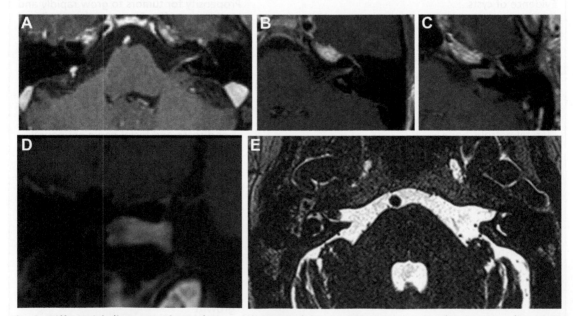

Fig. 8. Differential diagnosis of IAM lesion. (A) Post-gadolinium T1w axial images demonstrates linear IAM enhancement related to (A) neurosarcoid, (B) Lyme disease, and (C) adenoid cystic carcinoma perineural spread. (B) and (C) demonstrate extension in the *line* of the facial nerve. (D) Post-gadolinium T1w image also demonstrates an intracanalicular meningioma, whereas (E) CISS imaging demonstrates a focal abnormality in the IAM secondary to tympanomastoid inflammation.

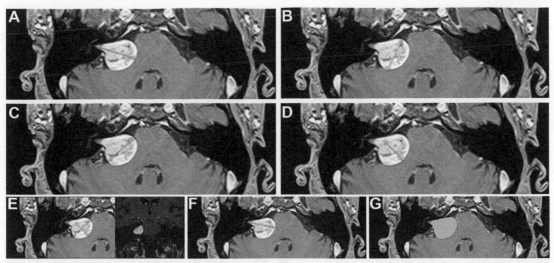

Fig. 9. Different VS measuring methods (indicated by double arrows). Post-gadolinium T1w axial images demonstrate previously described measurements for the documentation of VS size: (*A*) Longest axial dimension, (*B*) maximum extrameatal dimension, (*C*) maximum extrameatal dimension parallel to posterior petrous pyramid, (*D*) maximum extrameatal dimension perpendicular to posterior petrous pyramid, (*E*) combination of dimensions perpendicular and parallel to posterior petrous pyramid with a craniocaudal dimension (AAOHNS method), (*F*) longest axial dimension in the *line* of the IAM and (*G*) area dimension.

important to have some knowledge of their natural history. CPA VSs grow at a mean rate of 1 to 2 mm/y and approximately 33% of tumor volume/y, but this is variable, with growth varying over time. Larger tumors at presentation and cystic tumors have greater propensity to growth with approximately 10% of tumors demonstrating rapid growth of greater than 1 cm/y. Between 20% and 50% of tumors undergo a degree of growth which requires intervention, and this usually occurs in the first 2 to 3 years after diagnosis. The longer the VS has been observed to be stable, the lower the risk of subsequent growth is, but in 5% to 10% of patients, it should be noted that the growth first occurs after 5 years.[23,24] In 5% to 20% of tumors, it

has been observed that tumors will undergo spontaneous regression.

Therefore, as most significant growth occurs in the first 2 to 3 years after presentation, this should represent the most intensive period of monitoring; however, longer term follow-up is also required to detect growth. There is no standardized protocol, although most guidelines propose yearly imaging for 3 to 5 years before increasing the duration between MRI studies in the context of a stable tumor.

MRI sequences for "wait and scan" imaging follow-up

A series of studies have now shown that 3D T2w MRI sequences are equivalent to gadolinium-

Table 4
Staging systems for vestibular schwannoma

Tumor Size	House	Koos		Samii: Tumor Extent
Intracanalicular	Intracanalicular	Grade I	T1	Isolated to IAM
≤10 mm	Grade 1 (small)	Grade II	T2	Minor extrameatal extension
≤15 mm	Grade 2 (medium)		T3a	Extrameatal tumor without brain stem contact
≤20 mm				
≤30 mm	Grade 3 (moderately large)	Grade III	T3b	Tumor contacting brainstem without compression
≤40 mm	Grade 4 (large)	Grade IV	T4a	Tumor compressing brainstem
>40 mm	Grade 5 (giant)		T4b	Tumor severely compressing brainstem and fourth ventricle

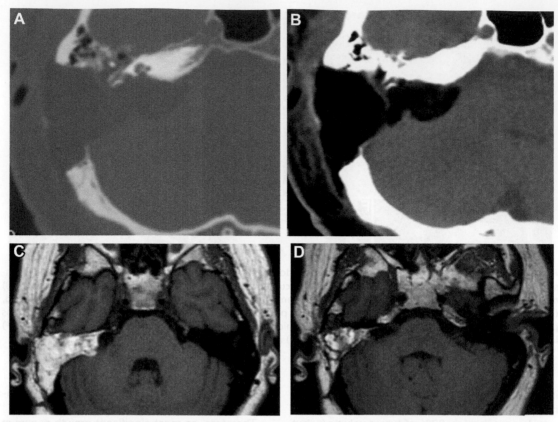

Fig. 10. Translabyrinthine postsurgical appearances. CT axial with (A) bone and (B) soft-tissue windows indicating the expected petro-mastoid bony defect and fat graft to the subtotal petrosectomy cavity. T1w axial images (C) 3 months after surgery and (D) 4 years after surgery demonstrate interval involution of the fat graft.

enhanced imaging in terms of their ability to predict tumor progression, with less than 0.5 mm mean difference in measurements obtained between the two different types of sequences. Although guidelines indicate that either MRI approach is acceptable, it is likely that 3D T2w sequences will be adopted because of concerns about the long-term safety of multiple administrations of gadolinium-based agents.[25]

Tumor growth and failure of "wait and scan" conservative management

Demonstration of tumor growth is critical for deciding whether a "wait and scan" conservative approach has failed and whether specific interventions are required, so "significant" growth needs to be defined. A recent position statement[26] specified growth as greater than 2 mm linear measurement compared with the index study, or alternatively a 1.2 mm^3 or greater than 20% increase in volume. The concept of growth rate, rather than absolute growth, was also introduced as a feature requiring a change in management strategy.[26] As the ability to define growth will depend on the imaging and

measurement technique, it could be argued that the smallest detectable difference between serial imaging studies should be calculated locally, on the basis of departmental agreement parameters. It is likely that future approaches will include advanced imaging paramaters and genetic alterations to help predict tumor behavior and a propensity for growth.[27]

It should be appreciated that growth is not the only factor to indicate whether surgery or radiotherapy is to be offered. Absolute tumor size is important, and it is noted that larger tumors are associated with younger patients, possibly reflecting a more aggressive tumor biology. In addition, patient preference, age, comorbidities, and clinical features (eg, hearing loss) are all considered by the multidisciplinary team.

IMAGING IN THE SURGICAL MANAGEMENT OF VESTIBULAR SCHWANNOMAS
Surgical Approaches for Vestibular Schwannoma

Surgery may be required to address large or growing CPA VSs, and the main surgical options are the

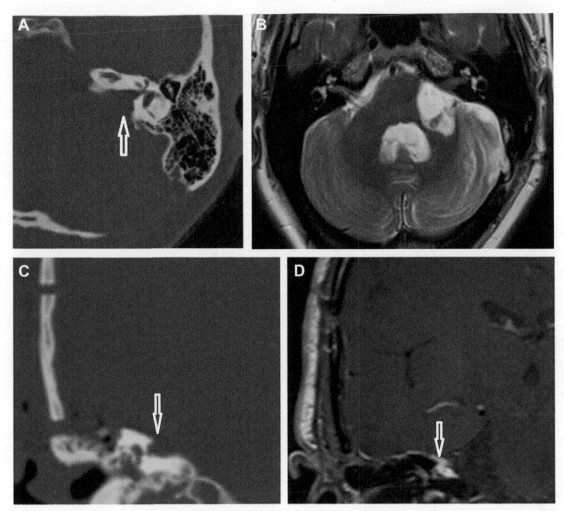

Fig. 11. Retrosigmoid and middle cranial fossa approach postsurgical appearances. Post retrosigmoid approach appearances: (*A*) axial CT demonstrates the expected occipito-mastoid and posterior porus acusticus (*arrow*) bony defects while the (*B*) T2w axial image reveals left cerebellar encephalomalacic changes and widening of the left CPA. Post-middle cranial fossa approach appearances: (*C*) Coronal CT demonstrates the temporal craniotomy and defect within the superior IAM (*arrow*) with (*D*) T1w coronal demonstrating a fat graft at the site of the IAM defect (*arrow*).

retro-sigmoid (suboccipital) or translabyrinthine surgical approaches (**Figs. 10** and **11**). The middle cranial fossa approach is less frequently used to remove intracanalicular tumors, or those with small extrameatal components. There is potential for hearing preservation with translabyrinthine and middle cranial fossa surgical routes. A summary of the surgical steps is listed in **Table 5**, together with the advantages and role of each operative approach.[5,28,29] Surgery is generally preferred to radiotherapy in younger patients, patients presenting with trigeminal neuralgia, and when there are significant cystic components. A surgical approach is also favored for larger tumors because of concerns about compressive ischemia of the facial nerve or brainstem due to tumor swelling with radiotherapy.

Preoperative imaging assessment
A check list for a radiological review of preoperative imaging is proposed in **Table 6** (**Fig. 12**), with the most relevant preoperative imaging features depending on the intended surgical approach. The key observations which should be identified include

- Venous variants which may encroach on the surgical pathway;
- Facial nerve location anterior to the VS which may lead to inadvertent injury;
- Extension of petro-mastoid air cells which will requires sealing to prevent CSF leak;
- Lateral extension of tumor within the IAM which may limit resection or result in increased morbidity;

Table 5
Surgical approaches for vestibular schwannoma resection

Surgical Approach	Stages of Surgical Technique	Advantages	Main Role	Risks/Potential Postoperative Complications
Middle cranial fossa	• Preauricular approach • Temporal craniotomy • Temporal lobe retraction • Medio-lateral decompression of the superior IAM and open dura • Remove tumor • Graft to dural defect	• Good access to fundus • May preserve hearing	Intracanalicular lesions or limited extrameatal component	• Slight increased risk of facial nerve injury • Temporal lobe seizures from temporal lobe retraction
Retrosigmoid (suboccipital)	• Postauricular approach • Retrosigmoid craniectomy inferior to transverse sinus • Seal any mastoid air cells • Dura incised and arachnoid opened • Drain CSF and retract cerebellum • Remove tumor • Facial nerve usually identified later at brainstem after debulking • Access IAM component by medio-lateral decompression posterior two-third (to avoid labyrinth) IAM	• Wide exposure to CPA • *Compared to trans-labyrinthine:* • May preserve hearing	CPA lesions of any size with view to preserving hearing Cannot preserve hearing if far lateral IAM extension	• CSF leak into petro-mastoid air cells • Aseptic meningitis • Cerebellar atrophy • Early postoperative headaches

| Trans-labyrinthine | • Postauricular approach
• Subtotal petrosectomy (anterior to sigmoid sinus)
• (Partial) labyrinthectomy
• Sigmoid sinus can be retracted and jugular bulb displaced inferiorly
• 270^0 removal of IAM
• Access CPA dorsal to porus acusticus
• Tumor removal
• Facial nerve identified early in IAM and lateral at brainstem
• Packing of middle ear
• Fat graft to subtotal petrosectomy | • Wide exposure to CPA
• Compared to retrosigmoid:
• Extradural bone drilling
• Identification of facial nerve early in IAM
• Less cerebellar retraction | CPA lesions of any size in patients without serviceable hearing or poor hearing prognosis
Can address intralabyrinthine extension | • Hearing eliminated
• Complications of fat harvesting
• Sigmoid sinus and jugular bulb thrombosis from retraction |

Table 6
Preoperative and postoperative imaging assessment

Surgical Approach	What the Surgeon Needs to Know? Preoperative Imaging Features of Surgical and Clinical Importance	What the Radiologist Should Expect to Find? Postoperative Imaging Features
Middle cranial fossa	• Far lateral extension below crista falciformis/cochlear aperture (reduces possibility of hearing preservation)	• Temporal craniotomy • Fat/fascial graft to roof of IAM
Retrosigmoid (suboccipital)	• Extensive petromastoid pneumatisation (risk of postoperative CSF leak if air cells not sealed with those adjacent to IAM particularly important) • High jugular bulb behind IAM (assess requirement for displacement and potential morbidity) • Inner ear signal change on T2w 3D/FLAIR (reduces possibility of hearing preservation) • Extension of tumor to fundus of IAM (may increase risk to facial nerve and result in fenestration when accessing lateral IAM so decreased possibility of hearing preservation) • Facial nerve location/deflection relative to tumor in CPA (increased risk of injury if surgeon unaware of rare anterior position relative to tumor)	• Retrosigmoid craniectomy • Absent posterior wall IAM • Cerebellar signal change and lateral flattening • Posterior fossa extra-axial collection • Linear enhancement at IAM
Translabyrinthine	• Anterior sigmoid sinus and high jugular bulb (assess requirement for retraction/displacement and potential morbidity) • Presence of intact torcula (to assess risk of postoperative sigmoid sinus or jugular bulb thrombosis due to retraction) • Facial nerve location/deflection relative to tumor in CPA (increased risk of injury if surgeon unaware of rare anterior facial nerve position relative to tumor)	• Subtotal petrosectomy • Triangular fat graft to cavity • May be feint enhancement at margins of graft • Fat graft involutes with time • Linear enhancement at IAM

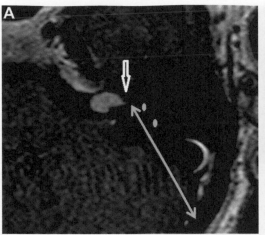
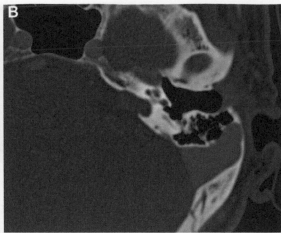

Fig. 12. Preoperative imaging assessment for VS surgery. (A) Post-gadolinium T1w image illustrates how to estimate the access to the fundus of the IAM via a retro-sigmoid route. An *arrowed line* extending from 2 cm posterior to the sigmoid sinus and medial to the line of the posterior semicircular canal (*dots*). The distance of the lesion from the fundus is also noted (*arrow*) (B) CT demonstrates a markedly anterolateral sigmoid sinus (*arrow*) which would impede access via a translabyrinthine route.

- Inner ear CISS or 3D FLAIR signal abnormality which indicates a poorer hearing outcome.[28–30]

There has been increased interest in the potential of MRI techniques to demonstrate the position of the cisternal facial nerve with respect to the tumor. Despite microscopic inspection and intraoperative monitoring, there remains only 50% to 70% preservation of facial nerve function when operating on tumors greater than 2 cm in size. Less than 10% of facial nerves lie along the anterior or inferior aspect of the tumor, and these are

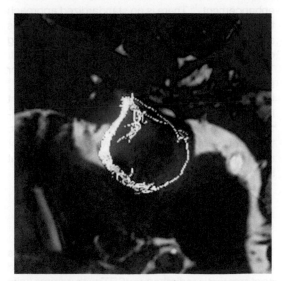

Fig. 13. Facial nerve tractography. Probabilistic DTI tractography fused with a T2 CISS image demonstrates the cochlear nerve lateral and the facial nerve medial to the vestibular schwannoma.

particularly important to identify preoperatively, as they will be encountered early in the resection.[31] As routine T2 3D sequences are less successful in demonstrating the interface with the flattened or attenuated facial nerve in the larger VS, the potential for facial nerve tractography to predict facial nerve position has been explored (Fig. 13). Technical aspects are reviewed in more detail later in this issue. A recent systematic review and pooled analysis of 14 studies (n = 234) has demonstrated the facial nerve to be verified and concordant with surgical findings in 87%.[32] Prospective blinded studies using probabilistic tractography are ongoing, and the potential for integration into neuro-navigation systems as well as the actual impact on preserving facial nerve function will require further evaluation.

Postoperative Imaging Assessment

The expected postoperative MRI appearances for each of the surgical approaches are described.[28,29] Imaging may be required to evaluate postoperative complications. Potential postoperative complications depend on the surgical approach (see Table 6) with imaging being required to assess those due to CSF leaks (and associated meningitis) or parenchymal injury. In the context of CSF leaks (1%–8%), CT and 3D T2w MRI may be used to identify breaches in unsealed petro-mastoid air cells, at the margins of the craniectomy or at the petrous apex, and the associated transgression of CSF (Fig. 14). Fat graft necrosis (1%) after translabyrinthine surgery may also predispose to CSF leak and manifests as fragmentation and fluid infiltration of the graft with potential lipoid meningitis and

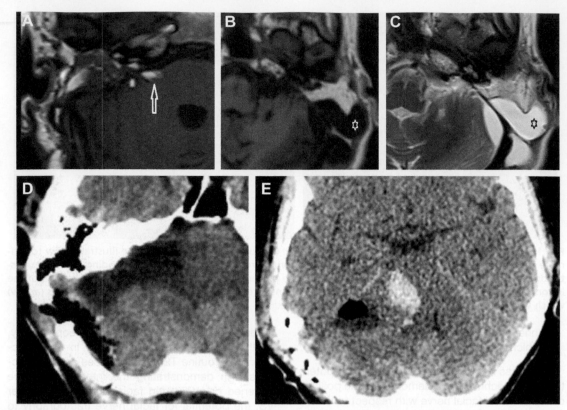

Fig. 14. Postoperative complications. (A) T1w axial demonstrates fragmentation of the fat graft with subarachnoid dissemination (arrow). (B) T1w post-gadolinium and (C) T2w images demonstrate fat graft necrosis with development of a pseudomeningocele (star). (D) and (E) CT axial images made early after surgery illustrate low-density bone wax mimicking air deep to the craniotomy (arrow) while acute hemorrhage is demonstrated in the surgical bed.

pseudomeningocele. Bone wax used to seal air cells or control bleeding from emissary veins should not be mistaken for intracranial air at the site of surgery or dural venous thrombus. Brain parenchymal injury may be secondary to arterial or venous ischemia, cerebritis, or retraction injury.[28] Postoperative hemorrhage (0.6%) may result from venous injury, with particular risk to bridging petrosal veins which are adherent to almost all large tumors. There is also a risk of ipsilateral dural venous sinus thrombosis (5%–6%).

Postoperative Imaging for Monitoring

Although a gross tumor resection (GTR) may be achieved, the goal of surgery has shifted from total resection to functional preservation. Near total resection (NTR) with less than 5% residuum, or subtotal resection (STR) with greater than 5% residuum, may be observed. In the context of a GTR, enhancement is still expected at the site of resection due to inflammation and early fibrosis. At 1 year after the surgery, it is possible to stratify the risks of recurrence according to the pattern of enhancement with linear enhancement (present in

3%) rarely progressing,[33] while there is a 6 to 16 times increased recurrence rate with nodular enhancement.[34] There is no standardized approach to the monitoring of GTR, but stable MRI changes are generally followed up for 3 to 5 years, depending on whether there is linear or nodular enhancement. The requirement for gadolinium enhancement for subsequent MRI in this setting is controversial.[35] In the context of NTR and STR, the tumor remnant is usually related to the facial nerve (Fig. 15). Monitoring MRI protocols for NTR and STR are similar to those for preoperative tumor; however, small tumor remnants are noted to demonstrate more indolent biological behavior.

RADIOTHERAPY FOR VESTIBULAR SCHWANNOMAS

The main alternative therapeutic intervention for VSs is radiotherapy, and this is most frequently delivered as stereotactic radiotherapy (SRT) with gamma knife or a linear accelerator. In most small- to medium-sized VSs (<3 cm), SRT is recognized as the primary treatment[36] and is more cost-effective. When

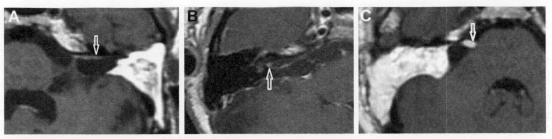

Fig. 15. Postoperative monitoring of the VS remnant. Post-gadolinium T1w axial images demonstrate (*A*) a linear pattern of enhancement (*arrow*) which is a normal postoperative finding and which (*B*) can sometimes appear more tumefactive and thicker (*arrow*), whereas (*C*) illustrates residual VS in the line of the facial nerve (*arrow*).

corrected for expected natural history of the tumor, there is a 75% control rate achieved with SRT[37] given at 11 to 13 Gy, and with similar long-term hearing outcomes.

Pretreatment MRI is principally required for the contouring of the tumor and to calculate accurate dose volume histogram. Effective tumor segmentation has now proven possible with 3D T2w imaging. Some imaging features may also prove useful in predicting outcomes, with maintained cochlear CISS signal being associated with hearing preservation,[38] while some texture feature parameters and lower pretreatment ADC values have correlated with response to radiotherapy.[39]

Expected changes after SRT include a transient enlargement which occurs in 25% to 60% of patients depending on the definition.[40,41] This should not be misinterpreted as tumor progression which is only observed in a small proportion of these enlarging tumors. Subsequent shrinkage of the tumor usually occurs within 2 years of treatment, with regression to a volume smaller than the original size occurring over 20 to 55 months.[40] The tumor swelling is often associated with reduced central enhancement (necrosis), but this does not correlate with success of treatment. Radiotherapy may also result in adjacent brain parenchymal signal change (30%) which usually resolves (**Fig. 16**). There are concerns about SRT inducing malignant transformation in schwannomas although there are

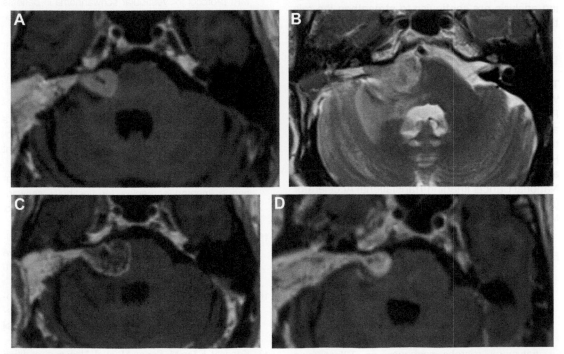

Fig. 16. Radiotherapy-related imaging changes. (*A*) Post-gadolinium T1w axial image demonstrates a recurrent VS after previous translabyrinthine surgery. (*B*) and (*C*) T2w and post-gadolinium T1w axial images at 6 months after SRT shows expansion ("pseudoprogression") of the VS with necrosis and adjacent parenchymal edema. At 2 years after SRT, the (*D*) post-gadolinium T1w image demonstrates regression of the VS.

only a few reports of definitively benign VSs becoming malignant after radiotherapy.

MEDICAL THERAPY FOR VESTIBULAR SCHWANNOMA

Bevacizumab (Avastin) is a vascular endothelial growth factor-binding antibody which has been reported to induce tumor shrinkage and improve hearing in 40% to 60% of NF2-related progressive VSs.[42] Additional biological therapeutics such as lapatinib (an ErbB2/EGFR inhibitor) are also being evaluated. Volumetric changes in tumor size are key to defining eligibility for initiation and continuing of treatment, while also providing robust outcome tools for clinical trials. Imaging may also play a future role in the prediction of response to these medical therapies, and a series of studies have already shown promising associations between response to bevacizumab and imaging markers such as Ktrans and mean ADC.[43]

SUMMARY

Imaging is integral to the diagnosis, treatment planning, and follow-up of VSs. MRI has led to increased detection of symptomatic and incidental small tumors,[44] which require long-term monitoring. Developments in MRI techniques and imaging analysis are continuing to strengthen the role that radiology plays in the management of the VS.

DISCLOSURE

The author acknowledges funding support from Wellcome/Engineering and Physical Sciences Research Council Centre for Medical Engineering at King's College London (WT 203148/Z/16/Z); National Institute for Health Research Biomedical Research Centre at Guy's & St Thomas' Hospitals and King's College London; Cancer Research UK National Cancer Imaging Translational Accelerator (A27066); the UK Research & Innovation London Medical Imaging and Artificial Intelligence Centre.

REFERENCES

1. Bonneville F, Savatovsky J, Chiras J. Imaging of cerebellopontine angle lesions: an update. Part 1: enhancing extra-axial lesions. Eur Radiol 2007;17: 2472–82.

2. Thamburaj k, Radhakrishnan VV, Thomas B, et al. Intratumoral microhaemorrhages on T2*-weighted gradient-echo imaging helps differentiate vestibular schwannoma from meningioma. AJNR Am J Neuroradiol 2008;29:552–7.

3. Yamakami I, Kobayashi E, iwadate Y, et al. Hypervascular vestibular schwannomas. Surg Neurol 2002;57:105–12.

4. Okamoto K, Furusawa T, Ishikawa K, et al. Focal T2 hyperintensity in the dorsal brain stem in patients with vestibular schwannoma. AJNR Am J Neuroradiol 2006;27:1307–11.

5. Lin EP, Crane BT. The management and Imaging of vestibuar schwannomas. AJNR Am J Neuroradiol 2017;38:2034–43.

6. Komatsuzaki A, Tsunoda A. Nerve origin of the acoustic neuroma. J Laryngol Otol 2001;115:375–9.

7. Scheich M, Hagen R, Ehrmann-Muller D, et al. Lesions mimicking small vestibular schwannomas. J Neurol Surg B 2017;78:447–53.

8. Sweeney AD, Carlson ML, Shepard NT, et al. Congress of Neurological Surgeons systematic review and evidence-based guidelines on otologic and audiological screening for patients with vestibular schwannomas. Neurosurgery 2018;82:E29–31.

9. Hearing loss in adults: assessment and management. NICE guideline [NG98].

10. Nouraei SAR, Huys QJM, Chatrath P, et al. Screening patients with sensorineural hearing loss for vestibular schwannoma using a Bayesian classifier. Clin Otolaryngol 2007;32:248–54.

11. Crowson MG, Rocke DJ, Hoang JK, et al. Cost-effectiveness analysis of a non-contrast screening MRI protocol for vestibular schwannoma in patients with asymmetric sensorineural hearing loss. Neuroradiology 2017;59:727–36.

12. Vandervelde C, Connor SE. Diagnostic yield of MRI for audiovestibular dysfunction using contemporary referral criteria: correlation with presenting symptoms and impact on clinical management. Clin Radiol 2009;64:156–63.

13. Harcourt JP, Vijaya-Sekaran S, Loney E, et al. The incidence of symptoms consistent with cerebellopontine angle lesions in a general ENT out-patient clinic. J Laryngol Otol 1999;113:518–22.

14. Obholzer RJ, Rea PA, Harcourt JP. Magnetic resonance imaging screening for vestibular schwannoma: analysis of published protocols. J Laryngol Otol 2004;118:329–32.

15. Reznitsky M, Petersen MM, West N, et al. Epidemiology Of Vestibular Schwannomas - Prospective 40-Year Data From An Unselected National Cohort. Clin Epidemiol 2019;11:981–6.

16. Li D, Tsimpas A, Germanwala AV. Analysis of vestibular schwannoma size: a literature review on consistency with measurement techniques. Clin Neurol Neurosurg 2015;138:72–7.

17. Kanzaki J, Tos M, Sanna M, et al. New and modified reporting systems from the consensus meeting on systems for reporting results in vestibular schwannoma. Otol Neurotol 2003;24:642–9.

18. Varughese JK, Wentzen-Larsen T, Vassbotn F, et al. Analysis of vestibular schwannoma size in multiple dimensions : a comparative cohort study of different measurement techniques. Clin Otolaryngol 2010;35: 97–103.

19. Mackeith SAC, Das T, Graves M, et al. A Comparison of Repeatability and Usability of Semi-Automated Volume Segmentation Tools for Measurement of Vestibular Schwannomas. Otol Neurotol 2018;39:e496–505.

20. Snell JW, Sheehan J, Stroila M, et al. Assessment of imaging studies used with radiosurgery: a volumetric algorithm and an estimation of its error. J Neurosurg 2006;104:157–62.

21. George-Jones NA, Wang K, Wang J, et al. Automated Detection of Vestibular Schwannoma Growth Using a Two-Dimensional U-Net Convolutional Neural Network. Laryngoscope 2021;131(2):E619–24.

22. Morris KA, Parry A, Pretorius PM. Comparing the sensitivity of linear and volumetric MRI measurements to detect changes in the size of vestibular schwannomas in patients with neurofibromatosis type 2 on bevacizumab treatment. Br J Radiol 2016;89:20160110.

23. Moffat DA, Kasbekar A, Axon PR, et al. Growth characteristics of vestibular schwannomas. Otol Neurotol 2012;33:1053–8.

24. Macielak RJ, Patel NS, Lees KA, et al. Delayed Tumor Growth in Vestibular Schwannoma: An Argument for Lifelong Surveillance. Otol Neurotol 2019 Oct;40(9):1224–9.

25. Ozgen B, Oguz B, Dolgun A. Diagnostic accuracy of the Constructive Interference in Steady State sequence alone for follow up Imaging of vestibular schwannomas. AJNR Am J Neuroradiol 2009;30:985–91.

26. Kania R, Verillaud B, Camous D, et al. EANO position statement on vestibular schwannoma: Imaging assessment question: How should growth of vestibular schwannoma be defined? J Int Adv Otol 2018;14:90–4.

27. Lewis D, Roncaroli F, Agushi E, et al. Inflammation and vascular permeability correlate with growth in sporadic vestibular schwannoma. Neuro-Oncology 2019;21:314–25.

28. Ginat DT, Martuza RL. Post operative imaging of vestibular schwannomas. Neurosurg Focus 2012;33:1–7.

29. Silk PS, Lane JI, Driscoll CL. Surgical approaches to vestibular schwannomas: What the radiologist needs to know. Radiographics 2009;29:1955–70.

30. Kim DY, Lee JH, Goh MJ, et al. Clinical Significance of an Increased Cochlear 3D Fluid-Attenuated Inversion Recovery Signal Intensity on an MR Imaging Examination in Patients with Acoustic Neuroma. AJNR Am J Neuroradiol 2014;35:1825–9.

31. Sampath P, Rini D, Long DM. Microanatomical variations in the cerebellopontine angle associated with vestibular schwannomas: a retrospective study of 1006 consecutive cases. J Neurosurg 2000;92:70–8.

32. Savardekar AR, Patra DP, Thakur JD, et al. Preoperative diffusion tensor imaging-fiber tracking for facial nerve identification in vestibular schwannoma: a systematic review on its evolution and current status with a pooled data analysis of surgical concordance rates. Neurosurg Focus 2018;44:E5.

33. Tysome JR, Moffat DA. Magnetic resonance imaging after translabyrinthine complete excision of verstibular schwannomas. J Neurol Surg B Skull Base 2012;73: 121–4.

34. Carlson ML, Van Abel KM, Driscoll CL, et al. Magnetic resonance imaging surveillance following vestibular schwannoma resection. Laryngoscope 2012;122:378–88.

35. Williams JC, Carr CM, Eckel LJ, et al. Utility of Noncontrast Magnetic Resonance Imaging for Detection of Recurrent Vestibular Schwannoma. Otol Neurotol 2018;39:372–7.

36. Wolbers JG, Dallenga AHG, Romero AM, et al. What intervention is best practice for vestibular schwannomas? A systematic review of controlled studies. BMJ Open 2013;3:e001345.

37. Tu A, Gooderham P, Mick P, et al. Stereotactic Radiosurgery versus Natural History in Patients with Growing Vestibular Schwannomas. J Neurol Surg B Skull Base 2015;76:286–90.

38. Prabhu V, Kondziolka D, Hill TC. Preserved Cochlear CISS Signal is a Predictor for Hearing Preservation in Patients Treated for Vestibular Schwannoma With Stereotactic Radiosurgery. Otol Neurotol 2018;39:628–31.

39. Camargo A, Schneider T, Liu J, et al. Pretreatment ADC Values Predict Response to Radiosurgery in Vestibular Schwannomas. Am J Neuroradiol AJNR 2017;38:1200–5.

40. Meijer OWM, Weijmans EJ, Knol DL, et al. Tumor-Volume Changes after Radiosurgery for Vestibular Schwannoma: Implications for Follow-Up MR Imaging Protocol. Am J Neuroradiol AJNR 2008;29: 906–10.

41. Mohammed FF, Schwartz ML, Lightstone A, et al. Pseudoprogression of vestibular schwannomas after fractionated stereotactic radiation therapy. J Rad Oncol 2013;2:15–20.

42. Plotkin SR, Merker VL, Halpin C, et al. Bevacizumab for progressive vestibular schwannoma in neurofibromatosis type 2: a retrospective review of 31 patients. Otol Neurotol 2012;33:1046–52.

43. Blakeley JO, Ye X, Halpin C, et al. Efficacy and Biomarker Study of Bevacizumab for Hearing Loss Resulting From Neurofibromatosis Type 2-Associated Vestibular Schwannomas. J Clin Oncol 2016; 10:1669–75.

44. Peris-Celda M, Graffeo CS, Perry, et al. Main symptom that led to medical evaluation and diagnosis of vestibular schwannoma and patient-reported tumor size: Cross sectional study in 1304 patients. J Neurol Surg B 2019;80:316–22.

Patterns of Perineural Skull Base Tumor Extension from Extracranial Tumors

Bernhard Schuknecht, MD

KEYWORDS

- Head and neck malignancy • Perineural invasion and extension • 3D MR submillimetric sequences
- Facial-trigeminal nerve anastomoses • Skull base

KEY POINTS

- Perineural extension may be present at an early stage of head and neck neoplasms.
- Cutaneous, mucosal, and salivary gland malignancies arising in the face, nose, oral cavity, and upper pharynx may lead to perineural extension.
- Trigeminal and facial nerve branches are affected most commonly.
- A dedicated imaging protocol encompassing MR imaging 3-dimensional contrast-enhanced submillimetric sequences of 0.5 to 0.8 mm is the mainstay for the recognition of the presence and extent of perineural extension.
- Categorizing extension into a zonal classification is mandatory for management decisions.

INTRODUCTION

Tumors of the head and neck may spread beyond their confines by direct extension, by hematogenous or lymphatic dissemination. Perineural extension is an additional and important pathway that rarely may represent the sole route of tumor extension.

The terms perineural invasion, perineural spread, and perineural extension in the literature are at times indiscriminately or synonymously applied, although they signify a different process or degree of neoplastic nerve involvement. Perineural invasion indicates nerve involvement by neoplastic cells at the primary site of the neoplasm. Batsakis'[1] broad definition encompassed "tumor cell invasion in, around, and through nerves." As a histologic finding, perineural invasion therefore is commonly indistinguishable from the primary tumor by imaging.

Perineural extension or spread, however, represents a pathway of growth along nerve conduits in direct continuity or dissolute from the primary tumor location and is much less common than perineural invasion. Perineural extension is commonly visible at the macroscopic scale and thus amenable to detection by imaging. In a review article, Liebig and colleagues[2] classified histologic findings as (A) infiltration into the epi-, peri-, or endoneurium and/or (B) infiltration surrounding more than 33% of the nerve circumference, regardless of intratumoral or extratumoral nerve involvement.

The location of intratumoral versus extratumoral nerve infiltration is relevant. In a novel classification aimed to subcategorize intratumoral central, intratumoral peripheral, and extratumoral perineural invasion, Miller and colleagues[3] found a trend of separation regarding time to recurrence and patient survival between negative and intratumoral nerve invasion; a worse prognosis was associated with tumor edge and extratumoral perineural extension. This study was the first to transfer the dichotomous variable of perineural positivity or

Medical Radiological Institute, Bahnhofplatz 3, Zürich 8001, Switzerland
E-mail address: bschuknecht@mri-roentgen.ch

Neuroimag Clin N Am 31 (2021) 473–483
https://doi.org/10.1016/j.nic.2021.05.007
1052-5149/21/© 2021 Elsevier Inc. All rights reserved.

negativity into a more differentiated classification that also distinguishes semantically between perineural invasion (intratumoral and purely histologic) and perineural extension (tumor edge and extratumoral and macroscopic spread). High-resolution MR imaging and/or computed tomography (CT) scans commonly allow for the identification of perineural extension.

TUMORS ASSOCIATED WITH PERINEURAL INVASION AND EXTENSION

Perineural invasion and extension are associated with different types of head and neck neoplasms. Because of their high incidence, mucosal squamous cell carcinomas are leading in frequency, followed by cutaneous neoplasms such as basal cell and squamous cell carcinoma or melanoma. Rates of perineural invasion and extension are 0.5% to 1.0% for basal cell carcinoma and 2% to 10% in cutaneous squamous cell carcinoma with a tendency to be more common in the desmoplastic variant of melanoma and in cases of recurrent skin carcinomas.

Adenoid cystic carcinoma of major and minor salivary glands constitutes only 1% to 3% of head and neck neoplasms, but has a known propensity for perineural extension with rates as high as 50% to 80%. Among 186 patients with parotid gland malignancies, 46.2% of the tumors showed perineural invasion on histology. Salivary duct carcinoma, mucoepidermoid carcinoma, and adenoid cystic carcinoma followed by adenocarcinoma were the most common histologic types. Malignancies with perineural invasion more often presented with facial pain and paresis and more likely harbored an advanced T and N classification.[4]

Head and neck lymphomas are rarely associated with perineural spread. The more common extranodal presentation renders non-Hodgkin lymphomas of the oral cavity or paranasal sinuses prone to perineural extension.

PROGNOSTIC IMPLICATIONS OF PERINEURAL INVASION AND EXTENSION

Perineural invasion was present at the time of staging in 57% (16/28 patients) and later developed at the time of recurrence in 43% in a series of patients with diverse primary head and neck neoplasms.[5] Regardless of the histologic type, an increasing risk of perineural extension is linked to progressive T stage and tumor recurrence after therapy. In particular, it constitutes an additional independent risk factor in squamous cell carcinoma.

The presence of perineural extension correlated with T stage, nodal positivity, and the number of positive nodes, as well as a reduced disease-free survival in 142 patients with noncutaneous head and neck squamous cell carcinoma.[3] Accordingly, a study focusing on squamous cell carcinoma of the oral cavity observed recurrence-free survival rates of 47.1% in patients with perineural invasion in comparison to 80.4% in a control group.[6] In the same study,[6] the pattern of perineural invasion corresponded to a mixed type of the Liebig classification (any of the 3 layers plus >33% circumference) in 53% of patients. Exclusive manifestations such as type A were less common with 29.5% and type B with 17.5% of resection specimens.

Perineural extension indicates a pathway of extension of malignancy that exerts significant impact on surgical resectability. Once perineural growth abuts the skull base the limits of radical (R0) surgical therapy are reached. Clear surgical margins does not exclude perineural dissemination. Involvement of the skull base and the cisternal segment of a cranial nerve implies surgery plus adjunctive treatment such as radiotherapy and/or chemotherapy or a combination of local radiation and systemic chemotherapy if a surgical approach is considered noncurative.

An imaging-based localizing system integrating therapeutic management aspects has been proposed by Williams and colleagues[7] and modified by Gandhi and Sommerville[8] (Table 1). This considers the—so far—limits of curative surgical resection and the impact of intracranial perineural tumor extension on therapy. Perineural extension is categorized into 3 zones: peripheral or zone 1, central/skull base or zone 2, and cisternal or zone 3. For the different trigeminal nerve divisions and the facial nerve, the transition to zone 2 is the superior orbital fissure, the foramen rotundum and ovale, and the stylomastoid foramen, respectively; zone 3 encompasses the cisternal segments to the brainstem.

PATTERNS OF PERINEURAL EXTENSION

Perineural extension most commonly involves the trigeminal and facial nerve. However, it may affect any cranial nerve that is in contact with mucosal and cutaneous surfaces or courses within the parotid gland or adjacent to major and minor salivary glands (Table 2). Perineural tumor extension involves distal cranial nerve branches, initially in a retrograde fashion from a peripheral to centripetal direction. As a tumor adheres to a nerve branch, segments of uninvolved or only microscopically affected nerves may be present that may give

Table 1
Categories of perineural extension

	Zone 1	Zone 2	Zone 3
V1	To superior orbital fissure	To gasserian ganglion cistern	Cisternal segment to brainstem
V2	To external aperture of foramen rotundum	To gasserian ganglion cistern	Cisternal segment to brainstem
V3	To external aperture of foramen ovale	To gasserian ganglion cistern	Cisternal segment to brainstem
VII	To external aperture of stylomastoid foramen	To fundus of interior auditory canal	Cisternal segment to brainstem

Adapted from Williams LS, Mancuso AA, Mendenhall WM. Perineural spread of cutaneous squamous and basal cell carcinoma: CT and MR detection and Its impact on patient management and prognosis. Int J Radiat Oncol Biol Phys 2001:49;1061–1069 and Gandhi M, Sommerville J. The imaging of large nerve perineural spread. J Neurol Surg B Skull Base 2016;77:113–23.

rise to skip areas, potentially impeding the identification of the full extent of perineural extension. Furthermore, retrograde extension may divert into an additional antegrade direction at branching points by preformed anastomoses between different cranial nerves or branches of the same nerve (**Box 1**). Bilateral perineural extension is more likely to represent multifocal cutaneous

squamous cell carcinoma[9] than to cross over via facial nerve and trigeminal interconnections.

IMAGING APPROACHES AND PROTOCOLS

High-resolution MR imaging and CT scans are required to raise the suspicion that a tumor infiltrates a nerve branch. Clinical clues such as

Table 2
The location of a neoplasm and the expected pathways of perineural extension to serve as a check list in order to perform a "guided" image analysis

Primary Malignancy Location	Nerve Branches at Risk for Perineural Extension	Nerve Involved
Cutaneous forehead	Supratrochlear, supraorbital branch of frontal nerve	V1
Cutaneous ear	Greater auricular nerve, auriculotemporal nerve	VII–V3
Cutaneous temporal fossa, zygoma	Zygomatic nerve, frontal nerve	V2, VII
Cutaneous cheek	Infraorbital + zygomatic nerve, facial nerve branches	V2, VII
Cutaneous nose	Infraorbital nerve	V2
Cutaneous upper lip	Infraorbital nerve, buccal branches of facial nerve	V2, VII
Cutaneous lower lip, chin	Mental nerve, marginal mandibular nerve	V3, VII
Floor of mouth	Lingual nerve	V3
Submandibular gland	Lingual nerve, hyoglossal nerve	V3, XII
Mandible	Inferior alveolar nerve	V3
Retromolar trigone	Lingual nerve, inferior alveolar nerve	V3
Buccal oral cavity	Buccal branches	V3, VII
Base of tongue	Hypoglossal nerve	XII
Palate	Greater and lesser palatine nerves	V2
Maxillary sinus	Superior alveolar nerve anterior/posterior	V2
Ethmoid sinus	Nasociliary nerve, optic nerve	V1, II, III, IV, VI
Frontal sinus	Supraorbital- supratrochlear nerve	V1
Parotid gland	Facial nerve + branches, auriculotemporal nerve	VII, V3
Nasal cavity	Superior palatine, infraorbital nerve	V2

Modified from Moonis G, Cunnane MB, Emerick K, Curtin H Patterns of Perineural Tumor Spread in Head and Neck Cancer. Magn Reson Imaging Clin N Am 2012; 20: 435–446.

Box 1

Anastomoses relevant to assessment of potential perineural spread from one nerve branch to another

Trigeminal–trigeminal nerve anastomoses

Auriculotemporal nerve (V3) - zygomatico-temporal branch - zygomatic branch (V2)

Auriculotemporal nerve (V3) - inferior alveolar nerve V3

Lacrimal nerve (V1) - zygomaticotemporal branch- zygomatic nerve (V2)

Facial – trigeminal nerve anastomoses:

Facial- auriculotemporal nerve - mandibular nerve >90%

Facial - chorda tympani - lingual nerve (V3)

Facial - communicating buccal nerve- buccal nerve (V3)

Facial – communicating marginal branch mental branch (V3)

Facial - greater superficial petrosal/deep petrosal - vidian - maxillary nerve (V2)

Facial –communicating temporal branch – lacrimal nerve (V1)

Facial – IX anastomoses

Facial – Jacobson's nerve (IX)

Facial - glossopharyngeal (Ansa of von Haller)

Facial - lesser petrosal nerve

Facial - X anastomoses

Facial- Arnolds (X) tympanic plexus

Facial - lesser petrosal nerve - auricular branch

Box 2

MR imaging protocols

MR imaging skull base and face: CN I – V

Hyoid Frontal sinus: axial T2 fat-saturated 512/3 mm, cor T1 noncontrast 2.5 mm

Skull base and face – brainstem: cor 3D T2 0.8 mm (CISS, T2 SPACE, THRIVE, CUBE Gd)

Axial 3D T1 fat-saturated Gd volume (eg, Star-VIBE 0.5–0.8 mm) 3 planes MPR 1 mm

Optional: axial DESS/PSIF cor. 3D STIR

Routine brain protocol: T2, T1 noncontrast, 3D FLAIR, T1MPRAGE Gd (DWI, SWI)

Neck protocol: cor STIR, DWI, axial T2 fat-saturated, VIBE Dixon Gd

MR imaging skull base and face (CN VI–XII)

Hyoid - Frontal sinus: axial T2 fat-saturated 512/3 mm, axial T1 noncontrast 2.5 mm

Hard palate – orbital roof: axial 3D T1 fat-saturated Gd volume (eg, StarVIBE 0.5–0.8 mm)

Axial 3D T2-weighted 0.5–8.0 mm (CISS, T2 SPACE, THRIVE, CUBE …post gd)

Optional: axial DESS, PSIF cor 3D STIR

Routine brain protocol: T2, (T1 noncontrast, 3D FLAIR, T1 MPRAGE Gd, DWI, SWI)

Neck protocol: cor STIR, DWI, axial T2 fat-saturated, VIBE Dixon Gd

Abbreviations: 3D, 3-dimensinal; CISS, common integration site; CN, cranial nerve; DESS, double echo steady state; DWI, diffusion-weighted imaging; FLAIR, fluid attenuation inversion recovery; Gd, gadolinium; MPR, multiplanar reconstruction; MPRAGE, magnetization prepared rapid acquisition gradient echo; PSIF, reversed FISP (Fast Imaging with Steady State Precession); STIR, short T1 inversion recovery; SWI, susceptibility weighted imaging.

---

pain, numbness, and dysesthesia along the course of the affected nerve, motor denervation, or rarely multiple cranial neuropathies are vague and ambiguous. Approximately 40% of patients with perineural extension do not have associated symptoms.

Therefore, a protocol needs to:

- Cover the area of interest with sufficient high resolution and extent,
- Recognize a primary tumor, and/or lymph node involvement,
- Detect perineural tumor extension *and* define the extent
- Distinguish perineural extension from entities such as infection, inflammation, or treatment induced changes, and
- Serve to standardize examinations for comparison on follow-up investigations.

MR imaging best meets these requirements based on the following dedicated protocol (**Box 2**) tailored to the clinical area of interest and occasionally supplemented by CT scan (**Box 3**). A CT scan rarely is the first examination in a patient with a suspected perineural tumor extension, but maybe useful when MR imaging is not available or feasible. Three-dimensional submillimetric MR sequences and spiral CT scan acquisitions in multiplanar reconstructions increase conspicuity and thus permit to better identify the primary pathology and its pathway of extension. High-resolution CT scanning facilitates the verification of the presence and extent of additional cortical bone involvement, whereas MR imaging recognizes cancellous bone invasion to better advantage.

Box 3
CT scan protocols

CT skull base/face/posterior fossa

Hyoid: Frontal sinus (reduce FOV according to clinical question!)

ax MPR 0.5 mm/0.7 mm spacing/thickness soft tissue/bone algorithm + window,

ax/cor soft tissue 2.5 mm thickness MPR

ax/cor/sg high resolution bone window 0.7 (ax) −1.0 mm (cor/sag) MPR 1 mm

optional routine brain protocol

Abbreviations: ax, axial; cor, coronal; FOV, field of view; MPR, multiplanar reconstruction; sag, sagittal.

An important goal of imaging is to support treatment planning. Therefore, the imaging data should be transmissible into a navigation system and/or a planning system for definition of the radiation target volume.

Fusion of MR imaging on CT scan bone algorithm images is an under-recognized method to enhance visualization of extracranial and intracranial perineural tumor growth and bone involvement. A combined assessment by MR imaging and CT scanning and fusion may facilitate to attribute perineural tumor extension to the zonal classification indicated in **Table 1** and thus ease the management and assign the patient to the appropriate treatment regimen.

MR IMAGING INDICATION FOR DETECTION AND LOCALIZING EXTENT

MR imaging is the modality of choice to identify the primary neoplasm and map the potential pathways of perineural tumor extension. In 30 patients with cutaneous malignancy,[9] MR imaging identified the presence of perineural spread in all 30 of the 30 patients. The sensitivity for mapping the tumor extent, however, was lower with 25 of 30 nerves (83.3%) correctly identified. In a similar study,[10] the correlation of MR imaging and histology yielded a sensitivity for detection of 95% in 19 patients and a sensitivity of 63% for imaging the exact extent. After resection for adenoid cystic carcinoma, the sensitivity and specificity for the detection of perineural extension—with histologic correlation—was 100% and 85%, respectively, in 25 cranial nerves affected in 26 patients.[11] Interestingly, apparent diffusion coefficient values acquired at the site of parotid malignancy were significantly lower in those 22 patients with perineural invasion (apparent diffusion coefficient

0.88 ± 0.08) compared with those without (apparent diffusion coefficient 1.01 ± 0.119).[12] Less favorable results for MR imaging (1.5 T) supplemented by diffusion-weighted imaging were reported by Schroeder and colleagues[13] in a recent analysis of 25 patients with residual or recurrent squamous cell carcinoma after chemoradiotherapy. For the detection of perineural spread, MR imaging had a sensitivity of 62% (5/8), specificity of 88% (15/17), a positive predictive value of 71%, and a negative predictive value of 83% (15/18), respectively. In a study based on 3T MR imaging, Baulch and colleagues[14] reported a higher sensitivity of 95% and a specificity of 84% for the detection of perineural spread in 36 of 38 nerves. Improved recognition of the zonal extent with 3T MR imaging was present, with an 89% detection rate, in comparison with a prior investigation with a 83% detection rate (9).

In the same study[14]—and despite 3T MR assessment—the sensitivity decreased from 95% to 87% and specificity from 84% to 79% when the clinical details were not available to the radiologist. This situation reminds the clinician to provide the symptoms and clinical findings and the radiologist to target the examination and focus the analysis accordingly. In any case, the radiologist should be vigilant not to miss an early case of asymptomatic perineural extension.[15]

MR IMAGING FEATURES OF PERINEURAL SPREAD

Criteria in favor of the diagnosis of perineural extension of malignancy on MR include loss or rarefaction of perineural and/or foraminal fat pads adjacent to a nerve course.[16,17] A direct sign is asymmetric thickening and increased contrast enhancement of a nerve or nerve segment in comparison with the supposedly healthy contralateral side (**Fig. 1**). T2-weighted images may show intermediate signal of the nerve and blurred margins affected owing to increased cellularity. Once perineural extension is present, it is commonly more prominent at the neural foramina and canal exit points with focal or nodular enlargement and corresponding signal increase on contrast enhanced sequences (see **Fig. 1**; **Fig. 2**). Skip lesions (eg, along the auriculotemporal nerve) may adopt an identical nodular and T2 short T1 inversion recovery high signal characteristic (see **Fig. 2A**). Sites that need additional specific assessment are areas of proximity of a nerve to periosteum and fascia, such as the superior muscular aponeurotic system.[18]

Enlargement of the orifice of the skull base foramina and canals caused by perineural extension may initially seem to be more expansile and

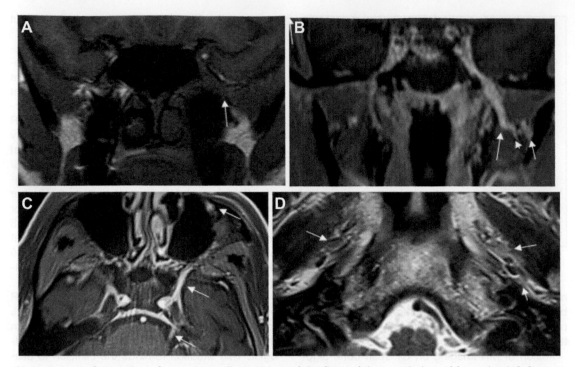

Fig. 1. Perineural extension of squamous cell carcinoma of the floor of the mouth: loss of fat pad at left foramen ovale. T1 noncontrast coronal image with loss of fat pad of left sphenoid (*long arrow*) (*A*). Increased contrast enhancement and thickened mandibular nerve (*long arrow*), inferior alveolar nerve (*short arrow*), and lingual nerve (*arrow head*) on a T1 contrast-enhanced 0.8 mm StarVIBE sequence (*B*). Axial T1 StarVIBE image depicts extension toward the cisternal segment of the trigeminal nerve, anterograde involvement of V2, pterygopalatine fossa, and infraorbital nerve (*C*). The V3 segment below the foramen ovale is blurred and enlarged, depicts intermediate T2 signal, and continues into an enlarged auriculotemporal branch (*short arrow*) (*D*).

less aggressive (**Fig. 3**; see **Fig. 6**). Additional linear to nodular contrast enhancement, however, favors perineural extension and is not indicative of a benign tumor, such as a schwannoma. Further intracranial extension is often associated with infiltration of cavernous sinus, Meckel's cave, the geniculate ganglion, and dural thickening adjacent to affected nerve segments (**Fig. 4**). Enhancement and/or thickening of cisternal segments ultimately indicate perineural extension toward the brainstem.

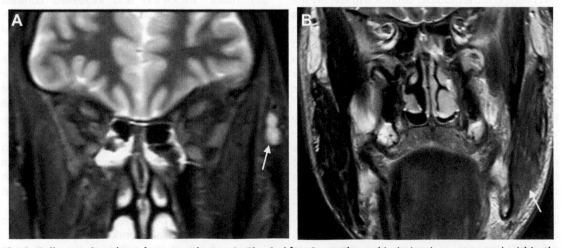

Fig. 2. Follow-up imaging of same patient as in **Fig. 1**. After 2 months, a skip lesion is encountered within the distribution of the left auriculotemporal nerve on coronal short T1 inversion recovery image (*A*) and muscular atrophy (masseter, temporal muscle) on coronal T2-weighted imaging (*B*).

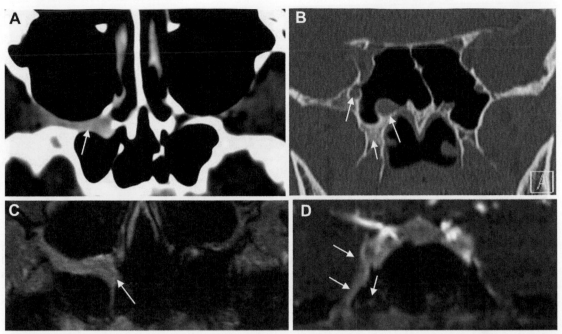

Fig. 3. A 36-year-old woman with progressive hypesthesia in right cheek. Histology-proven adenoid cystic cancer with a soft tissue lesion within the pterygopalatine fossa is hyperdense on contrast-enhanced soft tissue window axial CT scanning (*A*). Pressure erosion and widening of foramen rotundum and pterygoid canal (*arrows*) are present as well as sclerosis at the base of the pterygoid process on coronal bone window CT (*short arrow* in *B*). Axial contrast-enhanced T2-weighted SPACE sequence (0.5 mm) shows widening of the orifice and a prominent signal along the vidian nerve (*C*). Coronal T2-weighted SPACE contrast-enhanced multiplanar reconstruction image depicts thickening of maxillary nerve, lateral dural cavernous sinus and extension into foramen ovale (*D*).

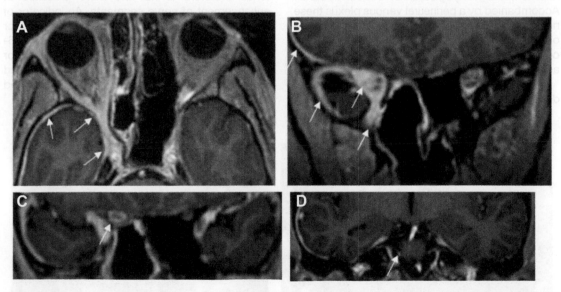

Fig. 4. Follow-up imaging of the same patient as in **Fig. 3** at 5 years after surgery and radiotherapy. Axial T1 Star-VIBE gadolinium-enhanced sequence 0.5 mm (*A*), and corresponding coronal multiplanar reconstruction 1 mm (*B*) depicts tumor progression into the orbital apex via inferior orbital fissure, extension into the superior orbital fissure and cavernous sinus invasion with marked thickening of V2 compared with the contralateral side. Dural invasion is present in the lateral middle cranial fossa and along the major sphenoid wing. Encasement of the right optic nerve is found on a coronal multiplanar reconstruction 1 mm of axial StarVIBE gadolinium sequence 0.5 mm (*arrow C*) and involvement of the cisternal segment of abducens nerve (*arrow D*).

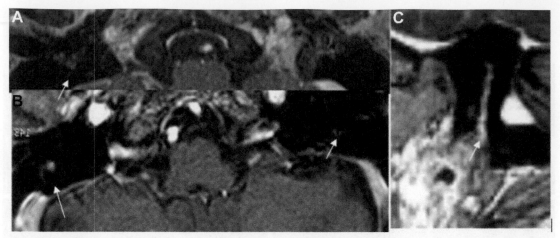

Fig. 5. Perineural tumor extension of salivary duct carcinoma of the right parotid gland. The facial nerve is shown as a dark dot target sign within the adjacent contrast-enhanced perineural venous plexus (*A*) and contralateral (*B*) on axial 3-dimensional contrast-enhanced 0.5 mm StarVIBE sequence. Perineural tumor extension shows loss of the target sign and thickening of the right facial nerve (*arrow* in *B*) and segmental thickening. Skipping segments macroscopically may occur and lead to a string of beads appearance of nerve segments on the sagittal multiplanar reconstruction 1 mm (*C*).

An additional sign is the loss of the physiologic target-like or tram-track–like contrast enhancement[19] on 3-dimensional submillimeter sequences perpendicular to a nerve's course (Fig. 5). As a sign of infiltration at the entrance to zone 2, it affects V2 at the foramen rotundum, V3 at the foramen ovale, the facial nerve at the stylomastoid foramen, and the hyoglossal nerve within its canal. Accompanied by a perineural venous plexus these nerves course through foramina or canals and once infiltrated loose their normal target (dotlike) or linear tram track–like appearance within the adjacent venous plexus (see Fig. 5; Fig. 6).

Secondary changes that occur late are signs of denervation within the muscles of mastication and facial expression (see Fig. 2B). These consist of increased muscle T2 signal, pronounced contrast enhancement, and in a later stage of progressive muscle atrophy and fatty transformation.

Even after radiochemotherapy, MR findings commonly persist indefinitely despite clinical signs of improvement. Evidence of radiographic persistence therefore is not the mere presence of enhancement of nerve segments. An indicator of a controlled tumor is a combination of stable or regressive imaging and/or clinical clues on the 6- to 12-month follow-up examinations. For adequate comparison, the same modality and preferentially an identical imaging protocol need to be applied.

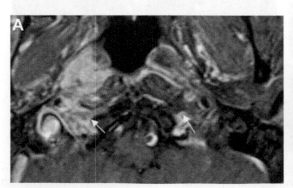
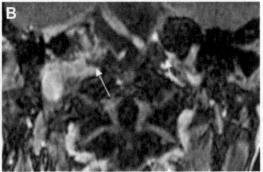

Fig. 6. Hypoglossal nerve involvement by infiltration of nasopharynx carcinoma into the carotid space through hiatus Morgagni. Perineural extension results in loss of tram track sign (*short arrow*; left hypoglossal nerve) on an axial contrast-enhanced fat-suppressed T1-weighted sequence (*A*) and coronal multiplanar reconstruction of 0.5 mm StarVIBE gadolinium sequence image (*B*). Smooth external orifice enlargement of hypoglossal by tumor extension (*long arrow*) that spares cisternal nerve segment.

Increased contrast enhancement and neural thickening are not specific for perineural extension. Benign nerve tumors and neuritis, fungal, granulomatous or IgG4-related disease are major differential diagnostic considerations to perineural extension.

COMPUTED TOMOGRAPHY INDICATIONS FOR DETECTION AND LOCALIZING EXTENT

Data regarding the capability of CT scans to detect perineural spread are scarce. In a retrospective study published in 2007,[11] the sensitivity and specificity of a CT scan for the detection of perineural invasion in 25 of 38 named nerves were 88% and 89% compared with MR imaging at with 100% and 85%, respectively. Since, then CT scanning has increasingly adopted a complementary role. A CT scan may add specificity to MR imaging findings once cortical bone involvement is suspected and/or serve treatment purposes to map the bony extent of a tumor for resective and reconstructive surgery. Furthermore, a CT scan may be used as guidance for a biopsy of equivocal cases, particularly if a lesion involves the foramen ovale.[8] An additional important aspect is that a CT scan is a commonly used modality in conjunction with PET. Despite the PET component, a CT scan requires a high index of suspicion and meticulous analysis not to miss perineural extension within the face and at the skull base.

COMPUTED TOMOGRAPHY FEATURES OF PERINEURAL INVASION

CT signs on soft tissue window images that should raise concern for perineural spread include obliteration of juxtaforaminal fat, replacement of fat along a nerve's course such as in the pterygopalatine fossa (see **Fig. 3**), retroantral fat, and fat within the orbit. On contrast-enhanced images, thickening of the fascia, periorbita, or dura are additional clues. Denervation atrophy of facial muscles and/or muscles of mastication represent late observations.

High-resolution bone window CT scan changes are late findings, because the nerve is small in relation to the osseous foramen or canal.[20] Pertinent signs include enlargement and irregular cortical erosion of skull base or midface foramina and nerve canals (**Fig. 7**). In the early stage, slight remodeling may precede irregular erosion of neural foramina (see **Fig. 3**) Osseous contour erosion is usually accompanied by soft tissue findings that in the context of perineural extension are relatively small compared with the often large size of a benign tumor.

PET SCANS

PET-CT scanning has evolved as a fundamental tool in the detection of unknown primary tumors, staging of head and neck neoplasms (especially lymph node involvement), and sensitive detection of tumor recurrence. Further advantages are exclusion of systemic metastases and synchronous primary malignancy. PET-CT scans and recently PET-MR imaging have become invaluable in the evaluation of treatment response on follow-up assessment. The sensitivity of PET/CT scan with fluorodeoxyglucose (FDG) for the detection of perineural spread, however, is considered low, proven by the fact that perineural spread was the least reported route of locoregional spread with only few case reports.[21] In a recent study of 25

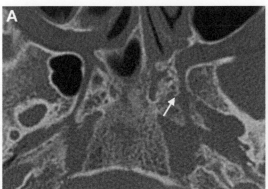
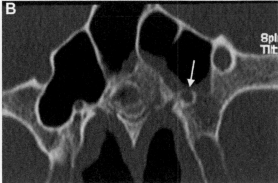

Fig. 7. Perineural extension of adenoid cystic carcinoma of the nasopharynx: typical enlargement and slightly irregular contour erosion is present along the vidian nerve canal more prominent along the medial wall and reaching toward foramen lacerum. (A) An axial CT 0.6 mm scan. A coronal CT multiplanar reconstruction 1 mm (B) depicts a slight enlargement, contour erosion, and cancellous bone sclerosis adjacent to soft tissue swelling indicative of adjacent bone infiltration as well.

patients with persistent or recurrent head and neck squamous cell carcinoma, histology confirmed perineural invasion in 8 patients proven by MR imaging in 5, whereas PET-CT scanning did not detect the perineural spread in any patient.[13] Failure to identify perineural extension on PET-CT scanning or PET/MR imaging may, however, also depend on the tumor's property not to display high tracer uptake such as in low-grade adenoid-cystic or mucoepidermoid carcinoma.

Based on fusion of FDG PET scans with contrast-enhanced MR imaging, however, Kuhn and colleagues[22] reported perineural extension in 7% (3/44) of head and neck malignancies. In a study of 58 patients with locally advanced squamous cell carcinomas and perineural extension in 13 patients (22%), a comparison of PET/MR imaging and PET/CT scanning yielded equally high accuracy in the detection for each modality (100% vs 98%).[23] With contrast-enhanced MR imaging as the reference correlation with PET-CT scanning provided an agreement of 100% in 28 patients with perineural spread proven by histology in 12 and clinical consensus in 16 patients.[5] This agreement was based on direct and indirect PET findings, such as linear or curvilinear increased FDG uptake (mean standardized uptake value, 15 ± 10), distribution along or within cranial nerves V and VII, heterogeneous uptake, and cranial nerve or foraminal enlargement. The authors admit, however, that this high correlation was a "consequence of a very sensitive reading by a pair of specialists trained in the detection of PNS in FDG-avid malignancies."[5]

SUMMARY

In general, a knowledge of the clinical findings is the essence for the radiologist to choose the correct imaging modality and to define the area of examination at the right spatial resolution. In the context of head and neck cancer, there should be a high index of suspicion for perineural extension, even in the absence of associated clinical features. Ideally, dedicated MR imaging protocols should cover the primary tumor location together with the entire extent of associated cranial nerve branches from the periphery to the brainstem. Keep in mind potential anastomoses between nerves and branches, not only on initial examinations but in particular on follow-up, because perineural extension is a dynamic process.

Note that, despite high-sensitivity imaging, there is a tendency to undercall the zonal extent owing to microscopic, radiologically occult tumor extension. Cisternal segments of smaller cranial nerves and the superficial portion of large named nerves remain difficult areas for detection of perineural spread and therefore should undergo a regular "check list control" on follow-up examinations.

MR imaging findings tend to persist after treatment; therefore, metabolic information by PET/MR imaging may occasionally yield greater diagnostic confidence when assessing therapeutic response.

CLINICS CARE POINTS

- Employ most sensitive technique (MR) with high resolution 3 D sequences (protocol Box 2) to identify primary tumor location, and extension (perineural included) at time of first examination.

- In case of suspected skull base involvement consider to supplement MR by targeted CT examination to render data for navigation and enable image fusion such as with submillimetric T1gd fat suppressed sequences.

- On follow up ensure to be knowledgeable about histology, mode and extent of treatment and to cover field of treatment based on identical protocol.

- Scrutinize images always for residual /recurrence at periphery of field of therapy.

- Ambiguous imaging findings may be correctly interpreted by addition of PET-CT or PET/MR.

DISCLOSURE

The author reports no conflicts of interest.

REFERENCES

1. Batsakis JG. Nerves and neurotropic carcinomas. Ann Otol Rhinol Laryngol 1985;94(4 Pt 1):42.
2. Liebig C, Ayala G, Wilks JA, et al. Perineural invasion in cancer: a review of the literature. Cancer 2009;115:3379–91.
3. Miller ME, Palla B, Qiaolin C, et al. A novel classification system for perineural invasion in noncutaneous head and neck squamous cell carcinoma: histologic subcategories and patient outcomes. Am J Otolaryngol 2012;33:212–5.
4. Huyett P, DuvvuriU, Ferris RL, et al. Perineural invasion in parotid gland malignancies. Otolaryngol Head Neck Surg 2018;158:1035–41.
5. Dercle L, Hartl D, Rozenblum-Beddok L, et al. Diagnostic and prognostic value of 18F-FDG PET, CT, and MRI in perineural spread of head

and neck malignancies. Eur Radiol 2018;28: 1761–70.

6. Laske RD, Scholz I, Ikenberg K, et al. Perineural invasion in squamous cell carcinoma of the oral cavity: histology, tumor stage, and outcome. Laryngoscope 2016;1:13–8.

7. Williams LS, Mancuso AA, Mendenhall WM. Perineural spread of cutaneous squamous and basal cell carcinoma: CT and MR detection and Its impact on patient management and prognosis. Int J Radiat Oncol Biol Phys 2001;49:1061–9.

8. Gandhi M, Sommerville J. The imaging of large nerve perineural spread. J Neurol Surg B Skull Base 2016;77:113–23.

9. Gandhi MR, Panizza B, Kennedy D. Detection and defining the anatomic extent of large nerve perineural spread of malignancy: comparing "Targeted" MRI with the histologic findings following surgery. Head Neck 2011;33:469–75.

10. Nemzek WR, Hecht S, Gandour-Edwards R, et al. Perineural spread of head and neck tumors: how accurate is MR imaging? AJNR Am J Neuroradiol 1998;19:701–6.

11. Hanna E, Vural E, Prokopakis E, et al. The sensitivity and specificity of high-resolution imaging in evaluating perineural spread of adenoid cystic carcinoma to the skull base. Arch Otolaryngol Head Neck Surg 2007;133:541–5.

12. Khalek Abdel Razek AA, Elkhamary SM, Nada N. Correlation of apparent diffusion coefficient with histopathological parameters of salivary gland cancer. Int J Oral Maxillofacial Surg 2019;48:995–1000.

13. Schroeder C, Jung-Hyun Lee J-H, Tetzner U, et al. Comparison of diffusion-weighted MR imaging and 18F fluorodeoxyglucose PET/CT in detection of residual or recurrent tumors and delineation of their local spread after (chemo) radiotherapy for head

and neck squamous cell carcinoma. Eur J Radiol 2020;130:10915.

14. Baulch J, Gandhi M, Sommerville J, et al. 3T MRI evaluation of large nerve perineural spread of head and neck cancers. J Med Imaging Radiat Oncol 2015;59:578–85.

15. Moonis G, Cunnane MB, Emerick K, et al. Patterns of perineural tumor spread in head and neck cancer. Magn Reson Imaging Clin N Am 2012;20:435–46.

16. Curtin HD. Detection of perineural spread: fat is a friend. AJNR Am J Neuroradiol 1998;19:1385–6.

17. Dankbaar JW, Pameijer FA, Hendrikse J, et al. Easily detected signs of perineural tumour spread in head and neck cancer. Insights Imaging 2018; 9:1089–95.

18. Kirsch CFE, Schmalfuss IM. Practical tips for MR imaging of perineural tumor spread. Magn Reson Imaging Clin N Am 2018;26:85–100.

19. Maroldi R, Farina D, Borghesi A, et al. Perineural tumor spread. Neuroim Clin N Am 2008;18:413–29.

20. Caldemeyer KS, Mathews VP, Righi PD, et al. Imaging features and clinical significance of perineural spread or extension of head and neck tumors. RadioGraphics 1998;18:97–110.

21. Paes FM, Singer AD, Checkver AN, et al. Perineural spread in head and neck malignancies: clinical significance and evaluation with 18F-FDG PET/CT. RadioGraphics 2013;33:1717–36.

22. Kuhn FP, Martin Hüllner M, Mader CE. Contrast-enhanced PET/MR imaging versus contrast-enhanced PET/CT in head and neck cancer: how much MR information is needed? J Nucl Med 2014;55:551–8.

23. Sekine T, Barbosa FG, Delso G, et al. Local resectability assessment of head and neck cancer: positron emission tomography/MRI versus positron emission tomography/CT. Head Neck 2017;39: 1550–8.

Imaging of Trigeminal Neuralgia and Other Facial Pain

Rudolf Boeddinghaus, MBChB, FCRad(D)SA, FRANZCR, FRCR[a,b,]*,
Andy Whyte, BDS(Hons), MBBCh, FFDRCSI, DDMFR, FRCR, FRANZCR[c,d]

KEYWORDS

- Trigeminal neuralgia • MR imaging • Glossopharyngeal neuralgia • Facial pain • Cranial neuropathy
- Nociceptive pain • Neuropathic pain • Referred otalgia

KEY POINTS

- Facial pain can be neuropathic or nociceptive and is best investigated using high-resolution MR imaging, with a role for computed tomography scans in nociceptive pain.
- Trigeminal neuralgia is an uncommon but severe facial pain disorder with distinctive clinical features.
- Trigeminal neuralgia is usually primary; this is designated classical if vascular compression deforms the trigeminal root, otherwise idiopathic. Secondary trigeminal neuralgia is rare.
- MR imaging should not be used to diagnose trigeminal neuralgia, but to exclude mimics and secondary causes and to aid treatment decisions in primary trigeminal neuralgia by showing neurovascular conflicts.
- MR imaging protocols for investigating facial pain should allow both detailed assessment of the trigeminal root and adjacent vessels, and detection of diverse other causes of facial pain.

INTRODUCTION

The many causes of facial pain can be divided into nociceptive pain (derived from pain receptors within the end organs such as the teeth, sinuses, salivary glands, and temporomandibular joints [TMJs]) and neuropathic pain, derived from the trigeminal nerve and other nerves supplying the facial region. Neuropathic pain can be further subdivided into the neuralgias (which have typical short paroxysmal episodes of severe pain) and painful cranial neuropathies (in which nerve damage causes pain as well as other symptoms such as decreased sensation). Other causes to consider include the trigeminal autonomic cephalgias, giant cell arteritis, and the entity of persistent idiopathic facial pain (**Table 1**).

Classical trigeminal neuralgia (TN) is caused by vascular (usually arterial) impingement on the root entry zone (REZ) of the trigeminal nerve in the prepontine cistern. This neurovascular impingement can be demonstrated on targeted high-resolution T2-weighted MR imaging. However, TN is relatively rare (lifetime prevalence of up to 0.3%[1]) compared with dental and other nociceptive causes of facial pain. Therefore, many patients with TN will have undergone treatment for a suspected dental cause of the pain[2] before a diagnosis of TN is eventually made. In contrast, clinicians may mistake odontogenic and other nociceptive facial pain for TN. Many asymptomatic individuals will have MR evidence of vascular contact with the cisternal segment of the trigeminal nerve.[3–6] Occasionally, no vascular contact (or

[a] Perth Radiological Clinic, 127 Hamersley Road, Subiaco, Western Australia 6008, Australia; [b] Department of Surgery, University of Western Australia, 35 Stirling Highway, Perth, Western Australia 6009, Australia; [c] Department of Medicine and Radiology, University of Melbourne, Grattan Street, Parkville, Victoria 3010, Australia; [d] Department of Dentistry, University of Western Australia, 35 Stirling Highway, Perth, Western Australia 6009, Australia
* Corresponding author.
E-mail address: rudolf.boeddinghaus@perthradclinic.com.au

Neuroimag Clin N Am 31 (2021) 485–508
https://doi.org/10.1016/j.nic.2021.05.008
1052-5149/21/© 2021 Elsevier Inc. All rights reserved.

Table 1
Overview of causes of facial pain

Neuropathic	Neuralgias	TN, Glossopharyngeal Neuralgia, Nervus Intermedius Neuralgia
	Painful neuropathies	Traumatic, neoplastic, inflammatory, postinflammatory
Nociceptive	End-organ pain	Teeth, sinuses, salivary glands, TMJ
	Referred otalgia	TMJ, upper cervical spine, teeth, oropharynx
Trigeminal autonomic cephalgias	Cluster headache SUNCT, SUNA Paroxysmal hemicrania Hemicrania continua	All may be primary or secondary
Vascular	Giant cell arteritis	Elderly, jaw claudication, temporal pain, elevated inflammatory markers
Other	Persistent idiopathic facial pain	Functional

Abbreviations: SUNA, short-lasting unilateral neuralgiform headache attacks with cranial autonomic features; SUNCT, short-lasting unilateral neuralgiform headache attacks with conjunctival injection and tearing.

secondary cause) is shown on MR imaging in a patient with TN. Therefore, the demonstration of neurovascular contact on MR imaging cannot be used to make a diagnosis of TN, but is used to help treatment decisions in clinically diagnosed TN.[1] Furthermore, radiologists investigating a patient with facial pain, whether TN is suspected or not, should ensure that the MR imaging protocol used covers the central and peripheral distribution of the trigeminal nerves and their end organs, and that all potential causes for facial pain, not just trigeminal neurovascular impingement, are identified and communicated.

RELEVANT ANATOMY
Trigeminal Nuclei

The trigeminal nerve (cranial nerve [CN] V), the largest CN, is predominantly sensory, with a lesser motor function. It has 4 nuclei (**Fig. 1, Table 2**), 3 of which (sensory) are in continuity with one another. This extensive central nuclear anatomy requires that MR imaging for trigeminal symptoms include coverage of the upper cervical spinal cord.

Trigeminal Cisternal Segment

The cisternal segment of the trigeminal nerve consists of a small motor root superomedially and a larger sensory root; these structures can often be resolved as separate on MR imaging (**Fig. 2**). The root entry point is on the lateral margin of the mid pons. The roots run anteriorly and slightly superiorly within the prepontine cistern before entering the cerebrospinal fluid–filled dural recess

of Meckel's cave (the trigeminal cave) at a narrow opening, the porus trigeminus, medial to the petrous apex.

In all cranial and spinal nerve roots, the transition from the central nervous system (CNS, myelinated by oligodendrocytes) to the peripheral nervous system (myelinated by Schwann cells) occurs a variable distance from the point at which the roots emerge from the surface of the brainstem (or spinal cord). The transition is not a sharp line, but a dome-shaped zone, the CNS portion extending further distally in the center of the root (**Fig. 3**). This zone is the transition zone (also known as the Obersteiner–Redlich zone). It is not synonymous with the term "root entry zone," which is widely used in the surgical and radiologic literature, but is rarely and variably defined.[5] There is evidence that the CNS portion of the root is more susceptible to demyelination by vascular compression. It has been shown that the CNS portion of the root varies in length between about the proximal one-fifth and the proximal one-half of the root[7] (in absolute terms from 0.1 to 2.5 mm anterior to the root entry point on the pons medially and from 0.17 to 6.75 mm laterally, the longer lateral distance owing to the oblique contour of the pons). Although recognizing that the CNS portion of the root is variable, and unknowable in an individual subject, it is reasonable to define the proximal (ie, posterior) half of the cisternal portion as the REZ.[8]

The sensory root has been described as having a somatotopic organization, with the ophthalmic (V1) fibers superomedially, the maxillary fibers

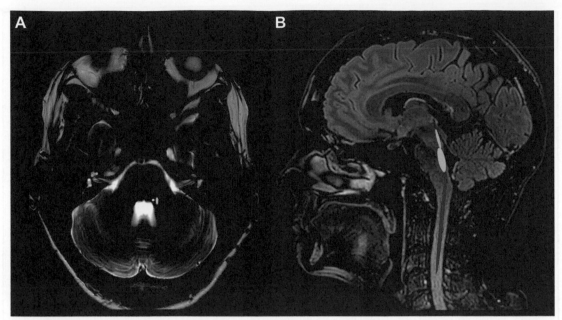

Fig. 1. Trigeminal nuclei. Axial T2-weighted (*A*), pontine level showing location of principal sensory nucleus (*orange*), with motor nucleus medial (*yellow*). Sagittal fluid attenuated inversion recovery image. (*B*) Levels of principal sensory (*orange*), mesencephalic (*green*), and spinal trigeminal (red) nuclei.

(V2) medially and the mandibular (V3) fibers inferolaterally. A weak association between the site of neurovascular compression around the diameter of the root and the symptomatic division/s has been shown,[9] supporting this somatotopic organization.

Trigeminal Dural Cave Segment, Ganglion, Divisions, and Branches

Within Meckel's cave, sensory rootlets fan out and enter the trigeminal (also known as semilunar or Gasserian) ganglion, which lies along the anteroinferior margin of Meckel's cave. The trigeminal ganglion consists of the cell bodies of the pseudounipolar sensory neurons subserving sensation from the face. The 3 separate sensory divisions of the trigeminal nerve (**Fig. 4**, **Table 3**) enter the ganglion (but the small motor root bypasses the ganglion and passes inferior to it to join the mandibular division). The U-shaped ganglion, unlike the other portions of the nerve, normally enhances after the administration of gadolinium-based contrast agents (see **Fig. 4**). The 3 dermatomes corresponding with the divisions of the trigeminal nerves curve posterosuperiorly (**Fig. 5**).

Glossopharyngeal and Vagus Nerves

The glossopharyngeal nerve (CN IX) carries general sensory fibers from the oropharynx and special sensory (taste) fibers from the tongue base. It

is the most superior of the group of 3 lower CNs (IX, X, and XI) running laterally from the medulla toward the jugular foramen. Its identity can be inferred from the marked lateral protrusion of the brainstem at this level.[10] It enters the smaller anteromedial pars nervosa of the jugular foramen. The vagus (CN X) supplies general sensation to the remainder of the pharynx as well as the larynx and it forms a neural complex with the accessory nerve (CN XI) in the larger pars vacularis of the jugular foramen, medial to the internal jugular vein.[11] CNs IX, X, and XI exit the jugular foramen to enter the carotid space.

The Cervical Plexus and the Innervation of the Ear

Sensory branches of the cervical plexus (formed by the ventral rami of C1–C4) are derived from C2 and C3: the great auricular and lesser occipital nerves innervate the pinna, skin situated anteroinferior to the pinna and the mastoid region. The greater occipital nerve, which is the larger medial branch of the dorsal ramus of C2, supplies the occipital region and scalp overlying the posterior cranium extending superiorly toward the vertex (see Fig. 5).

Sensory innervation of the ear is complex (**Fig. 6**), with contributions from several CNs as well as C2 and C3. The auriculotemporal branch of V3 innervates skin overlying the posterior two-thirds of the

Table 2
Anatomy of the trigeminal nuclei

Nucleus	Location	Function	Comments
Principal sensory nucleus	Lateral aspect of pontine tegmentum, anterolateral to the fourth ventricle	Tactile stimuli	
Spinal trigeminal nucleus	Elongated, extends down from inferior pons, through medulla into superior cervical spinal cord	Incorporates sensory information from different CNs, including the 3 divisions of CN V and the facial (CN VII), glossopharyngeal (CN IX), and vagus (CN X) nerves	Superior one-third: orofacial tactile Middle one-third: dental pain Inferior third: facial pain and temperature, which explains the loss of ipsilateral facial pain and temperature sensation—but not light touch sensation—in the lateral medullary syndrome
Mesencephalic nucleus	Extends superior from principal sensory nucleus into midbrain, lateral margin of periaqueductal gray matter to level of superior colliculus	Proprioception	
Motor nucleus	Small, medial to principal sensory nucleus in pons	Motor to muscles of mastication, mylohyoid and anterior belly of digastric, tensor tympani and tensor veli palatini	The supplied 8 muscles are those derived from the first pharyngeal (branchial) arch

temporal fossa, the pre-auricular region and tragus, the TMJ and the anterior wall of the external auditory canal and tympanic membrane. The nervus intermedius division of CN VII, and CN X, also supply skin of the concha, the external auditory canal and the lateral aspect of the tympanic membrane. Sensory supply to the middle ear and mastoid air cells is primarily from CN IX.

TRIGEMINAL NEURALGIA
Clinical Features

TN is characterized by short (<1 second to several seconds) episodes of paroxysmal intense lancinating facial pain in the distribution of one or more of the trigeminal nerve divisions (most commonly V2 and/or V3), including intraoral pain. Paroxysms of pain may be so severe that they

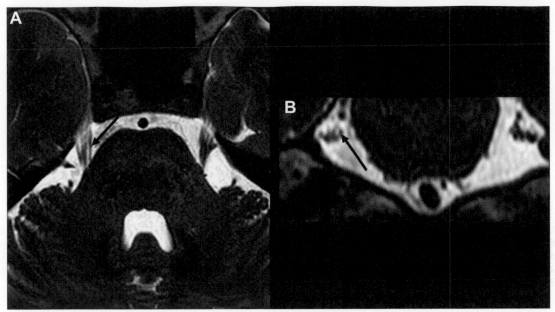

Fig. 2. Trigeminal motor root. Axial (*A*) volumetric T2-weighted, coronal reconstruction (*B*) showing a small motor root (*black arrows*) of trigeminal nerve, superomedial to larger sensory root.

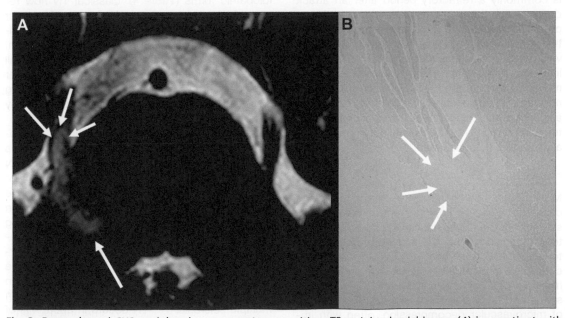

Fig. 3. Dome-shaped CNS–peripheral nervous system transition. T2-weighted axial image (*A*) in a patient with right facial parasthesia and MR features of multiple sclerosis. (*A*) Swelling and hyperintensity in keeping with demyelinating plaque affecting centrally myelinated portion of trigeminal root, extending along parenchymal fascicular segment of the nerve within lateral pons (*arrows*). Photomicrograph (*B*) of a trigeminal nerve root section showing dome-shaped transition zone (*arrows*). ([B] Courtesy Prof Selçuk Peker, Istanbul, Turkey.)

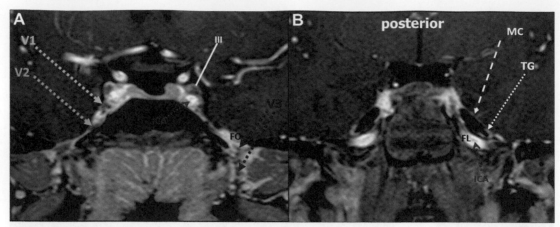

Fig. 4. Cavernous sinus, Meckel's cave. Postgadolinium gradient echo coronal T1-weighted fat-saturated image showing the right V1 and V2 divisions within right cavernous sinus (*A*) and left V3 division in and below foramen ovale (FO). Left intracavernous oculomotor nerve (III), internal carotid artery (ICA) also indicated. Posteriorly (*B*), inferiorly situated, U-shaped enhancing trigeminal ganglion (TG) is shown within Meckel's cave (MC). The ICA is indicated in the foramen lacerum (FL).

are accompanied by involuntary contraction of the facial muscles, accounting for the older name of "tic douloureux." Painful episodes are usually and characteristically triggered by light touch of the skin within this distribution or by other innocuous sensory (including intraoral) stimuli, such as brushing the teeth, eating, talking, shaving or applying make-up, or even by draughts of cold wind. The pain is almost always unilateral. There is commonly a refractory period after an attack during which the pain cannot be triggered. Up to one-half of patients report persistent dull ache between episodes, but the dominant feature is of severe short-lasting episodes of stabbing pain. TN increases in incidence with age and is more common in women. Autonomic symptoms such as rhinorrhea and conjunctival injection may occur, but are not a dominant feature[12]; when autonomic features are prominent, a trigeminal autonomic cephalgia should be considered.[13]

Etiology and Classification

Most TN is now generally accepted as being caused by vascular impingement on the cisternal segment of the trigeminal nerve, usually by an artery (most commonly the superior cerebellar artery) but commonly ($\leq$56%) combined compression by an artery and a vein, and uncommonly ($\leq$12%) by a vein alone.[14,15] The vessel itself is normal or only mildly ectatic. The success of microvascular decompression, often with immediate relief of symptoms, supports vascular impingement as the cause, although lingering doubts remain,[16] because in a minority of patients no compressing vessel is seen, neurovascular

conflict is extremely common in asymptomatic individuals, and there is a small but predictable rate of recurrence after successful microvascular decompression. There is interest in the role of voltage-gated sodium channels in the etiology of TN[17] and a central role of the superior portion of the spinal trigeminal nucleus.[18]

Recent (2018) classifications from international societies[1,19] divide primary TN into classical and idiopathic forms (**Table 4**): classical TN now requires MR imaging or surgical evidence of vascular compression with morphologic changes of the trigeminal nerve root; if no root deformity is shown, it is considered idiopathic TN. This change will result in many more cases, where there is vascular contact with the root but no root distortion, being classified as idiopathic TN (which would formerly have been classified as classical TN).

Secondary (previously also known as "symptomatic") TN refers to the minority of cases ($\leq$15%) where the typical clinical syndrome of TN is present, but a cause other than impingement on the nerve by a normal vessel is shown. The cause may be either an intra-axial, central lesion or an extra-axial space-occupying lesion along the nerve root. A central lesion, typically demyelination (**Fig. 7**), rarely an infarct (**Fig. 8**) or a cavernoma, may cause secondary TN by involving the nuclei within the brainstem. Vascular compression of the trigeminal root in the cistern can coexist with multiple sclerosis.[20,21] TN occurs in about 4% of patients with multiple sclerosis.[21] Compressive extra-axial lesions include neoplasm (**Fig. 9**) (typically schwannoma or meningioma) or cyst (eg, an epidermoid cyst). In these cases, it has been

Table 3
Anatomy of trigeminal divisions and branches

Division	Course	Branches and Supplied Territories
Ophthalmic (V1)	Runs anteriorly along the lateral wall of the cavernous sinus (inferior to CN III and IV and lateral to CN VI), branching into 3 before entering the orbit Two of the branches enter orbit via superior orbital fissure, the nasociliary nerve enters via the common tendinous ring	*Frontal nerve*: runs anteriorly in superior margin of the orbit between superior muscle group and orbital roof. Divides into *supra-orbital nerve*, exiting orbit via the supra-orbital notch or foramen to supply skin of forehead and scalp almost as far posteriorly as lambdoid suture; *supratrochlear nerve* medially for the inferomedial forehead *Lacrimal nerve*: small lateral nerve *Nasociliary nerve*: medial; crosses obliquely below the superior rectus and superior oblique muscles to reach the medial orbital wall, and gives rise to the anterior and posterior ethmoidal nerves and the infratrochlear nerve
Maxillary (V2)	Lies inferior to V1 in lateral margin of cavernous sinus (most inferior nerve seen within it). Passes anteriorly within foramen rotundum (actually a short canal), enters superior aspect of pterygopalatine fossa. It continues, after a lateral and anterior bayonet bend, as the infraorbital nerve	*Infraorbital nerve*: main continuation of V2, runs anteriorly in orbital floor, in infraorbital groove and/or canal and through infraorbital foramen to supply skin of anterior cheek and upper lip[a] *Posterior superior alveolar nerve* (supplying posterior maxillary teeth) *Zygomaticofacial* and *zygomaticotemporal nerves*, running in lateral orbit, exiting orbit through canals of the same names to supply the skin over the malar eminence and anterior temporal fossa, respectively *Greater* and *lesser palatine nerves*: course inferiorly from pterygopalatine fossa within canals of the same names to supply mucosa of palate
Mandibular (V3)	Descends from trigeminal cave to exit cranial compartment via foramen ovale, entering masticator space where it is visible in a plane of fat between medial and lateral pterygoid muscles	*Inferior alveolar nerve*: enters mandibular foramen on medial surface of mandibular ramus, supplying lower teeth, gingiva and lip *Lingual nerve*: visible medial to mandibular ramus in narrow fat-containing pterygomandibular space, supplying sensation to the tongue *Auriculotemporal nerve*: communicates with CN VII within parotid gland, posterior to the condylar neck, supplying TMJ and preauricular skin, anterior wall of the external auditory canal

[a] The *anterior superior alveolar nerve*, for the anterior teeth and gingiva, is a branch of the infraorbital nerve: its canal, the canalis sinuosus, can be seen curving anteroinferiorly within the frontal process of the maxilla.

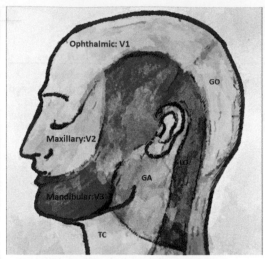

Fig. 5. Craniomaxillofacial sensory innervation. Face and anterior scalp are supplied by the 3 trigeminal divisions (V1–V3). The pinna, parotid, and retroauricular regions, submental region and anterior upper neck are supplied by cervical plexus (C2/3) branches: the great auricular (GA), lesser occipital (LO), and transverse cervical (TC) nerves. The posterior scalp is supplied by the greater occipital (GO) nerve, the medial branch of dorsal ramus of C2. (Courtesy Dr Amanda Phoon-Nguyen, Perth, Australia.)

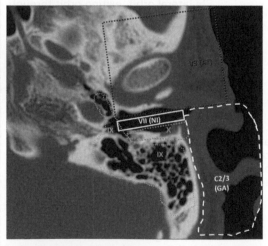

Fig. 6. Ear innervation. Preauricular skin, TMJ, anterior wall of external auditory canal supplied by the auriculotemporal branch of V3 (red square, V3 [AT]). The skin of the pinna and retroauricular region supplied by great auricular from cervical plexus (C2/3 [GA], white outline). Sensation to central portion of the external auditory canal supplied by nervus intermedius branch of facial (yellow rectangle, VII [NI]) and posterior wall by vagus (X, dotted green outline). Sensation to middle ear, mastoid air cells from glossopharyngeal (IX; dotted blue outline).

reported that a vessel is present between the lesion and the nerve, compressing the nerve.[14] Rarely, a vascular lesion such as an aneurysm or vascular malformation (Fig. 10) compresses the nerve.

In general, the symptoms are identical in the classical, idiopathic, and secondary types of TN. Clinical clues to secondary TN include younger patient age, bilaterality of symptoms (especially in multiple sclerosis), and additional neurologic symptoms and signs (eg, sensorineural hearing loss).

Pathophysiology

Histologic examination of trigeminal nerve roots resected from patients with TN caused by arterial compression demonstrate focal demyelination at the site of vascular indentation of the nerve, with close apposition of demyelinated axons.[22] The loss of the myelin sheath separating adjacent axons allows abnormal transmission of neural impulses between adjacent axons, known as ephaptic transmission (from the ancient Greek ephapsis, meaning touching). This loss is thought to allow cross-talk between fibers, subserving light touch and those transmitting the sensation of pain, accounting for painful paroxysms being triggered by innocuous stimuli. It is also hypothesized that the spontaneous generation of nerve impulses is induced by mechanical pulsatile indentation of the root, accounting for the rapid resolution of symptoms after microvascular decompression, which is observed in most patients.[22]

Treatment

The treatment (Table 5) of primary TN is initially medical. In medically refractory cases, treatment options are ablative procedures and neurosurgical microvascular decompression. Microvascular decompression is the first choice in classical TN (ie, where the MR imaging shows neurovascular compression with morphologic changes of the root). It is performed via a suboccipital craniectomy and a retrosigmoid approach, with placement of a pledget of polytetrafluoroethylene (Teflon) foam between the nerve and the offending vessel: the same operation is used for glossopharyngeal neuralgia (Fig. 11) and for hemifacial spasm. The pledget can be shown on CT scans and MR imaging (Fig. 12).

In patients refractory to medical treatment and unsuitable for an open neurosurgical procedure, an ablative procedure may be used. Ablative procedures are also considered the first choice where the MR imaging shows no neurovascular contact.[1] In those cases of idiopathic TN where MR imaging shows neurovascular contact without morphologic

Table 4
Current classification of TN

Primary TN	Classical	Neurovascular contact *with morphologic root changes*
	Idiopathic	No neurovascular contact, or neurovascular contact without change in root morphology
Secondary TN		Intra-axial lesion (demyelination, infarct, cavernoma)
		Space-occupying lesion (neoplastic mass, aneurysm, vascular malformation)

root changes, microvascular decompression and ablative procedures are considered equal first choices. Ablative procedures include stereotactic radiotherapy (gamma knife surgery), targeting the cisternal segment,[23] which shows enhancement after this procedure (**Fig. 13**), and percutaneous rhizotomy, in which the ganglion is approached under imaging guidance via the foramen ovale.[24] After rhizotomy, clumping of nerve rootlets in Meckel's cave may be visible on MR imaging[25] (**Fig. 14**).

Imaging

MR imaging is performed to confirm and demonstrate the neurovascular contact, and to exclude less common secondary causes of TN (**Table 6**). The critical MR sequence to demonstrate neurovascular contact is a heavily T2-weighted high-resolution volumetric sequence, demonstrating the nerve and the offending vessel(s) as hypointense structures surrounded by the markedly hyperintense cerebrospinal fluid (**Fig. 15**). Time of flight MR angiography is also usually performed, but does not improve accuracy,[8] although it has a role demonstrating rare vascular secondary

causes of TN (see **Fig. 10**). Contrast-enhanced CISS sequences have been used to improve the detection of neural compression by a vessel.[4]

A high prevalence of vascular contact with the trigeminal nerve root is present in individuals without TN[3–6,15] and this MR imaging finding has poor specificity. In contrast, higher grades of neurovascular contact, including indentation, displacement, or compression and flattening of the root, have been shown to be highly specific for TN, but have a low sensitivity (about 50%). The superior cerebellar artery is the commonest vessel to cause significant neurovascular contact, followed by the anterior inferior cerebellar artery. In many cases (>50%), venous (ascending petrosal or transverse pontine) contact with the trigeminal root is present (**Fig. 16**), but it is uncommon for a vein to be the only vessel implicated in causing TN.[14] The site of neurovascular contact is commonly in the proximal (posterior) one-half of the root in the expected location of centrally myelinated fibers.[8] However, in a large series[26] neurovascular contact was seen in the mid-cisternal portion in more than one-half and in the juxtapetrosal anterior portion of the root adjacent

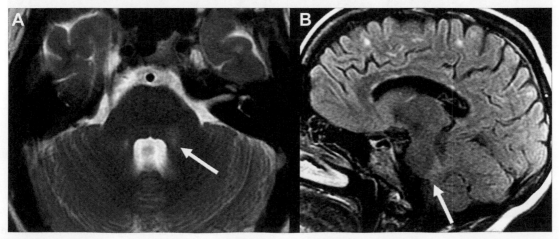

Fig. 7. TN secondary to multiple sclerosis. Axial T2-weighted image (*A*) and fluid attenuated inversion recovery sagittal image (*B*) showing new subacute demyelination (*arrows*) involving trigeminal main sensory nucleus in known multiple sclerosis patient presenting with left TN. Pericallosal and juxtacortical lesions noted in (*B*).

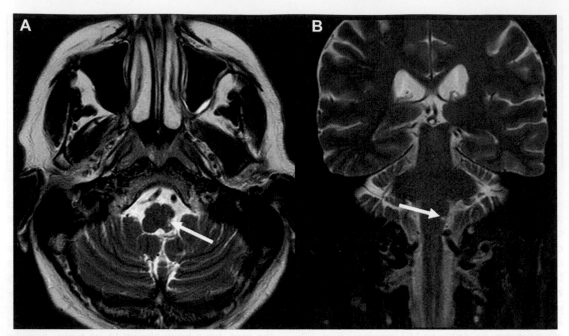

Fig. 8. Facial pain caused by prior lateral medullary infarct. Axial (*A*) and coronal (*B*) T2-weighted images in a patient with longstanding paroxysmal left facial pain; focal gliosis in the lateral aspect of medulla is consistent with a chronic lateral medullary infarct.

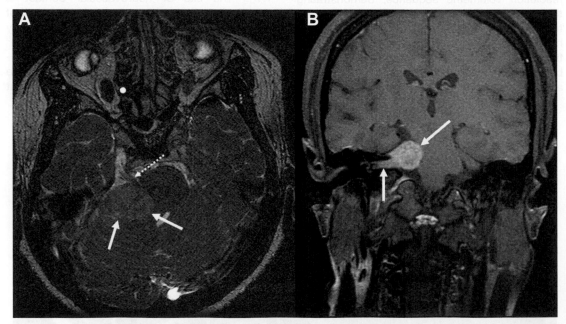

Fig. 9. TN secondary to cisternal mass. Volumetric T2-weighted axial image (*A*) and postgadolinium T1-weighted fat-saturated coronal image (*B*) in a patient with severe paroxysmal right facial pain triggered by chewing. An enhancing mass (*arrows*) typical of a vestibular schwannoma in the cerebellopontine angle cistern and internal auditory canal compresses the trigeminal REZ (*dotted arrow*).

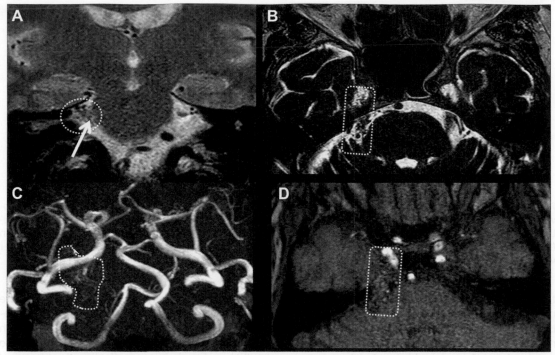

Fig. 10. TN secondary to vascular malformation. T2-weighted coronal (A) and volumetric axial (B) images showing an enlarged, hyperintense cisternal trigeminal nerve (arrow) surrounded by multiple punctate flow voids (dotted outlines) extending into Meckel's cave, in patient with right TN. The maximum image projection (C) and source data (D) from MR angiography confirm a dural arteriovenous fistula (dotted outlines).

Table 5 Treatment options for primary TN		
Medical	Carbamazepine/ Oxcarbazepine, Sometimes in Conjunction with Other Anticonvulsants	Excellent Control but High Side Effect Rate at Doses Required for the Control of Pain
Ablative	Percutaneous rhizotomy	Mechanical (balloon) Chemical (glycerol) Thermal (radiofrequency)
	Stereotactic radiotherapy	Gamma knife
Open Surgery	Microvascular decompression	High success rate (often immediate); low recurrence rates
	Surgical partial sensory rhizotomy	If no neurovascular contact found at surgery (traditionally 15%, should be rare with good pre-operative MR imaging)

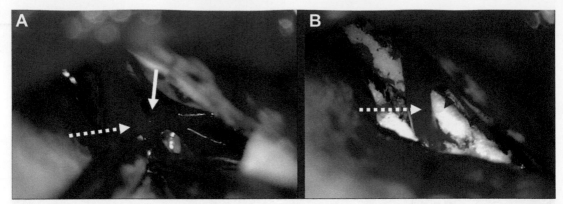

Fig. 11. Microvascular decompression for glossopharyngeal neuralgia. Intraoperative photographs during microvascular decompression for glossopharyngeal neuralgia. An arterial loop (*arrow*) of the posterior inferior cerebellar artery abuts REZ of glossopharyngeal nerve (*dotted arrow*) in (*A*). After microvascular decompression (*B*), a pledget (*arrowheads*) of polytetrafluoroethylene (PTFE) separates nerve from artery, which is no longer visible. (*Courtesy* Prof Stephen Lewis, Perth, Australia.)

to the porus trigeminus in nearly 10%. High-grade neurovascular contact (indentation, displacement) is usually proximal and always arterial, whereas milder neurovascular contact (mere contact) also occurred distally and could be arterial, venous or both.[15]

In patients with multiple sclerosis causing TN, MR imaging may show plaques affecting the REZ and/or nuclei (see **Fig. 7**), but are not always visible.[20] In contrast, hyperintense lesions involving the trigeminal nuclei and root are commonly seen on 3T MR imaging in multiple sclerosis patients and do not necessarily correlate with symptoms of TN.[27] Rarely, demyelination owing to multiple sclerosis is seen affecting the trigeminal root itself, even in patients without clinical TN (see **Fig. 3**).

Apart from its value in treatment decisions, MR imaging also has prognostic value. Atrophy of the trigeminal root (reduced cross-sectional

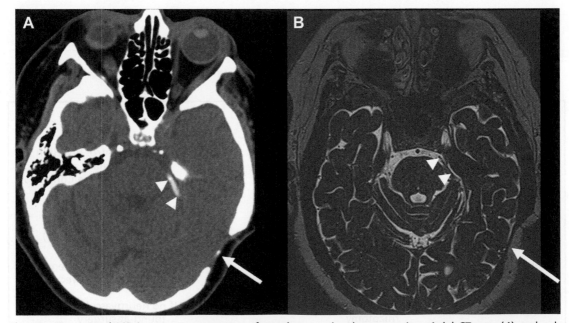

Fig. 12. CT scan and MR imaging appearances after microvascular decompression. Axial CT scan (*A*) and volumetric T2-weighted MR imaging (*B*) after successful microvascular decompression for left TN. Left suboccipital craniectomy (*arrows*). Polytetrafluoroethylene pledget (*arrowheads*) appears as hyperdense rectilinear structure on the CT scan, with a signal void on MR imaging.

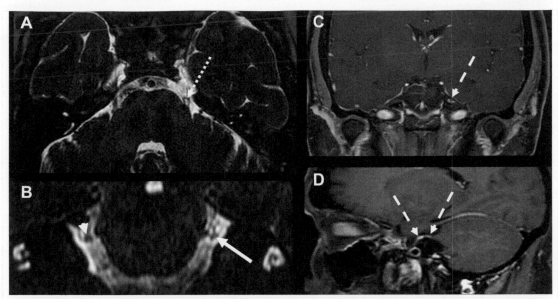

Fig. 13. MR imaging appearance after stereotactic radiotherapy. Volumetric T2-weighted axial (A), coronal reconstruction (B), postgadolinium gradient echo T1-weighted fat-saturated coronal, (C) and fast spin echo T1-weighted fat-saturated sagittal (D) images 18 months after stereotactic radiotherapy for refractory left TN. Arterial impression on superior surface of trigeminal REZ by the superior cerebellar artery (dotted arrow); the trigeminal root is atrophic (arrow) compared with the right side (arrowhead). Abnormal enhancement of left nerve at and posterior to porus trigeminus (dashed arrows).

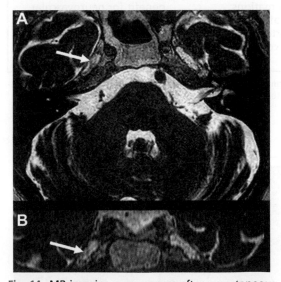

Fig. 14. MR imaging appearances after percutaneous rhizotomy. Volumetric T2-weighted axial image (A) and coronal reconstruction (B) in patient with recurrent right TN 5 years after trigeminal rhizotomy. Reduced T2 hyperintensity, clumping of trigeminal rootlets in Meckel's cave (arrows) compared with left side. Arterial impingement on right trigeminal REZ was present (not shown).

area and volume) correlated with high degrees of neurovascular contact and with the success of microvascular decompression.[28] In a small series, it was suggested that although proximal root atrophy is a good prognostic factor, distal root atrophy may predict a poor outcome after microvascular decompression.[29]

Diffusion tensor imaging uses anisotropic diffusion to estimate the axonal (white matter) organization of the brain and also large CNs, such as the cisternal segment of the trigeminal nerve.[30,31] Demyelination, loss of axonal membranes, axonal disorganization, and inflammation owing to neurovascular contact are hypothesized to account for the decreased fractional anisotropy and elevated apparent diffusion coefficient of the affected trigeminal nerve (and ipsilateral cerebral white matter tracts) in patients with TN. There is evidence that these changes are at least partially reversible after successful treatment with surgical decompression or radiosurgery.[30,31] Similar changes are seen in patients with secondary TN owing to multiple sclerosis, also involving the clinically unaffected root.[21]

Table 6
Suggested MR imaging sequences for investigation of facial pain

Sequence	Rationale	Additional Comments
Heavily T2W volume prepontine	Critical sequence for showing neurovascular conflict	If volumetric, only one plane required (typically axial), with coronal, sagittal and oblique reconstructions as required Extend above tip of basilar so that the superior cerebellar arteries can be confidently traced
FLAIR volume sagittal whole brain	Detection of multiple sclerosis and other intra-axial pathology	Should extend to C4 level for detection of upper cervical cord lesions (spinal trigeminal root)
T2W and DWI axial whole brain	Detection of infarcts, demyelination, cavernomas	Should extend to upper cord
Coronal high resolution T1W, T2W (with and without FS), post-Gd T1W (with FS):	Detection of painful trigeminal neuropathies, skull base pathology and nociceptive (end-organ) causes of facial pain, referred otalgia, secondary trigeminal autonomic cephalgia	Coverage anterior face to posterior pons Dixon technique useful for obtaining images without and with fat saturation Gradient echo post-Gd T1WFS useful for showing hyperintense signal from flow-related enhancement of vessels, which can improve grading of neural compression
Time-of-flight *MR angiography* intracranial arteries	Detection of aneurysms, vascular malformations; identification of compressing arteries in neurovascular contact	Some authors report no extra benefit for neurovascular compression in classical TN Important in investigation of trigeminal autonomic cephalgias

Abbreviations: DWI, diffusion-weighted imaging; Gd, gadolinium; FLAIR; fluid attenuated inversion recovery; T1W, T1-weighted; T1WFS, T1-weighted fat saturated; T2W, T2-weighted.

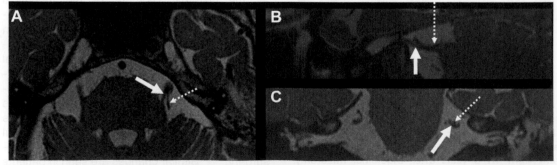

Fig. 15. Neurovascular compression causing TN. Volumetric T2-weighted axial (*A*), sagittal (*B*), and coronal (*C*) re-constructions in patient with left TN. Arterial loop (*dotted arrow*), shown by following images superiorly to represent left superior cerebellar artery, indents superior surface of proximal left trigeminal root (*arrow*) indenting and flattening its superior surface.

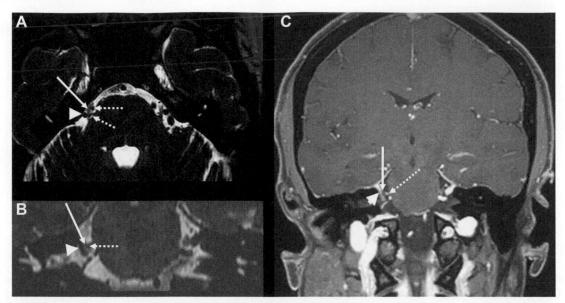

Fig. 16. Arterial and venous compression causing TN. Volumetric T2-weighted axial (*A*), coronal reconstruction (*B*), and volumetric gradient echo T1-weighted fat-saturated coronal (*C*) images in a patient with right V3 TN, showing right trigeminal nerve (*arrow*) compressed between vein laterally (*arrowhead*) and inferior loop of superior cerebellar artery (*dotted arrow*) medially. The vessels are more hypointense than nerve on T2-weighted imaging. Vessels enhance on the gradient echo ("bright blood") T1 sequence. Both sequences show flattening of the nerve.

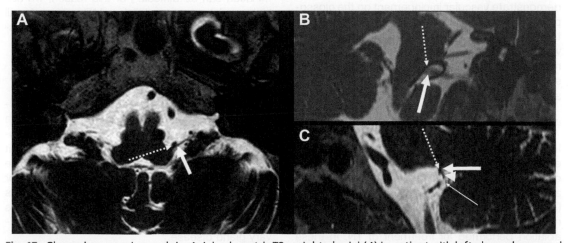

Fig. 17. Glossopharyngeal neuralgia. Axial volumetric T2-weighted axial (*A*) in patient with left glossopharyngeal neuralgia showing artery (*dotted arrow*), identified as the left posterior inferior cerebellar artery (PICA), contacting the glossopharyngeal REZ (*arrow*), the most superior of lower CNs (IX, X, and XI). Note the lateral bulge of medulla at this level, immediately below the pons. Oblique coronal minimum intensity projection (MinIP) (*B*) shows a PICA loop (*dotted arrow*) crossing cisternal portions of lower CNs (*arrow*) immediately lateral to brainstem and again further laterally. The lower CNs, appearing hypointense (not as signal void), cannot be resolved as separate structures on MinIP. Oblique sagittal (*C*) reconstruction demonstrates the PICA (*dotted arrow*) abutting CN IX (*arrow*). CN X (largest of the lower CNs, *arrowhead*) and CN XI (*narrow arrow*) are shown inferiorly.

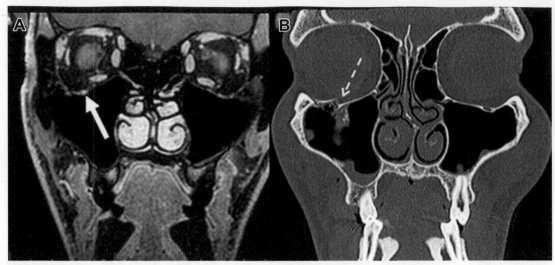

Fig. 18. Painful post-traumatic trigeminal neuropathy. Postgadolinium T1-weighted fat-saturated coronal image (A) in patient with right cheek pain and hypoesthesia. There is a subtle asymmetric enhancement and thickening of infraorbital nerve (arrow). He recalled facial injury months earlier (declined surgery). Coronal bone algorithm reconstruction from a CT scan at time of injury (B). Comminuted orbital floor fracture involving the infraorbital canal (dashed arrow).

GLOSSOPHARYNGEAL NEURALGIA

Glossopharyngeal neuralgia is rare and is characterized by severe short-lived lancinating bursts of pain, similar to those of TN, but occurring in the pharynx. Episodes may be provoked by swallowing or chewing. High-resolution MR imaging may demonstrate vascular impingement on the glossopharyngeal nerve near the brainstem (Fig. 17), and treatment is similar to that for TN: initially medical, with microvascular decompression (see Fig. 11) reserved for patients with medically refractory symptoms. MR imaging is also used to exclude a secondary cause.

PAINFUL CRANIAL NEUROPATHIES

In contradistinction to the neuralgias described elsewhere in this article, painful trigeminal (and other CN) neuropathies occur when there is a lesion affecting the nerve. Examples include trauma (Fig. 18), inflammation, skull base neoplasm, large nerve perineural tumor spread (Fig. 19), or previous ablation performed for treatment of TN. In these cases, there is loss of nerve function (anesthesia, hypoesthesia or paresthesia), which is accompanied by pain in the distribution of the nerve, hence the term anesthesia dolorosa. Unlike the paroxysmal lancinating pain of the neuralgias, the quality of this pain is usually persistent and may be described as burning or dull. Inflammatory causes

include acute herpes zoster, postherpetic neuralgia (Fig. 20), and inflammatory demyelinating polyneuropathy. Although the nature of the pain and the accompanying sensory deficit should make the clinical distinction between painful trigeminal neuropathy and TN possible, in some cases this determination can be difficult. For this reason, we use high-resolution postgadolinium MR imaging for all patients with facial pain, even when the clinical suspicion is TN.

NOCICEPTIVE FACIAL PAIN

The end organs within the trigeminal nerve distribution may be affected by painful lesions, which can frequently be mistaken for TN or other neuropathic facial pain. Nociceptive pain has a different quality to neuropathic pain. It responds to simple analgesics and changes with load or position or movement. The commonest causative lesions are dental periapical inflammatory lesions (Fig. 21), TMJ pathology, sinus disease, and salivary gland disease.

Many of the nociceptive causes of facial pain are better assessed with CT scans than with MR imaging (eg odontogenic, sinugenic) or as well assessed with CT scans as with MR imaging (eg, TMJ, upper aerodigestive tract malignancy), and where nociceptive pain is suspected rather than neuropathic pain it may be reasonable to use

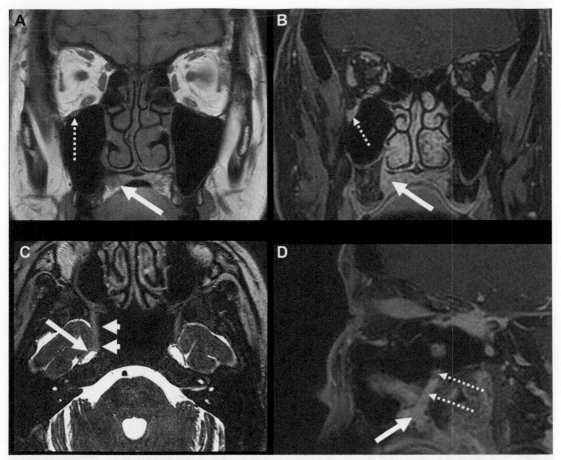

Fig. 19. Facial pain caused by perineural tumor. T1W coronal image (*A*) in patient with right periorbital pain and parasthesia for months. Loss of submucosal fat in hard palate owing to nodule (*arrow*), and subtle thickening of the infraorbital nerve (*dotted arrow*). Volumetric postgadolinium T1-weighted fat-saturated coronal image. (*B*) Thickened, enhancing infraorbital nerve (*dotted arrow*), enhancing tissue at the greater palatine foramen (*arrow*). Volumetric T2-weighted axial scan (*C*). A thickened hyperintense V2 division in foramen rotundum (*arrowheads*) and thickened trigeminal ganglion (*arrow*). Sagittal reconstruction (*D*) from volumetric postgadolinium T1-weighted fat-saturated image: enhancing lesion in posterior hard palate (*arrow*), thickened enhancing greater palatine nerve (dotted *arrows*). There is a minor salivary gland adenoid cystic carcinoma.

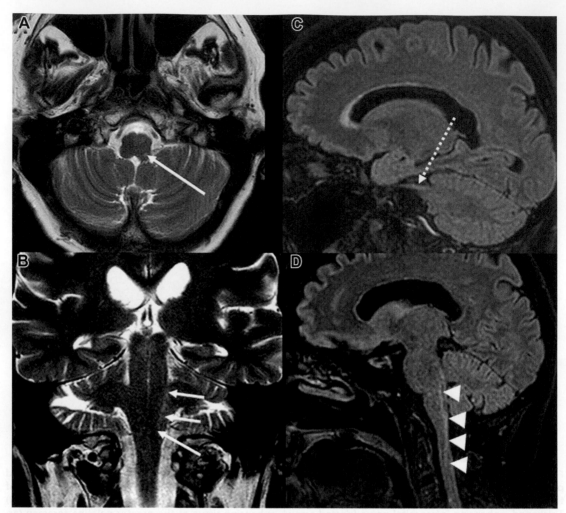

Fig. 20. Postherpetic neuralgia. T2-weighted axial (*A*) and coronal (*B*) images in a patient with persistent left facial pain after shingles in V3 distribution 1 month previously: subtle hyperintensity in medulla and pons (*arrows*). Volumetric fluid attenuated inversion recovery sagittal (*C*) and (*D*). Hyperintensity of trigeminal root (*dotted arrow*) and extending from the pons into the upper cervical spinal cord (*arrowheads*).

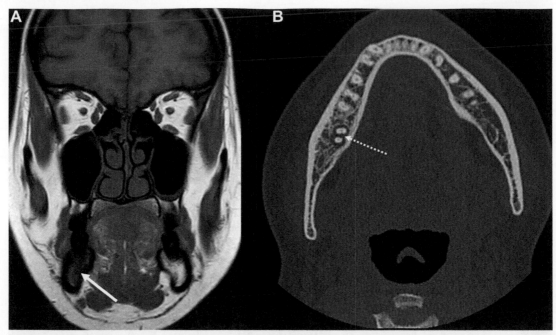

Fig. 21. Dental inflammation presenting as TN. Young adult referred for MR imaging with right V3 TN not responding to carbamazepine. MR imaging showed no neurovascular conflict. T1W coronal image (*A*) shows a loss of normal marrow fat signal in mandibular body (*arrow*). CT scan (*B*) shows periapical inflammatory lucency (*dotted arrow*) around the molar roots and surrounding reactive sclerosis.

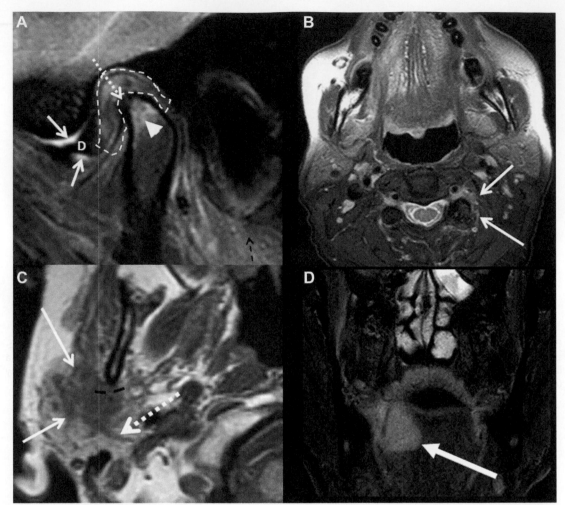

Fig. 22. Benign and malignant causes of referred otalgia. (*A*) TMJ pathology. T2-weighted fat-saturated oblique sagittal image: the anteriorly displaced articular disc (*D*), small effusions in both joint spaces (*arrows*), intra-articular (including retrodiscal) synovitis (*dashed outline*), small erosion of condyle (*dotted arrow*), and marrow edema (*arrowhead*). (*B*) Facet arthritis causing left referred otalgia. T2-weighted fat-saturated axial image: active arthritis C2/3 facet joint (*arrows*), with marrow edema, and capsulitis. (*C*) Parotid malignancy. T1-weighted axial image in a patient with right otalgia and mild facial weakness: an irregular mass (*arrows*) in the parotid and thickened facial nerve (*dotted arrow*). Expected position of involved auriculotemporal nerve (*black dashes*). Un-differentiated carcinoma with perineural spread. (*D*) Tongue base malignancy. Coronal T2-weighted fat-saturated image in patient with right otalgia and jaw pain, recent negative nasendoscopy and CT scan: large mass (*arrow*) in right side of tongue base. Oropharyngeal squamous cell carcinoma.

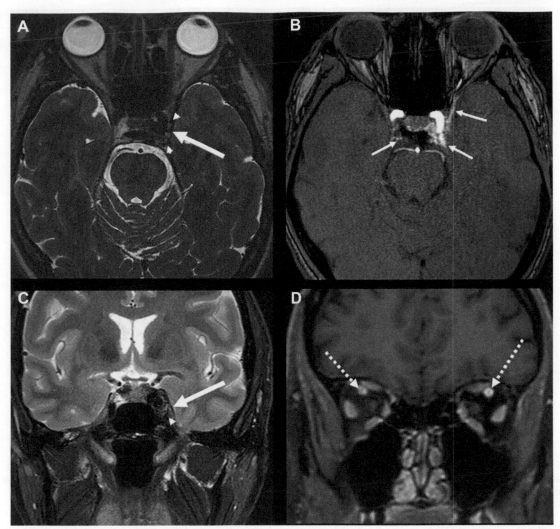

Fig. 23. Secondary trigeminal autonomic cephalgia owing to indirect carotid-cavernous fistula. Volumetric T2-weighted axial (A), T2-wighted fat-saturated coronal image (B) in a patient with left trigeminal autonomic cephalgia (left hemicrania, ptosis and conjunctival injection): asymmetric fullness of cavernous sinus (arrows), serpiginous signal voids (arrowheads). Source image time-of-flight MR angiography (C): flow-related enhancement in the left cavernous sinus, extending anteriorly toward the superior orbital fissure and involving the right cavernous sinus (small arrows). Postgadolinium volumetric turbo spin echo T1-weighted fat-saturated coronal reconstruction (D): enlargement of superior ophthalmic veins (dotted arrows).

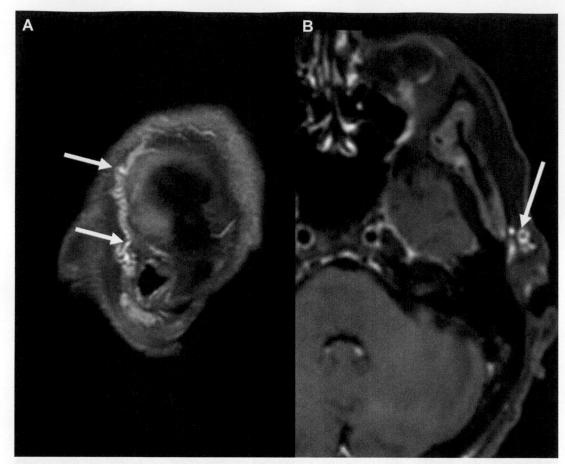

Fig. 24. Giant cell arteritis. Volumetric postgadolinium turbo spin echo T1-weighted fat-saturated sagittal (*A*), axial reconstruction (*B*) in patient with left periorbital pain of abrupt onset: mural thickening and periadventitial enhancement (*arrows*) of the superficial temporal artery.

contrast-enhanced CT scans as the first imaging modality.[32]

REFERRED OTALGIA

Neoplastic and inflammatory processes involving the sensory distribution of CNs V, VII, IX, and X as well as C2 and C3 may refer to the ear and TMJ, causing referred otalgia.[33] Periapical dental sepsis (via V2 and V3), TMJ disorders (via auriculo-temporal nerve), and active upper cervical facet joint arthritis (via cervical plexus) are common causes. Malignant causes including pharyngeal carcinoma and perineural tumor spread also require exclusion (**Fig. 22**). However, a recent study[34] has found a very low yield of imaging in the absence of a history of head and neck cancer.

TRIGEMINAL AUTONOMIC CEPHALGIAS

This group of uncommon primary headache disorders, comprising cluster headache, paroxysmal

hemicrania, and the short-lasting unilateral neural-giform headache attacks, as well as hemicrania continua, may be primary or secondary, and imaging (including vascular and sellar imaging) is always recommended to exclude causative underlying pathology[13] (**Fig. 23**).

OTHER CAUSES OF FACIAL PAIN

Giant cell arteritis (**Fig. 24**) occurs in patients who are older than 50 years of age. Its onset may be sudden, but the pain is typically constant and in the temporal region, although it may be frontal or occipital. Inflammatory markers are usually elevated. Prompt recognition is vital because it can cause blindness and is readily treatable with corticosteroids. Although the reference standard for diagnosis is temporal artery biopsy, ultrasound examination[35] and MR imaging[36,37] have high sensitivity.

Persistent idiopathic facial pain (formerly known as atypical facial pain) is a chronic orofacial pain disorder distinct from TN, commoner in women, sometimes bilateral and uncommonly stabbing in nature or with triggered episodes of pain or periods of remission. This has no correlation with neurovascular contact[38]

SUMMARY

Facial pain can be caused by a wide variety of different entities, ranging from intra-axial lesions such as multiple sclerosis to local pathology of the teeth, TMJs, sinuses, and salivary glands. MR imaging should include high resolution T2-weighted images to show the trigeminal nerve roots in the prepontine cistern, coverage of brain parenchyma and the upper cervical cord, and dedicated coverage to detect pathology in the skull base and end-organs. CT scanning is useful where nociceptive dental or sinus pain is suspected. TN is diagnosed clinically; MR imaging is used to exclude secondary causes and to demonstrate neurovascular contact and distortion, displacement or atrophy of the trigeminal root, which has prognostic implications and may influence choice of treatment.

CLINICS CARE POINTS

- Trigeminal neuralgia is an uncommon disorder with distinctive clinical features including short paroxysms of intense unilateral facial pain, often triggered by light touch.

- MR imaging is used to exclude secondary trigeminal neuralgia (for example caused by multiple sclerosis or a mass), and to distinguish between classical (neurovascular contact with root deformation) and idiopathic (no neurovascular contact, or contact but no abnormal root morphology) subtypes of primary trigeminal neuralgia. This can affect management decisions.

- MR imaging protocols should also be designed to exclude other causes of facial pain which can mimic trigeminal neuralgia, including nociceptive pain from end-organs innervated by the trigeminal nerve.

DISCLOSURE

Neither author has a funding source or any commercial or financial conflicts of interest to disclose.

REFERENCES

1. Bendtsen L, Zakrzewska JM, Heinskou TB, et al. Advances in diagnosis, classification, pathophysiology, and management of trigeminal neuralgia. Lancet Neurol 2020;19(9):784–96.
2. Zakrzewska JM. Differential diagnosis of facial pain and guidelines for management. Br J Anaesth 2013;111(1):95–104.
3. Peker S, Dinçer A, Necmettin Pamir M. Vascular compression of the trigeminal nerve is a frequent finding in asymptomatic individuals: 3-T MR imaging of 200 trigeminal nerves using 3D CISS sequences. Acta Neurochir (Wien) 2009;151(9):1081–8.
4. Blitz AM, Northcutt B, Shin J, et al. Contrast-enhanced CISS imaging for evaluation of neurovascular compression in trigeminal neuralgia: improved correlation with symptoms and prediction of surgical outcomes. Am J Neuroradiol 2018;39(9):1724–32.
5. Maarbjerg S, Wolfram F, Gozalov A, et al. Significance of neurovascular contact in classical trigeminal neuralgia. Brain 2015;138(2):311–9.
6. Antonini G, Di Pasquale A, Cruccu G, et al. Magnetic resonance imaging contribution in the diagnosis of neurovascular contact in classical trigeminal neuralgia. A blinded case-control study and meta-analysis. Pain 2014;155(8):1464–71.
7. Peker S, Kurtkaya Ö, Üzün I, et al. Microanatomy of the central myelin-peripheral myelin transition zone of the trigeminal nerve. Neurosurgery 2006;59(2):354–8.
8. Hughes MA, Frederickson AM, Branstetter BF, et al. MRI of the trigeminal nerve in patients with trigeminal neuralgia secondary to vascular compression. Am J Roentgenol 2016;206(3):595–600.
9. Sindou M, Brinzeu A. Topography of the pain in classical trigeminal neuralgia: insights into somatotopic organization. Brain 2020;143(2):531–40.
10. Casselman J, Mermuys K, Delanote J, et al. MRI of the cranial nerves-more than meets the eye: technical considerations and advanced anatomy. Neuroimaging Clin N Am 2008;18(2):197–231.
11. Linn J, Moriggl B, Schwarz F, et al. Cisternal segments of the glossopharyngeal, vagus, and accessory nerves: detailed magnetic resonance imaging-demonstrated anatomy and neurovascular relationships - Clinical article. J Neurosurg 2009;110(5):1026–41.
12. Maarbjerg S, Di Stefano G, Bendtsen L, et al. Trigeminal neuralgia - Diagnosis and treatment. Cephalalgia 2017;37(7):648–57.
13. Benoliel R. Trigeminal autonomic cephalgias. Br J Pain 2012;6(3):106–23.
14. Barker FG, Janetta PJ, Bissonette DJ, et al. The long-term outcome of microvascular decompression for trigeminal neuralgia. N Engl J Med 1996;334(17):1077–83.
15. Leal PRL, Hermier M, Souza MA, et al. Visualization of vascular compression of the trigeminal nerve with high-resolution 3T MRI: a prospective study comparing preoperative imaging analysis to

surgical findings in 40 consecutive patients who underwent microvascular decompression for trigeminal neuralgia. Neurosurgery 2011;69:15–26.

16. Burchiel KJ. Trigeminal neuralgia: new evidence for origins and surgical treatment. Neurosurgery 2016; 63(1):52–5.

17. Dib-Hajj SD, Geha P, Waxman SG. Sodium channels in pain disorders. Pain 2017;158(Suppl 1):S97–107.

18. Peker S, Sirin A. Primary trigeminal neuralgia and the role of pars oralis of the spinal trigeminal nucleus. Med Hypotheses 2017;100:15–8.

19. Cruccu G, Finnerup NB, Jensen TS, et al. Trigeminal neuralgia. New classification and diagnostic grading for practice and research. Neurology 2016;87(2):220–8.

20. Meaney JFM, Watt JWG, Eldridge PR, et al. Association between trigeminal neuralgia and multiple sclerosis: role of magnetic resonance imaging. J Neurol Neurosurg Psychiatry 1995;59(3):253–9.

21. Lummel N, Mehrkens JH, Linn J, et al. Diffusion tensor imaging of the trigeminal nerve in patients with trigeminal neuralgia due to multiple sclerosis. Neuroradiology 2015;57(3):259–67.

22. Love S, Coakham HB. Trigeminal neuralgia: pathology and pathogenesis. Brain 2001;124(12): 2347–60.

23. Wolf A, Kondziolka D. Gamma knife surgery in trigeminal neuralgia. Neurosurg Clin N Am 2016; 27(3):297–304.

24. Wang JY, Bender MT, Bettegowda C. Percutaneous procedures for the treatment of trigeminal neuralgia. Neurosurg Clin N Am 2016;27(3):277–95.

25. Northcutt BG, Seeburg DP, Shin J, et al. High-resolution MRI findings following trigeminal rhizotomy. Am J Neuroradiol 2016;37(10):1920–4.

26. Sindou M, Howeidy T, Acevedo G. Anatomical observations during microvascular decompression for idiopathic trigeminal neuralgia (with correlations between topography of pain and site of the neurovascular conflict). Prospective study in a series of 579 patients. Acta Neurochir(Wien) 2002;144(1):1–12.

27. Mills RJ, Young CA, Smith ET. Central trigeminal involvement in multiple sclerosis using high-

resolution MRI at 3T. Br J Radiol 2010;83(990): 493–8.

28. Leal PRL, Barbier C, Hermier M, et al. Atrophic changes in the trigeminal nerves of patients with trigeminal neuralgia due to neurovascular compression and their association with the severity of compression and clinical outcomes. J Neurosurg 2014;120(6):1484–95.

29. Duan Y, Sweet J, Munyon C, et al. Degree of distal trigeminal nerve atrophy predicts outcome after microvascular decompression for Type 1a trigeminal neuralgia. J Neurosurg 2015;123(6):1512–8.

30. De Souza DD, Davis KD, Hodaie M. Reversal of insular and microstructural nerve abnormalities following effective surgical treatment for trigeminal neuralgia. Pain 2015;156(6):1112–23.

31. Leal PRL. Fraction of anisotropy and apparent diffusion coefficient as diagnostic tools in trigeminal neuralgia. Acta Neurochir (Wien) 2019;161(7):1403–5.

32. Whyte A, Matias MATJ. Imaging of orofacial pain. J Oral Pathol Med 2020;49(6):490–8.

33. Chen RC, Khorsandi AS, Shatzkes DR, et al. The radiology of referred otalgia. Am J Neuroradiol 2009;30(10):1817–23.

34. Ainsworth E, Pai I, Kathirgamanathan M, et al. Diagnostic yield and therapeutic impact of face and neck imaging in patients referred with otalgia without clinically overt disease. Am J Neuroradiol Am 2020; 41(11):2126–31. https://doi.org/10.3174/ajnr.A6760.

35. Schmidt WA. Ultrasound in the diagnosis and management of giant cell arteritis. Rheumatol (United Kingdom) 2018;57:ii22–31.

36. Klink T, Geiger J, Ness T, et al. Giant cell arteritis: MR diagnostic accuracy. Neuroradiology 2014;273(3).

37. Rhéaume M, Rebello R, Pagnoux C, et al. High-resolution magnetic resonance imaging of scalp arteries for the diagnosis of giant cell arteritis: results of a prospective cohort study. Arthritis Rheumatol 2017;69(1):161–8.

38. Maarbjerg S, Wolfram F, Heinskou TB, et al. Persistent idiopathic facial pain – a prospective systematic study of clinical characteristics and neuroanatomical findings at 3.0 Tesla MRI. Cephalalgia 2017;37(13): 1231–40.

Imaging of Acquired Skull Base Cerebrospinal Fluid Leaks

Daniel J. Scoffings, MBBS, MRCP, FRCR

KEYWORDS

- CSF leak • CSF rhinorrhea • CSF otorrhea • Cisternography • Idiopathic intercranial hypertension

KEY POINTS

- Imaging of patients with suspected rhinorrhea or otorrhea from a suspected skull base leak should only be undertaken once there has been biochemical confirmation that the fluid is CSF.
- High resolution CT is the preferred initial investigation and is often the only imaging that is needed.
- Intrathecal contrast cisternography, either by CT or MRI, is indicated for patients with multiple skull base defects to determine which is leaking.
- Spontaneous skull base CSF leaks may be the result of idiopathic intracranial hypertension and imaging features that suggest this should be sought in these patients.

INTRODUCTION

Skull base cerebrospinal fluid (CSF) leaks occur when there is an abnormal communication between the subarachnoid space and an air space in the paranasal sinuses, nasal cavity, middle ear, or mastoid air cells. Such leaks require that there is a defect in the bone of the skull base and the adjacent dura mater. There may be associated herniation of meninges (a meningocele) or of brain and meninges (a meningoencephalocele) through the defect. Congenital skull base defects are beyond the scope of this article and are covered elsewhere in this edition.

Acquired osteodural defects can be broadly classified as traumatic (including iatrogenic) and nontraumatic,[1] with nontraumatic causes including tumors and spontaneous leaks in the context of intracranial hypertension. Patients typically present with intermittent unilateral CSF rhinorrhea or otorrhea, frequently positional in nature. It is important to note, however, that skull base CSF leaks do not cause spontaneous intracranial hypotension.[2]

Although skull base CSF leaks caused by craniofacial trauma often close spontaneously, the presence of a persistent osteodural defect in the skull base places the patient at risk of meningitis through the intracranial entry of sinonasal flora. The risk of ascending meningitis ranges from 5% to 30%[3–5] and is lower for spontaneous skull base CSF leaks than for other causes.[6] The risks of the morbidity and mortality of bacterial meningitis in patients with persistent CSF leaks necessitate surgical closure of the causative defect, which in turn requires accurate localization of its site and measurement of its dimensions. While patients who have extensive or highly comminuted anterior skull base fractures may need to be repaired via craniotomy, an endonasal endoscopic approach is increasingly favored for simple defects in the anterior and central skull base in view of the low morbidity and high rates of success.[7]

SKULL BASE ANATOMY

The skull base anatomy pertinent to a discussion of CSF leaks is that which interfaces with the sinonasal and petromastoid air spaces.

The anterior skull base is formed by parts of the frontal, ethmoid, and sphenoid bones and separates the nasal cavity, ethmoid air cells, and frontal sinuses from the anterior cranial fossa. The fovea ethmoidalis forms the roof of the ethmoid air cells

Department of Radiology, Cambridge University Hospitals NHS Foundation Trust, Hills Road, Cambridge CB2 0QQ, UK
E-mail address: daniel.scoffings@addenbrookes.nhs.uk

Neuroimag Clin N Am 31 (2021) 509–522
https://doi.org/10.1016/j.nic.2021.05.009
1052-5149/21/Crown Copyright © 2021 Published by Elsevier Inc. All rights reserved.

neuroimaging.theclinics.com

and is a medial extension of the orbital plate of the frontal bone. Medially this articulates with the lateral lamella of the cribriform plate, part of the ethmoid bone. The lateral lamella of the cribriform plate is the thinnest bone in the skull base and as such is prone to both traumatic and spontaneous CSF leaks. The Keros classification divides the lateral lamellae by height into type I (1–3 mm), type II (4–7 mm), and type III (8–16 mm). Asymmetry in the height of the lateral lamellae is common and predisposes patients to iatrogenic injury during endoscopic sinus surgery (ESS) on the deeper side. The horizontal part of the cribriform plate separates the olfactory grooves intracranially from the olfactory clefts of the nasal cavity and is perforated by numerous olfactory foramina, which are visible on high-resolution CT and should not be mistaken for abnormal defects. The planum ethmoidale and planum sphenoidale form the roofs of the posterior ethmoid air cells and sphenoid sinus, respectively.

The central and posterolateral skull base is formed by the sphenoid bone and paired petrous temporal bones. The paired sphenoid sinuses show variable pneumatization, which affects the thickness of bone covering the adjacent optic nerves, internal carotid arteries, and vidian and maxillary nerves and, when the intervening bone is thin or absent, increases the risk of traumatic and spontaneous CSF leaks. Pneumatization of the pterygoid processes, extending inferolateral to a plane through the vidian canal and foramen rotundum, occurs in up to 44%,[8] the dorsum sellae is pneumatized in up to 33%, and the anterior clinoid processes are pneumatized in up to 20%.[9] In the temporal bones, the air spaces of the middle ear cavity and mastoid air cells are separated from the intracranial cavity by thin plates of bone called the tegmen tympani and tegmen mastoideum, respectively.

IMAGING TECHNIQUES

A range of imaging techniques are available to investigate patients with skull base CSF leaks, and their advantages and disadvantages are summarized in **Table 1**.

Computed Tomography

CT is the preferred initial investigation for localizing skull base CSF leaks, and it is often the only imaging investigation that is necessary. Images are acquired as a three-dimensional data set using the narrowest slice thickness possible and a reconstruction field of view that covers from the anterior wall of the frontal sinuses to the posterior margins of the mastoid air cells to maximize in-plane spatial resolution. The axial data are reconstructed using an edge-enhancing ('bone') reconstruction kernel to improve the demonstration of the fine bony anatomy and reformatted in the sagittal and coronal planes.

CT depicts the bony components of osteodural defects with high accuracy. Ancillary findings of CSF leaks include sinonasal or petromastoid fluid levels and intracranial air. When there are multiple skull base fractures or defects, CT is unable to precisely locate the site of the dural defect required for CSF leakage.

Computed Tomography Cisternography

In this technique, nonionic iodinated contrast, typically 8 to 10 mL, is injected intrathecally at lumbar puncture and distributed to the intracranial subarachnoid space by means of Trendelenburg positioning. Computed tomography of the skull base is then obtained in the same manner as outlined previously for conventional CT without intrathecal contrast. A CT cisternogram is considered positive when contrast medium passes from the subarachnoid space through an osteodural defect into an adjacent sinonasal or petromastoid air space, producing an increase in the attenuation of an opacified air space by more than 50% when compared with a prior noncontrast CT.

CT cisternography is generally now used only in cases where noncontrast CT shows a patient to have multiple osseous defects, and it is unclear which is leaking. Potential complications include those related to the lumbar puncture (bleeding, infection, postdural puncture headache) and adverse reactions to iodinated contrast medium, including anaphylactoid reactions and seizures.

Magnetic Resonance Imaging

By using heavily T2-weighted sequences, MRI can demonstrate leaking CSF as high signal intensity extending from the subarachnoid space through a skull base defect into an adjacent air space. Thin slice imaging can be acquired as a 3D data set using balanced steady-state free precession sequences (eg, CISS, Siemens; FIESTA-C, GE; and DRIVE, Philips). More recently introduced 3D fast spin echo sequences with very long echo trains and variable flip angles can also be used to obtain cisternographic T2-weighted images without the potential for "banding artifacts" (eg, SPACE, Siemens; Cube, GE; and VISTA, Philips). T2-weighted images alone may not distinguish air space opacification caused by CSF from that because of mucus or inflammatory mucosal thickening as both will appear hyperintense. The addition of a fluid attenuated inversion recovery (FLAIR) sequence can resolve this as CSF will be hyperintense on T2-weighted images but suppress on the FLAIR sequence, while inflammatory changes

Table 1
Imaging techniques for investigation of skull base CSF leaks

	HRCT	CT Cisternography	MRI	IT-Gd MRC	RNC
Invasive	No	Yes	No	Yes	Yes
Requires active leak	No	Yes	No	Yes	Yes
Able to perform delayed imaging	N/A	No	N/A	Yes	Yes
Bony anatomy	+++	+++	+	+	-
Able to distinguish causes of air space opacification	-	+	+++	+++	-
Spatial resolution	+++	+++	++	++	-
Sensitivity	58.8%–100%	37.5%–72.3%	74.7%–100%	56%–100%	62%–76%
Indication	First-line investigation	Multiple osseous defects	Suspected encephalocele Usually used in conjunction with HRCT	Multiple osseous defects	Diagnostic test slow/ intermittent leaks rather than localizing investigation

Abbreviations: HRCT, high-resolution computed tomography; IT-Gd MRC, intrathecal gadolinium magnetic resonance cisternography; RNC, radionuclide cisternography.

will be hyperintense on both sequences.[10] MRI can also demonstrate brain herniation through osteodural defects into the sinonasal cavity or petromastoid air spaces and can show associated changes of encephalomalacia and gliosis. Gadolinium enhancement may be required if an inflammatory or neoplastic cause for the CSF leak is suspected.

Intrathecal Gadolinium Magnetic Resonance Cisternography

Analogous to CT cisternography, in this technique, a small volume (0.2–0.5 mL) of gadolinium-based contrast agent (GBCA) is injected intrathecally and distributed intracranially by Trendelenburg positioning. Thin section fat-suppressed T1-weighted spin echo images are then acquired in axial, coronal, and sagittal planes or alternatively a 3D fat-supressed T1-weighted spoiled gradient echo sequence (eg, VIBE, Siemens; LAVA-Flex, GE; and THRIVE, Philips) or a fat-suppressed T1-weighted 3D fast spin echo sequence (eg, SPACE, Cube, or VISTA) can be obtained and then reformatted into orthogonal planes.[11,12] A positive study is denoted by T1-hyperintense contrast-enhanced CSF passing from the subarachnoid space into an air space adjacent to the skull base (Fig. 1).

An advantage of this technique over CT cisternography is the ability to perform delayed imaging up to 24 hours after the injection of GBCA,[13] which can increase the sensitivity for slow or intermittent

CSF leaks. In addition, MRI depicts the T1 hyperintense CSF separately from hypointense bone, in contrast to CT in which both contrast-opacified CSF and bone are hyperattenuating. It should be noted that GBCAs are not licenced for intrathecal injection by the US Food and Drug Administration, and patients should be informed of this during the consent process. Although cases of encephalopathy and even death have been reported after the intrathecal injection of GBCA at high doses,[14,15] when administered at the minimum doses necessary for adequate contrast enhancement of the CSF, they are well tolerated, with reported adverse reactions including nausea, vomiting, and headache—the latter of which could equally well be attributed to the lumbar puncture.[16,17] As in the case of repeated intravenous injections of GBCA, there are reports of increased T1 signal intensity in the dentate nuclei and globus pallidi of patients who have undergone intrathecal GBCA injection. This has been recorded after intrathecal injection of gadopentetate dimeglumine, a linear GBCA, but has not been seen after administration of the macrocyclic agent gadoterate meglumine.[18,19]

Radionuclide Cisternography

The patient is injected intrathecally with a technetium-99m or indium-111 labeled diethylene triamine pentaacetic acid via lumbar puncture and placed in the Trendelenburg position to distribute

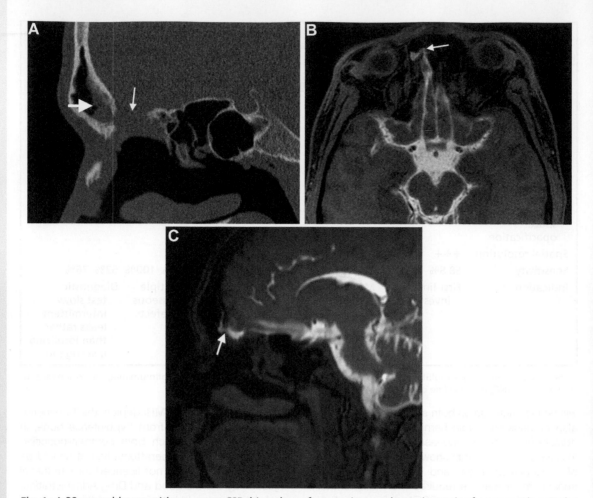

Fig. 1. A 28-year-old man with recurrent CSF rhinorrhea after previous endoscopic repair of a traumatic anterior skull base CSF leak. (*A*) Sagittal bone algorithm CT shows a defect in the ethmoid roof (*thin arrow*) and fluid in the right frontal sinus (*short arrow*), but the site of leakage is not clear. (*B*) Axial and (*C*) sagittal intrathecal gadolinium MR cisternography locates the precise site of the leak into the frontal sinus (*arrows*).

the tracer intracranially. Scintigraphic imaging at 2, 6, and 24 hours is evaluated for the presence of tracer in the nasal cavity or nasopharynx, indicating a positive study. Cotton pledgets may be placed in both sides of the nasal cavity at various locations before the injection of tracer and then removed at 24 to 48 hours to measure the level of radioactivity compared with serum, a pledget-to-serum ratio of more than 1.5 being considered indicative of an active leak.[20]

The low spatial resolution of planar scintigraphic images mixing of nasal secretions within the nasal cavity, and potential for labeled CSF to reach the nasal cavity via the eustachian tube in patients with a temporal bone CSF leak, often prevent accurate localization of CSF leaks. There is also a propensity of pledgets to move location or be poorly tolerated. It is seldom used except in cases where a fluid sample cannot be collected or tested

for beta-2 transferrin or beta trace protein or sometimes for slow or intermittent leaks[21]

IMAGING FINDINGS
Traumatic Leaks

Skull base CSF leaks are the result of head trauma in 80% to 90% of cases, with CSF leaks occurring in 1% to 3% patients experiencing closed head injury.[22,23] In 80% of cases, the leak manifests as CSF rhinorrhea or otorrhea within 48 hours of injury, but most resolve spontaneously, and it is only present in 5% of patients after the initial 3 months (24,25). The prevalence of CSF leaks is greatest with fractures through the temporal bones (11%–45%) and frontal sinus (30.8%) while it is less frequent in fractures of the sphenoid sinus (11.4%–30.8%), ethmoid air cells (15.4%–19.1%), cribriform plate (7.7%), fronto-ethmoid region (7.7%), and spheno-ethmoid region (7.7%).[24]

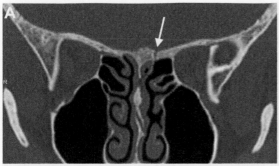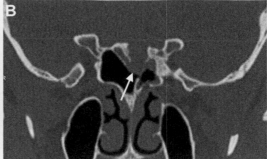

Fig. 2. A 37-year-old woman with CSF rhinorrhea and recurrent episodes of meningitis 1 year after traumatic head injury. (*A*) Coronal bone algorithm CT shows a well-corticated defect in the left ethmoid roof (*arrow*). (*B*) Coronal bone algorithm CT shows a meningoencephalocele protruding into the right sphenoid sinus (*arrow*) through a wide traumatic defect in its roof.

Imaging shows fractures through the affected region of the skull base, with opacification of the adjacent nasal cavity, paranasal sinus, middle ear cavity, or mastoid air cells (**Fig. 2**). There may be pneumocephalus, ranging from a few air bubbles to larger collections of air that can accumulate under tension and compress the brain. With fractures through the temporal bone that are associated with CSF leaks, bubbles of air may accumulate within the osseous labyrinth. Traumatic osteodural defects may be sealed temporarily by blood clots, bone fragments, herniated brain, or mucosal edema so that the patient does not present with overt CSF rhinorrhea, but the finding of a fracture of 3 mm or wider in conjunction with pneumocephalus is strongly suggestive of a skull base CSF leak.[25] With chronic or late-presenting leaks, the brain adjacent to the osteodural defect may show posttraumatic encephalomalacia (**Fig. 3**).

Iatrogenic Leaks

The inadvertent creation of osteodural defects at the skull base can occur during ESS, endoscopic endonasal approaches to the skull base and pituitary fossa, craniotomy (bifrontal, retrosigmoid, or middle fossa), or during tympanomastoid surgery. Anatomic variations that can predispose patients to iatrogenic CSF leaks at ESS include a low height of the cribriform plate relative to the ethmoid roof, a steeper angle of slope of the anterior skull base in the sagittal plane, and greater lateral slope of the ethmoid roof in the coronal plane.[26] The most frequently occurring sites of iatrogenic CSF leak as a result of ESS are the lateral lamella of the cribriform plate, the posterior part of the ethmoid roof, the frontal recess, and the sphenoid sinus.[27] The incidence of clinically apparent skull base CSF leaks after ESS is low, ranging from 0.13% to 0.5%,[28,29] although testing for beta trace protein indicates that occult leaks may occur in up to 2.9%.[30]

Intraoperative CSF leaks during endoscopic pituitary surgery necessitating repair with autologous fat, fascia, or a pedicled nasoseptal flap have been reported to occur in up to 37.4% cases.[31] Risk factors for intraoperative visualization of CSF include increasing tumor height, supraclinoidal extension of tumor, and invasion of the third ventricle.[32] Subsequent failure of such repairs, or failure to recognize a CSF leak at the time of surgery, lead to postoperative CSF leaks (**Fig. 4**), which occur with an incidence of 0.5% to 15%.[33]

Open neurosurgical skull base procedures may also lead to CSF rhinorrhea. Breach of the posterior wall of the frontal sinuses during bifrontal craniotomy can cause CSF rhinorrhea if not recognized and repaired. A pneumatized anterior clinoid process is present in 9.6% of patients,[34] and postoperative CSF rhinorrhea may develop if anterior clinoidectomy is required to expose and clip internal carotid artery aneurysms.

Tumor-Related Leaks

Erosion of the bone of the skull base and adjacent dura by tumors can result in CSF rhinorrhea or otorrhea as a presenting symptom. It can also occur when the tumor shrinks in response to medical treatment of radiotherapy, such that it no longer plugs the osteodural defect it had produced. Such CSF leaks have been reported in patients with pituitary adenomas treated with dopamine agonists (**Fig. 5**) or somatostatin analogs[35,36] and in an atypical meningioma treated with the tyrosine kinase inhibitor sunitinib.[37]

Spontaneous Leaks

CSF leaks that are not caused by accidental or iatrogenic trauma, or which are unrelated to a tumor or its treatment, have historically been classified as

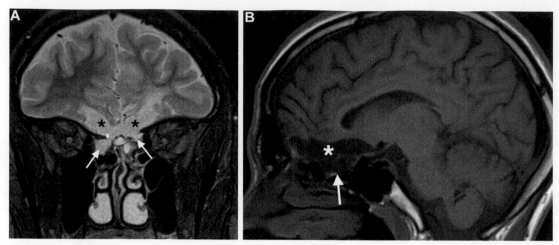

Fig. 3. An 18-year-old man with recurrent episodes of CSF rhinorrhea 1 year after traumatic brain injury. (*A*) Coronal short tau inversion recovery (STIR) and (*B*) sagittal T1w MRI show posttraumatic encephalomalacia of the gyri recti (*asterisks*) and meningoceles (*arrows*) in the superior nasal cavity adjacent to defects in the cribriform plate. (*Courtesy of* Dr L Carlton Jones, King's College Hospital, London UK.)

spontaneous leaks. More recently it has been increasingly recognized that many patients with spontaneous CSF leaks share similar demographic, clinical, and imaging characteristics to those with idiopathic intracranial hypertension (IIH), and moreover that chronically raised intracranial pressure may be the cause of these leaks.[38–40] Patients with spontaneous CSF leaks are most often found in overweight or obese, middle-aged women. The incidence of spontaneous CSF leaks

has increased in parallel with the prevalence of obesity in the United States, while the rate of occurrence of nonspontaneous leaks has been static.[41] Over a period of many years, raised intracranial pressure can cause thinning and eventually erosion of the bone of the skull base with herniation and rupture of the attenuated dura through the resulting bony defect.

Computed tomography of obese patients with spontaneous CSF leaks shows significantly

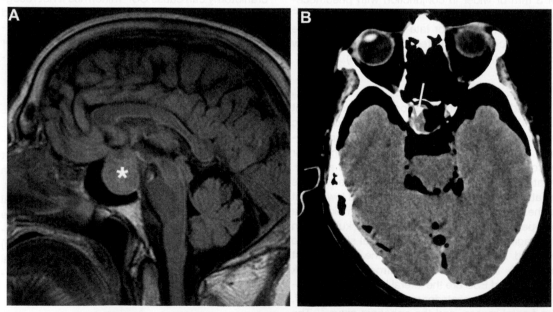

Fig. 4. A 76-year-old man who developed a postoperative CSF leak after transsphenoidal endoscopic debulking of a pituitary macroadenoma. (*A*) Sagittal FLAIR MRI shows a pituitary macroadenoma (*asterisk*) with suprasellar extension. The sphenoid sinus shows a sellar pattern of pneumatization. (*B*) Postoperative axial noncontrast CT shows residual tumor in the right side of the sella (*arrow*) and extensive pneumocephalus as a result of a persistent CSF leak.

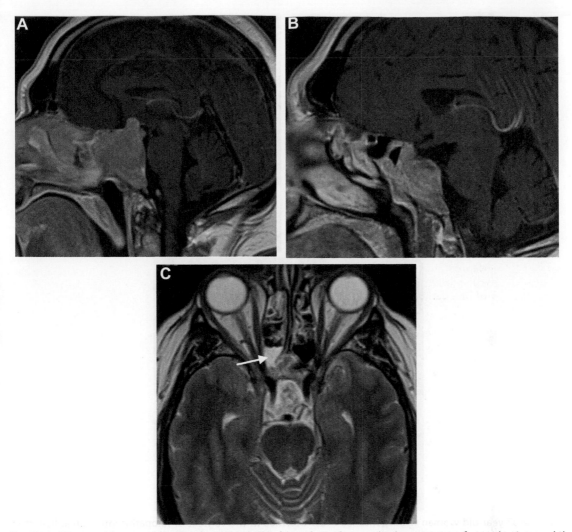

Fig. 5. A 57-year-old man with who developed CSF rhinorrhea after medical treatment of a prolactinoma (*A*) Baseline sagittal postcontrast T1w MRI shows a large prolactinoma that invades the clivus and sphenoid sinus, with suprasellar extension. (*B*) Sagittal postcontrast T1w MRI 1 year after commencing cabergoline therapy shows significant decrease in tumor size. (*C*) Axial T2w MRI shows a fluid level in the right posterior ethmoid air cells (*arrow*) secondary to the development of a CSF leak.

thinner bone at the tegmen tympani and tegmen mastoideum than in obese controls and nonobese controls (**Fig. 6**).[42] Leaks can also occur at so-called arachnoid pits, small defects in the floor of the middle cranial fossa which develop at the sites of arachnoid granulations that are progressively enlarged by the pulsatile hydrostatic forces of raised intracranial pressure (**Fig. 7**). These pits can contain herniated brain tissue, arachnoid, or dura and may lead to a CSF leak if they occur adjacent to a pneumatized part of the skull base.[43,44]

Most spontaneous CSF leaks occur at the cribriform plate (**Fig. 8**), reported to be the location in 39% to 51% cases, the ethmoid roof in 42.8%, the sphenoid sinus in 28% to 46.4%, the temporal bone in 39%, and the frontal sinus in 10%.[43,45,46]

Acquired sphenoid sinus CSF leaks are most commonly reported to occur lateral to foramen rotundum into the lateral recess (**Fig. 9**).

Magnetic resonance imaging of patients with spontaneous CSF leaks may show indirect features suggestive of underlying IIH (**Fig. 10**), including intrasellar herniation of arachnoid (producing partially empty sella or empty sella), optic nerve sheath dilatation, increased vertical tortuosity of the optic nerves, scleral flattening of the globes at the insertion of the optic nerves, arachnoid pits, enlargement of Meckel caves, enlargement of skull base foramina, and venous sinus stenoses.[45,47–49] Compared with patients with clinically definite IIH, patients with spontaneous CSF leaks more often show bony changes such

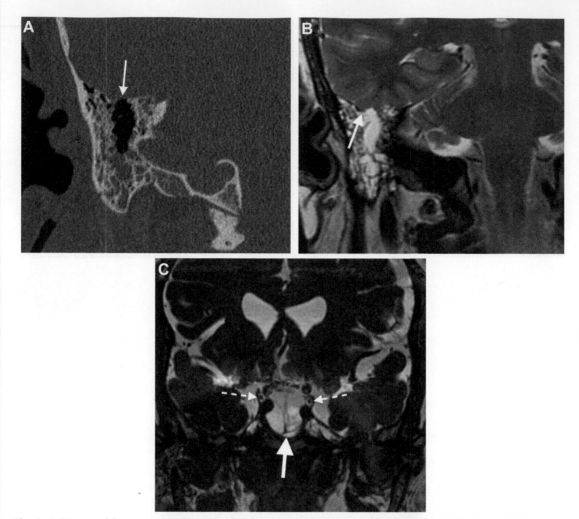

Fig. 6. A 57-year-old woman with spontaneous CSF otorrhea in the context of idiopathic intracranial hypertension. (*A*) Coronal bone algorithm CT shows a defect of the right tegmen mastoideum (*arrow*) with opacification of mastoid air cells. (*B*) Coronal T2w MRI shows a small encephalocele of the inferior temporal gyrus (*arrow*). (*C*) Coronal 3D FIESTA shows a partially empty sella (*arrow*) and distension of the oculomotor nerve sheaths (*dashed arrows*), features of idiopathic intracranial hypertension.

as empty sella and cephaloceles while orbital changes and venous sinus stenoses are less common. This is likely a reflection of the development of a CSF leak in the context of chronically elevated ICP allowing reduction in intracranial pressure and resolution of reversible soft-tissue changes while the chronic osseous erosive features are fixed.[45]

The association with increased intracranial pressure means that patients with spontaneous skull case CSF leaks may develop symptomatic intracranial hypertension after surgical repair and represent with headache and visual defects. Perioperative measures to reduce intracranial pressure, such as acetazolamide and lumbar drain insertion, may therefore be necessary.[10]

DIAGNOSTIC CRITERIA
Clinical Diagnosis

Before embarking on a search for the site of a skull base CSF leak in a patient with suspected CSF rhinorrhea or otorrhea, it is necessary to confirm that the fluid in question is CSF. Clinical features, such as rhinorrhea, that is, postural, or that tastes salty are not sufficiently specific, and laboratory testing of a sample of the fluid is required. Beta-2 transferrin is a glycoprotein found in CSF and perilymph but not in nasal secretions or blood and so can be used as a marker for CSF leak in patients with rhinorrhea. In cases of otorrhea, it cannot distinguish a CSF leak from a perilymphatic fistula.[50] Assays for beta-2 transferrin can detect 100 µL of CSF in

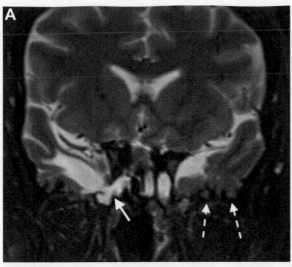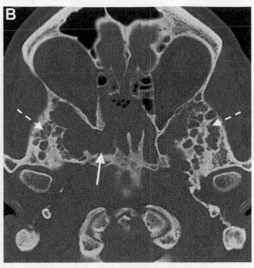

Fig. 7. A 61-year-old woman with spontaneous CSF rhinorrhea in the context of idiopathic intracranial hypertension. (*A*) Coronal fat-suppressed T2w MRI shows a meningoencephalocele with herniation of the medial part of the right temporal lobe into the sphenoid sinus (*arrow*) and traction gliosis in the right temporal pole. There are multiple arachnoid pits on the floor of the left middle cranial fossa containing protrusions of the inferior surface of the left temporal lobe (*dashed arrows*). (*B*) Axial bone algorithm CT shows the bony defect in the lateral wall of the right sphenoid sinus (*arrow*) and numerous well-defined defects in the floors of the middle cranial fossae at the sites of the arachnoid pits (*dashed arrows*).

1 mL of nasal secretions, with reported sensitivities ranging from 87% to 100% and specificities from 71% to 100%.[21] Beta trace protein, also known as prostaglandin D synthase, is secreted by the leptomeninges and choroid plexus. It is a more sensitive test than beta-2 transferrin, able to detect 5 μL of CSF in 1 mL of fluid and has reported sensitivity of 91% to 100% and specificity of 87% to 100%.[21] Beta trace protein is faster and cheaper to process than beta-2 transferrin, but it is less widely available.[10] Levels of beta trace protein in the serum are increased in renal insufficiency, and CSF levels are decreased in bacterial meningitis, so it is recommended that it should not be used as a test for CSF leak in these patient groups.[51]

Visualization of the skull base may be limited in patients who have not previously undergone sinonasal surgery; however, it may possible to directly see clear fluid leaking from the skull base at nasendoscopy, or a bluish-gray mass if there is a meningocele. Endoscopic localization of the site of the leak can be augmented by the intrathecal injection of fluorescein dye with or without the additional use of ultraviolet light, which results in yellow-green coloration of CSF.[52] Potential risks of intrathecal fluorescein include seizures, radiculopathy, and transient weakness, and it is an off-label use of the product in the United States.

Imaging Diagnosis

Once it has been confirmed that the fluid in the nasal cavity or middle ear is CSF, then imaging is undertaken to localize the site of the leak and

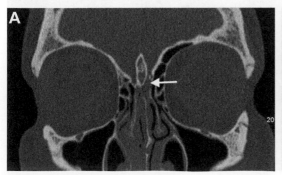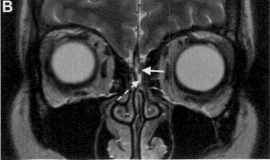

Fig. 8. A 42-year-old woman with recurrent episodes of spontaneous CSF rhinorrhea and meningitis in the context of idiopathic intracranial hypertension. (*A*) Coronal bone algorithm CT shows a defect in the left cribriform plate with opacification of the adjacent olfactory recess of the nasal cavity. (*B*) Coronal T2w MRI shows a meningoencephalocele containing CSF (*dashed arrow*) and inferiorly herniated olfactory bulb (*arrow*).

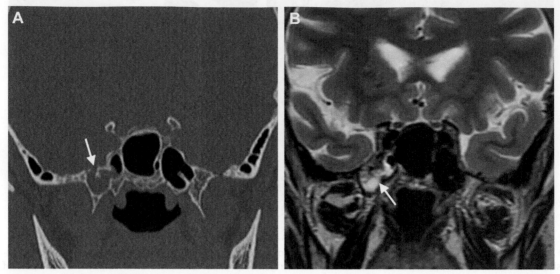

Fig. 9. A 62-year-old woman with spontaneous CSF rhinorrhea in the context of idiopathic intracranial hypertension. (*A*) Coronal bone algorithm CT shows a defect in the roof of the opacified lateral recess of the right sphenoid sinus (*arrow*). (*B*) Axial T2w MRI shows CSF opacifying the right lateral recess of the sphenoid sinus.

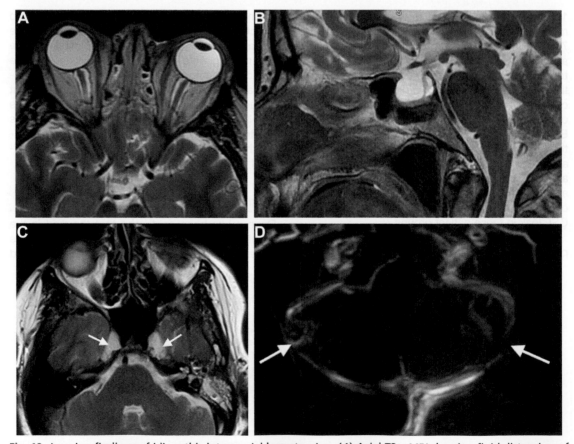

Fig. 10. Imaging findings of idiopathic intracranial hypertension. (*A*) Axial T2w MRI showing fluid distension of the optic nerve subarachnoid spaces. (*B*) Sagittal T2w MRI intrasellar protrusion of arachnoid producing a 'partially empty sella'. (*C*) Axial T2w MRI showing enlargement of Meckel's caves (*arrows*). (*D*) Maximum intensity projection of phase contrast MR venogram showing bilateral transverse sinus stenoses.

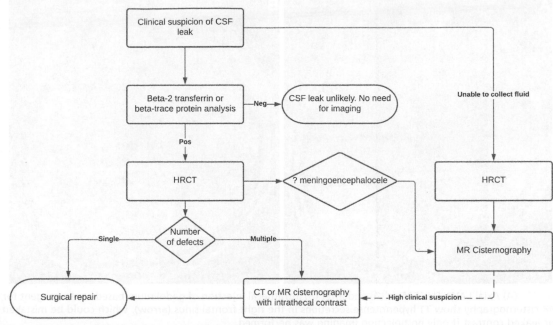

Fig. 11. Imaging algorithm for suspected skull base CSF leaks.

assess the relevant surrounding anatomy for the planning of surgical repair. An algorithmic approach to the use of imaging is shown in **Fig. 11**.

Noncontrast CT of the skull base can show an osseous defect with opacification of adjacent paranasal sinuses or temporal bone air spaces. An area of nondependent soft tissue with a polypoidal contour may be present adjacent to the defect if there is an associated cephalocele. If a CSF leak has been confirmed and CT shows a single osseous defect, then no further imaging is required before surgical repair. If no defect is identified, or if there is suspicion for a cephalocele on CT, then MRI may detect CSF signal intensity traversing the skull base. The radiologist may be directed to the presence of brain tissue herniating through a skull base by the presence of adjacent cerebral traction gliosis. In cases where there are multiple defects, then a cisternographic study with intrathecal contrast, either CT or MRI, is indicated. In either case, any actively leaking defects will show an uninterrupted column of contrast-opacified CSF extending from the subarachnoid space through the osteodural defect into the adjacent sinonasal or tympanomastoid air spaces.

DIFFERENTIAL DIAGNOSIS

The finding of opacification or a fluid level within the paranasal sinuses, middle ear cavity, or mastoid or

---

Box 1
Differential diagnoses

Paranasal sinus/middle ear fluid level or opacification

- CSF leak
- Hemosinus/hemotympanum
- Inflammatory/infective secretions

Sinonasal nondependent soft tissue

- Meningocele/pseudomeningocele
- Inflammatory polyps
- Ethesioneuroblastoma
- Respiratory epithelial adenomatoid hyperplasia

Box 2
Pitfalls in the diagnosis of skull base CSF leaks

- Normal skull base dehiscences and neurovascular channels: do not mistake for acquired osteodural defects. Examples around the cribriform plate include the nasal slit, which lies anterior to the crista galli and the foramen cecum, which is located between the crista galli and crest of the falx.

- Previous episodes of meningitis: may cause subarachnoid adhesions that prevent cisternographic contrast from reaching the an osteodural defect.

- Proteinaceous secretions: can be hyperintense on T1w MRI and could be misinterpreted as contrast-opacified leaked CSF at intrathecal gadolinium MR cisternography if precontrast T1w images are not acquired for comparison (**Fig. 12**).

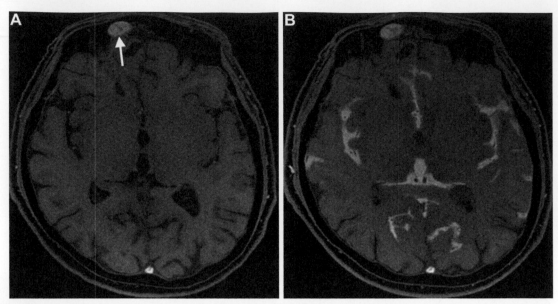

Fig. 12. (A) Axial LAVA-Flex before (A) and after (B) intrathecal injection of gadolinium-based contrast agent for MR cisternography show T1 hyperintense secretions in the right frontal sinus (arrow), which could be mistaken for leaked contrast if only postinjection imaging was performed.

the presence of soft tissue within the olfactory recess of the nasal cavity on CT are nonspecific and have a differential diagnosis (Box 1). MRI can be helpful for demonstrating fluid to be isointense to CSF and for distinguishing a cephalocele from inflammatory polyp or tumor. Equally, MRI should always be considered for the demonstration of a cephalocele when CT demonstrates a polypoid lesion extending to the nasoethmoid roof or a tegmen defect.

PITFALLS

There are several potential pitfalls in the interpretation of imaging studies obtained to localize a CSF leak, which are summarized in Box 2.

Box 3
What the referring physician needs to know

- Site of the osteodural defect. If multiple defects, which are leaking actively at cisternography?
- Transverse and anteroposterior dimensions of defect.
- Variant sinonasal anatomy that may influence the surgical approach (septal deviation, Onodi cells, degree of sphenoid sinus pneumatisation, including extension into the lateral recess or greater wing).
- Imaging features that suggest idiopathic intracranial hypertension.
- Presence of any meningoencephalocele and if adjacent brain is also gliotic.

WHAT THE REFERRING PHYSICIAN NEEDS TO KNOW

Factors that need to be considered and addressed to produce a clinically relevant report are given in Box 3.

SUMMARY

Acquired skull base CSF leaks typically present clinically with rhinorrhea or otorrhea. Once a CSF leak has been proven biochemically, imaging is undertaken to localize the causative osteodural defect and may require a stepwise approach. Interpretation of these studies requires detailed knowledge of normal and variant skull base anatomy, and reports should highlight features pertinent to surgical planning.

CLINICS CARE POINTS

- Traumatic skull base CSF leaks often close spontaneously.
- Many patients with spontaneous leaks show imaging findings in common with patients with idiopathic intracranial hypertension.
- High resolution CT is the best first investigation, once it has been confirmed that rhinorrhea or otorrhea is CSF.
- CT or MR cisternography with intrathecal contrast material requires the leak to be active at the time of scanning.

DISCLOSURE

The author has no commercial or financial conflicts of interests to disclose.

REFERENCES

1. Ommaya AK, Di Chiro G, Baldwin M, et al. Non-traumatic cerebrospinal fluid rhinorrhoea. J Neurol Neurosurg Psychiatry 1968;31(3):214–25.
2. Schievink WI, Schwartz MS, Maya MM, et al. Lack of causal association between spontaneous intracranial hypotension and cranial cerebrospinal fluid leaks: Clinical article. J Neurosurg 2012;116(4): 749–54.
3. Sonig A, Thakur JD, iboina PC, et al. Is posttraumatic cerebrospinal fluid fistula a predictor of posttraumatic meningitis? A US Nationwide Inpatient Sample database study. Neurosurg Focus 2012;32(6):E4.
4. Daudia A, Biswas D, Jones NS. Risk of meningitis with cerebrospinal fluid rhinorrhea. Ann Otol Rhinol Laryngol 2007;116(12):902–5.
5. Eljamel MS, Foy PM. Acute traumatic CSF fistulae: The risk of intracranial infection. Br J Neurosurg 1990;4(5):381–5.
6. Poletti-Muringaseril SC, Rufibach K, Ruef C, et al. Low meningitis-incidence in primary spontaneous compared to secondary cerebrospinal fluid rhinorrhoea. Rhinology 2012;50(1):73–9.
7. Thapa AJ, Lei BX, Zheng MG, et al. The Surgical Treatment of Posttraumatic Skull Base Defects with Cerebrospinal Fluid Leak. J Neurol Surg B Skull Base 2018;79(2):205–16.
8. Bolger WE, Butzin CA, Parsons DS. Paranasal Sinus Bony Anatomic Variations and Mucosal Abnormalities. Laryngoscope 1991;101(1):56–64.
9. Gibelli D, Cellina M, Gibelli S, et al. Anatomical variants of sphenoid sinuses pneumatisation: a CT scan study on a Northern Italian population. Radiol Med 2017;122(8):575–80.
10. Georgalas C, Oostra A, Ahmed S, et al. International consensus statement: spontaneous cerebrospinal fluid rhinorrhea. Int Forum Allergy Rhinol 2020;11(4):794–803.
11. Nacar Dogan S, Kizilkilic O, Kocak B, et al. Intrathecal gadolinium-enhanced MR cisternography in patients with otorhinorrhea: 10-year experience of a tertiary referral center. Neuroradiology 2018;60(5):471–7.
12. Duman IE, Demerath T, Stadler A, et al. High-Resolution Gadolinium-Enhanced MR Cisternography Using Compressed-Sensing T1 SPACE Technique for Detection of Intracranial CSF Leaks. AJNR Am J Neuroradiol 2020;42(1):116–8.
13. Delgaudio JM, Baugnon KL, Wise SK, et al. Magnetic resonance cisternogram with intrathecal gadolinium with delayed imaging for difficult to diagnose cerebrospinal fluid leaks of anterior skull base. Int Forum Allergy Rhinol 2015;5(4):333–8.
14. Gordin V, Kapoor R, Liu J, et al. Gadolinium encephalopathy after intrathecal gadolinium injection. Pain Physician 2010;13(5):E321–6.
15. Provenzano DA, Pellis Z, Deriggi L. Fatal gadolinium-induced encephalopathy following accidental intrathecal administration: A case report and a comprehensive evidence-based review. Reg Anesth Pain Med 2019;44(7):721–9.
16. Halvorsen M, Edeklev CS, Fraser-Green J, et al. Off-label intrathecal use of gadobutrol: safety study and comparison of administration protocols. Neuroradiology 2020;63(1):51–61.
17. Patel M, Atyani A, Salameh JP, et al. Safety of intrathecal administration of gadolinium-based contrast agents: A systematic review and meta-Analysis. Radiology 2020;297(1):75–83.
18. Öner AY, Barutcu B, Aykol Ş, et al. Intrathecal Contrast-Enhanced Magnetic Resonance Imaging-Related Brain Signal Changes: Residual Gadolinium Deposition? Invest Radiol 2017;52(4):195–7.
19. Ozturk K, Nas OF, Soylu E, et al. Signal Changes in the Dentate Nucleus and Globus Pallidus on Unenhanced T1-Weighted Magnetic Resonance Images after Intrathecal Administration of Macrocyclic Gadolinium Contrast Agent. Invest Radiol 2018;53(9):535–40.
20. Stone JA, Castillo M, Neelon B, et al. Evaluation of CSF leaks: High-resolution CT compared with contrast- enhanced CT and radionuclide cisternography. AJNR Am J Neuroradiol 1999;20(4):706–12.
21. Oakley GM, Alt JA, Schlosser RJ, et al. Diagnosis of cerebrospinal fluid rhinorrhea: An evidence-based review with recommendations. Int Forum Allergy Rhinol 2016;6(1):8–16.
22. Yilmazlar S, Arslan E, Kocaeli H, et al. Cerebrospinal fluid leakage complicating skull base fractures: Analysis of 81 cases. Neurosurg Rev 2006;29(1):64–71.
23. Schlosser RJ, Bolger WE. Nasal Cerebrospinal Fluid Leaks: Critical Review and Surgical Considerations. Laryngoscope 2004;114(2):255–65.
24. Banks CA, Palmer JN, Chiu AG, et al. Endoscopic closure of CSF rhinorrhea: 193 cases over 21 years. Otolaryngol Head Neck Surg 2009;140(6): 826–33.
25. Meco C, Oberascher G. Comprehensive algorithm for skull base dural lesion and cerebriospinal fluid fistula diagnosis. Laryngoscope 2004;114(6):991–9.
26. Heaton CM, Goldberg AN, Pletcher SD, et al. Sinus anatomy associated with inadvertent cerebrospinal fluid leak during functional endoscopic sinus surgery. Laryngoscope 2012;122(7):1446–9.
27. Gray ST, Wu AW. Pathophysiology of iatrogenic and traumatic skull base injury. In: Bleier BS, editor. Comprehensive techniques in CSF leak repair and skull base reconstruction, vol. 74. Basel: S. Karger AG; 2012. p. 12–23.
28. Krings JG, Kallogjeri D, Wineland A, et al. Complications of primary and revision functional endoscopic

sinus surgery for chronic rhinosinusitis. Laryngoscope 2014;124(4):838–45.

29. May M, Levine HL, Mester SJ, et al. Complications of endoscopic sinus surgery. Laryngoscope 1994; 104(9):1080–3.

30. Bachmann G, Djenabi U, Jungehülsing M, et al. Incidence of occult cerebrospinal fluid fistula during paranasal sinus surgery. Arch Otolaryngol Head Neck Surg 2002;128(11):1299–302.

31. Strickland BA, Lucas J, Harris B, et al. Identification and repair of intraoperative cerebrospinal fluid leaks in endonasal transsphenoidal pituitary surgery: Surgical experience in a series of 1002 patients. J Neurosurg 2018;129(2):425–9.

32. Rotman LE, Alford EN, Davis MC, et al. Preoperative radiographic and clinical factors associated with the visualization of intraoperative cerebrospinal fluid during endoscopic transsphenoidal resection of pituitary adenomas. Surg Neurol Int 2020;11:59.

33. Shiley SG, Limonadi F, Delashaw JB, et al. Incidence, etiology, and management of cerebrospinal fluid leaks following trans-sphenoidal surgery. Laryngoscope 2003;113(8):1283–8.

34. Abuzayed B, Tanriover N, Biceroglu H, et al. Pneumatization degree of the anterior clinoid process: A new classification. Neurosurg Rev 2010;33(3):367–74.

35. Česák T, Poczos P, Adamkov J, et al. Medically induced CSF rhinorrhea following treatment of macroprolactinoma: case series and literature review. Pituitary 2018;21(6):561–70.

36. Lam G, Mehta V, Zada G. Spontaneous and medically induced cerebrospinal fluid leakage in the setting of pituitary adenomas: Review of the literature. Neurosurg Focus 2012;32(6):E2. https://doi.org/10.3171/2012.4.FOCUS1268.

37. Raheja A, Colman H, Palmer CA, et al. Dramatic radiographic response resulting in cerebrospinal fluid rhinorrhea associated with sunitinib therapy in recurrent atypical meningioma: Case report. J Neurosurg 2017;127(5):965–70.

38. Tam EK, Gilbert AL. Spontaneous cerebrospinal fluid leak and idiopathic intracranial hypertension. Curr Opin Ophthalmol 2019;30(6):467–71.

39. Quatre R, Attye A, Righini CA, et al. Spontaneous Cerebrospinal Fluid Rhinorrhea: Association with Body Weight and Imaging Data. J Neurol Surg B Skull Base 2017;78(5):419–24. d.

40. Bidot S, Levy JM, Saindane AM, et al. Do most patients with a spontaneous cerebrospinal fluid leak have idiopathic intracranial hypertension? J Neuro Ophthalmol 2019;39(4):487–95.

41. Nelson RF, Gantz BJ, Hansen MR. The Rising Incidence of Spontaneous Cerebrospinal Fluid Leaks in the United States and the Association with Obesity and Obstructive Sleep Apnea. Otol Neurotol 2015;36(3):476–80.

42. Stevens SM, Lambert PR, Rizk H, et al. Novel radiographic measurement algorithm demonstrating a link between obesity and lateral skull base attenuation. Otolaryngol Head Neck Surg 2015;152(1):172–9.

43. Schuknecht B, Simmen D, Briner HR, et al. Nontraumatic skull base defects with spontaneous CSF rhinorrhea and arachnoid herniation: Imaging findings and correlation with endoscopic sinus surgery in 27 patients. AJNR Am J Neuroradiol 2008;29(3):542–9.

44. Shetty PG, Shroff MM, Fatterpekar GM, et al. A retrospective analysis of spontaneous sphenoid sinus fistula: MR and CT findings. AJNR Am J Neuroradiol 2000;21(2):337–42.

45. Bidot S, Levy JM, Saindane AM, et al. Spontaneous skull base cerebrospinal fluid leaks and their relationship to idiopathic intracranial hypertension. Am J Rhinol Allergy 2020;35(1):36–43.

46. Martínez-Capoccioni G, Serramito-García R, Martín-Bailón M, et al. Spontaneous cerebrospinal fluid leaks in the anterior skull base secondary to idiopathic intracranial hypertension. Eur Arch Otorhinolaryngol 2017;274(5):2175–81.

47. Bidot S, Saindane AM, Peragallo JH, et al. Brain Imaging in Idiopathic Intracranial Hypertension. J Neuro Ophthalmol 2015;35(4):400–11.

48. Dallan I, Cambi C, Emanuelli E, et al. Multiple spontaneous skull base cerebrospinal fluid leaks: some insights from an international retrospective collaborative study. Eur Arch Otorhinolaryngol 2020;277(12): 3357–63.

49. Bedarida V, Labeyrie MA, Eliezer M, et al. Association of spontaneous cerebrospinal fluid rhinorrhea with transverse venous sinus stenosis: a retrospective matched case-control study. Int Forum Allergy Rhinol 2020;10(12):1295–9.

50. Skedros DG, Cass SP, Hirsch BE, et al. Beta-2 transferrin assay in clinical management of cerebral spinal fluid and perilymphatic fluid leaks. J Otolaryngol 1993;22(5):341–4.

51. Meco C, Oberascher G, Arrer E, et al. β-trace protein test: New guidelines for the reliable diagnosis of cerebrospinal fluid fistula. Otolaryngol Head Neck Surg 2003;129(5):508–17.

52. Seth R, Rajasekaran K, Benninger MS, et al. The utility of intrathecal fluorescein in cerebrospinal fluid leak repair. Otolaryngol Head Neck Surg 2010; 143(5):626–32.

Imaging of Petrous Apex Lesions

Gillian M. Potter, MBChB, MD, MRCP, FRCR*, Rekha Siripurapu, MBBS, MRCP, FRCR

KEYWORDS

- Petrous apex • Skull base • Computed tomography • MRI • Paraganglioma • Chondrosarcoma
- Proton beam

KEY POINTS

- The petrous apex may be affected by a variety range of pathology, many with characteristic CT and MR imaging appearances in association with suggestive clinical presentations.
- Petrous apex lesions are commonly asymptomatic and encountered as incidental findings on imaging performed for other clinical reasons.
- In patients with petrous apex lesions, CT and MRI play a key role in lesion characterization, imaging, surveillance, surgical planning and oncological contouring.
- Postcontrast T1-weighted imaging performed as part of a skull base MRI protocol for petrous apex lesions should ideally be fat-suppressed to optimize lesion delineation.

INTRODUCTION

Petrous apex lesions are commonly encountered as incidental and asymptomatic findings on CT and MRI performed for other clinical reasons. In addition to several common intrinsic lesions with characteristic appearances on cross-sectional imaging, the petrous apex may be involved by a range of disease processes from closely related structures, including pathology of the adjacent temporal bone, sinonasal cavity, intracranial compartment, and nasopharynx.[1–5] In symptomatic patients, clinical presentation varies depending on site and extent of disease, with symptoms typically relating to mass effect and/or to direct involvement of closely adjacent structures, including the brainstem, petrous internal carotid artery, trigeminal nerve (CN5), and abducens nerve (CN6). Petrous apex lesions are optimally assessed on imaging using a combination of high-resolution CT and MRI. The management of petrous apex lesions varies widely, reflecting the wide range of possible pathologies. In surgical candidates, imaging plays a critical role in

preoperative planning, with the surgical approach (open, endoscopic, or combined techniques) determined by the nature of the pathology and location relative to vital structures and other surrounding structures.[6] Imaging also plays a central role in surveillance of patients with petrous apex pathology, and in oncological contouring for lesions such as postoperative chordoma and chondrosarcoma with petrous apex extension. The integration of artificial intelligence technology may herald potential for patients with petrous apex and other skull base lesions, including neoplastic lesions.[7–9]

NORMAL ANATOMY

The petrous apex is a pyramidal, medial projection of the petrous temporal bone, lying anteromedial to the inner ear (Fig. 1). The petrosphenoidal fissure, petrous carotid canal, and foramen lacerum lie anteriorly and laterally, the posterior cranial fossa posteriorly and medially, and the jugular bulb (transmitting CN9-11; see Fig. 1) and inferior petrosal sinus inferiorly. The anterior

Department of Neuroradiology, Manchester Centre for Clinical Neurosciences, Salford NHS Foundation Trust, Greater Manchester, England M6 8HD, UK
* Corresponding author.
E-mail address: gillian.potter@srft.nhs.uk
Twitter: @GillianPotter7 (G.M.P.)

Neuroimag Clin N Am 31 (2021) 523–540
https://doi.org/10.1016/j.nic.2021.06.005
1052-5149/21/Crown Copyright © 2021 Published by Elsevier Inc. All rights reserved.

surface forms the posterior part of the middle cranial fossa, while the posterior surface forms the anterior part of the posterior cranial fossa. The inferior surface forms part of the skull base. The internal auditory canal divides the petrous apex into a larger anterior compartment, consisting of bone marrow and/or a variable degree of pneumatized air cells, and a smaller posterior compartment, derived from the dense bone of the otic capsule, or bony labyrinth, surrounding the inner ear (see **Fig. 1**). In close proximity is the trigeminal ganglion in Meckel cave (**Fig. 2**). The petrosphenoidal ligament (Gruber ligament) arises from the tip of the petrous apex and crosses the petro-occipital fissure to the posterior clinoid process. The petrosphenoidal ligament demarcates the superior margin of Dorello canal, an anatomic channel from the dura along the petroclival junction to the posterior cavernous sinus, containing inferior petrosal sinus, the dorsal meningeal branch of the meningohypophyseal trunk, and portions of the basilar plexus and CN6 as it courses toward the cavernous sinus (see **Fig. 2**). The foramen lacerum lies at the anteromedial margin of the petrous apex and contains dense fibrous tissue and cartilage that merge with the cartilaginous portion of the Eustachian tube.

IMAGING FINDINGS AND PATHOLOGY

Imaging characteristics of common petrous apex lesions are summarized in **Table 1**.

NORMAL VARIANT ANATOMY AND PSEUDOLESIONS

The petrous apex is pneumatized in approximately 33% of individuals.[11] Petrous apex pneumatization is found in 21% of children, with prevalence and degree increasing with age.[12] Normal variations in extent and pattern of pneumatization (**Fig. 3**) can give rise to diagnostic confusion. An effusion within an asymmetrically pneumatized petrous apex (typically following otitis media) may be mistaken for a lesion on that side (**Fig. 3**). Petrous apex effusions with high T1 signal on MRI caused by proteinaceous content may be mistaken for cholesterol granuloma (see **Fig. 3**), CT will usually distinguish between trapped fluid (demonstrating intact bony margins and preserved trabeculae without expansion) and cholesterol granuloma (showing bony expansion with trabecular destruction and bony thinning/erosion). On MRI, normal high T1 marrow signal relating to an asymmetrically nonpneumatized or less pneumatized petrous apex may be mistaken for a cholesterol granuloma (see **Fig. 3**); however, the absence

of mass effect and the addition of either fat-suppressed T1-weighted MRI or CT skull base should enable a correct diagnosis in most cases (see **Fig. 3**), avoiding unnecessary further imaging or treatment. Where diagnostic uncertainty persists despite CT and MRI, follow-up imaging is often helpful in confirming stability. Normal anatomic structures in the petrous apex such as the subarcuate (or petromastoid) canal, which connects the mastoid antrum with the intracranial cavity, may be mistaken for a fracture (**Fig. 4**).[13]

DEVELOPMENTAL LESIONS
Cephalocele

Petrous apex cephaloceles are relatively rare congenital or acquired lesions that represent focal protrusion of dura, typically from Meckel cave, into the petrous apex, without brain tissue. They are considered to occur because of chronically increased intracranial pressure transmitted into Meckel cave through a patent porus trigeminus[3] and may be bilateral (**Fig. 5**). Petrous apex cephaloceles are most often asymptomatic and detected as incidental findings on CT or MRI; however, they may produce symptoms, including trigeminal neuralgia, sensorineural hearing loss, headache, and cerebrospinal fluid (CSF) otorrhea. They are associated with empty sella syndrome[14] and Usher syndrome.[15] They follow CSF signal on MRI and on CT show nondestructive erosion with a smooth or scalloped border.

Congenital Cholesteatoma

Congenital cholesteatomas (epidermoid cysts) of the petrous apex are intraosseous inclusions of ectoderm, comprising keratinous debris and cholesterol. On MRI, congenital cholesteatomas appear as well-defined lesions, usually isointense to CSF on T1- and T2-weighted imaging and with restricted diffusion (**Fig. 6**). They are usually nonattenuating on FLAIR imaging; however, partial attenuation may occur. On postcontrast imaging, thin rim enhancement may be seen. On CT, benign bony expansion and erosion is seen. Cholesteatoma may be distinguished from a cholesterol granuloma by the presence of low T1-weighted signal, from a mucocele by the presence of restricted diffusion, and from a benign bone tumor by the absence of enhancement.[5] Nonecho planar diffusion-weighted imaging provides the optimal means for assessment, similar to assessment of (typically acquired) cholesteatoma of the middle ear.[16] Diagnostic difficulty may arise in differentiation of white epidermoid from cholesterol granuloma, as both demonstrate high T1- and T2-weighted signal intensity on MRI.

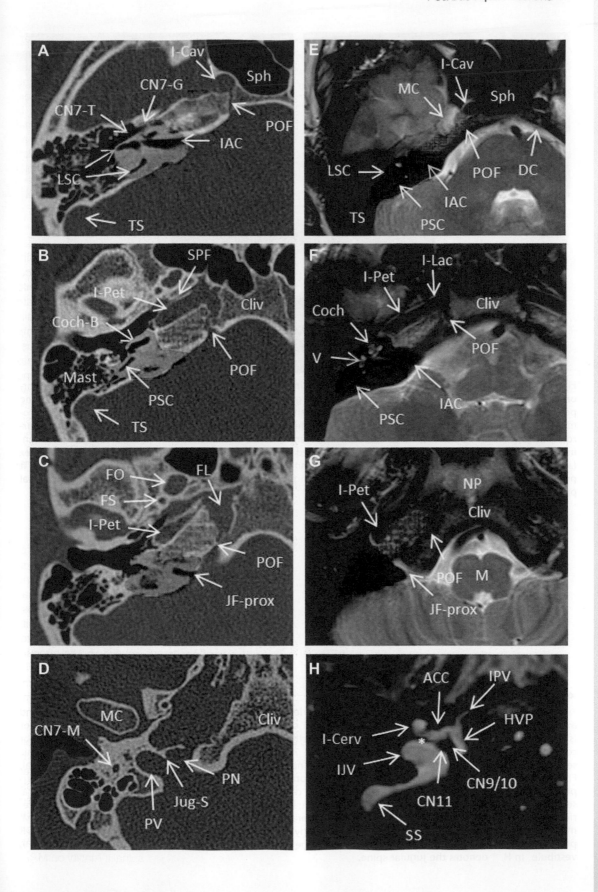

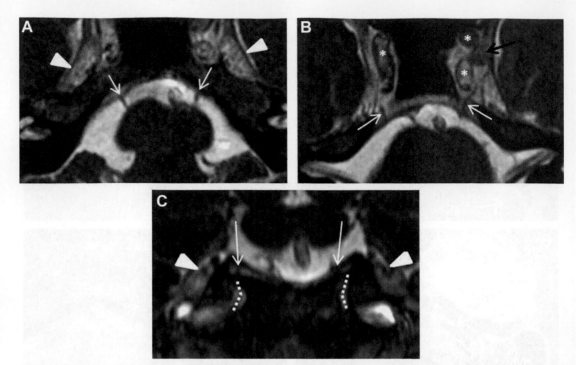

Fig. 2. Postcontrast FIESTA MRI showing the close proximity of CN6 to the petrous apex on axial (*A*, *B*) and coronal (*C*) imaging. (*A*) Cisternal segment of CN6 emerging from the pontomedullary junction, medial to the petrous apex, and crossing the prepontine cistern toward the dorsal clivus (*arrows*). Meckel cave is seen anteromedial to the petrous apex (*arrowheads*). (*B,C*) CN6 within Dorello canal on axial (*B*) and coronal (*C*) imaging (*arrows*). In (*B*), the cavernous internal carotid arteries (*asterisks*) and a CN3 schwannoma (*black arrow*) are also seen. In (*C*), the petro-occipital fissures are depicted by dotted lines with Meckel cave seen lateral to the petrous apex (*arrowheads*). The long subarachnoid course of CN6 and its relatively fixed position in Dorello canal make it prone to stretching, with CN6 palsy the most common false localizing sign in patients with raised intracranial pressure.

Fig. 1. (*A–D*) Normal axial CT of the petrous apex (superior to inferior). (*E–H*) Normal axial T2-weighted (*E–G*) and axial postcontrast fat-suppressed T1-weighted (*H*) MRI of the petrous apex (superior to inferior). The anterior (*shaded blue*) and posterior (*shaded purple*) compartments of the petrous apex are shown. ACC, anterior condylar confluence; Cliv, clivus; CN7-G, cranial nerve 7-geniculate ganglion; CN7-T, cranial nerve 7-typmanic segment; CN9/10, cranial nerves 9 and 10; CN11, cranial nerve 11; Coch-B, basal turn of cochlea; DC, Dorello canal; FL, foramen lacerum; FO, foramen ovale; FR, foramen rotundum; FS, foramen spinosum; HVP, hypoglossal venous plexus; IAC, internal auditory canal; I-Cav, internal carotid artery-cavernous segment; I-Cerv, ICA, cervical segment; I-Lac, internal carotid artery-lacerum segment; I-Pet, internal carotid artery-petrous segment; IPV, inferior petroclival vein; JB, jugular bulb; JG-prox, jugular foramen-proximal aspect; LSC, lateral semicircular canal; M, medulla; Mast, mastoid air cells; MC, mandibular condyle; NP, nasopharyngeal mucosa; PN, pars nervosa; POF, petro-occipital fissure; PV, pars vascularis; SPF, sphenopetrosal suture; Sph, sphenoid sinus; SS, sigmoid sinus; V, vestibule. In H, * denotes the jugular spine.

Table 1
Imaging characteristics of common petrous apex lesions

	Computed Tomography	T1-Weighted MRI	T2-Weighted MRI	Diffusion Restriction	Enhancement
Trapped fluid (effusion)	Preserved trabeculae and cortical margins with no expansion	Low-high – depending on content[a]	High (low if proteinaceous content)[a]	No	No
Mucocele	Benign bony expansion, benign trabecular erosion, cortical thinning/ erosion	Low (intermediate-high if proteinaceous content)	High	No[b]	No
Cholesterol granuloma	Benign bony expansion	High	High, often with focal areas of low signal	No	No[c]
Petrous apicitis	Aggressive bony destruction	Low	High	Common	Yes
Cholesteatoma	Early, trabecular erosion; later, bony expansion and erosion	Low-intermediate	High	Yes[d]	No
Cephalocele	Expansion with cortical thinning	Cerebrospinal fluid (CSF) (low)	CSF (high)	No	No

[a] Relative to brain parenchyma.
[b] Pseudorestriction if proteinaceous content.
[c] Difficult to assess because of intrinsic high T1 signal.
[d] Best assessed on non-EPI DWI.[10]

INFLAMMATORY/INFECTIOUS LESIONS
Cholesterol Granuloma

Cholesterol granulomas are rare, benign, expansile, cystic lesions containing cholesterol crystals, multinucleated body giant cells, red blood cells, and blood breakdown products, all within a thick fibrous capsule (Fig. 7).[17] They can occur in any aerated part of the temporal bone, including the petrous apex when pneumatized, and they often occur after otitis media. When present, symptoms can occur relating to local mass effect, including headaches, hearing loss, diplopia, and vertigo. On CT, cholesterol granulomas are seen as expansile masses with smooth bony remodeling, and on MRI, they demonstrate characteristic increased signal on T1-and T2-weighted imaging with a low T1-weighted signal rim and no enhancement. The aims of surgery are decompression of mass effect and the creation of a conduit for drainage of the petrous apex air cells. Surgery may be undertaken via transcranial or endoscopic endonasal approach.

Petrous Apicitis

Petrous apicitis, referring to infection of the pneumatized petrous apex, is usually the result of acute otomastoiditis.[18] Osteomyelitis, referring to infection of the nonpneumatized petrous apex, most often relating to necrotizing otitis externa or suppurative otitis media, is rare.[19] Gradenigo syndrome, relatively rare in the postantibiotic era, describes the triad of petrous apicitis, CN6 palsy caused by extension into Dorello canal, and pain in the distribution of the ophthalmic and maxillary divisions of the trigeminal nerve (from involvement of Meckel cave). In the early stages, only fluid may be seen on CT and MRI, and in later stages, CT shows aggressive bony destruction, with enhancement visible on MRI. Petrous apicitis may be seen in neurosarcoidosis (occurring in

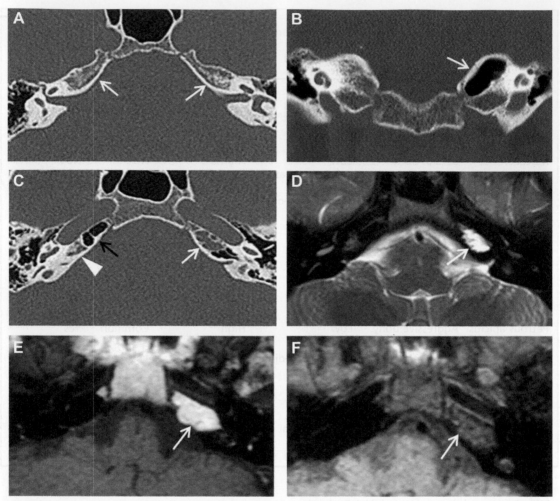

Fig. 3. Patterns of petrous apex pneumatization. (*A*) Normal marrow in a patient with nonpneumatized petrous apices (*arrows*) on axial CT in bone algorithm. (*B*) Coronal CT showing asymmetric pneumatization of the left petrous apex with a large solitary air cell (*arrow*). (*C,D*) Pseudolesion caused by trapped fluid in an asymmetrically pneumatized left petrous apex on axial CT (*C, white arrow*) and axial T2-weighted MRI (*D, white arrow*). In (*C*), the right petrous apex is partially pneumatized (*black arrow*) with normal marrow density in the nonpneumatized anterior compartment more posteriorly (*arrowhead*). (*E, F*) A pseudolesion on axial T1-weighted MRI caused by normal marrow signal in the nonpneumatized left petrous apex (*E, arrow*), showing complete fat suppression on subsequent fat-suppressed T1 imaging (*F, arrow*).

approximately 10% of patients with systemic sarcoidosis), which may affect bone (**Fig. 8**)[20] in addition to the leptomeninges, pachymeninges and brain parenchyma, with symptoms (when present) dependent on the site of disease.[21] The petrous apex may also be involved in granulomatous polyangiitis,[3] Immunoglobulin G-4 (IgG-4)-related disease[22,23] and intracranial xanthoma.[24]

NEOPLASMS
Chondrosarcoma and Chordoma

Chondrosarcoma and chordoma of the skull base are rare, typically slow-growing malignancies; however, they may be locally aggressive,

extending to closely related areas such as the petrous apex, pituitary fossa, middle fossa, retroclival region, cavernous sinus, sphenoid sinus, prevertebral space, foramen magnum, and upper cervical spine (**Figs. 9** and **10**).[25,26] Clinical presentation varies widely depending on location and proximity to critical structures. Histopathological and imaging features of skull base chondrosarcoma and chordoma are shown in (**Table 2**); however, both tumors may show a wide variation in tumor site, as well as pattern and extent of invasive growth. The use of axial high-resolution heavily T2-weighted MRI in addition to standard pre- and postcontrast MRI skull base sequences may be of value for assessing tumor residuum in

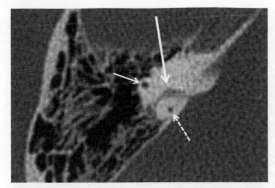

Fig. 4. Subarcuate (or petromastoid) canal (*long white arrow*) on axial CT in bone algorithm. The subarcuate canal courses between the anterior (*short white arrow*) and posterior (*dashed arrow*) limbs of the superior semicircular canal and transmits the subarcuate artery (supplying the bony labyrinth, facial canal, and mastoid antrum) and the subarcuate vein.

intraoperative and postoperative settings, including patients being considered for proton beam therapy (ie, with minimum residual tumor after maximal safe surgical resection), in whom adequate clearance between tumor residuum

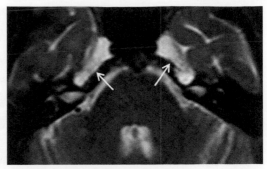

Fig. 5. Bilateral petrous apex cephaloceles. Axial T2-weighted MRI showing bilateral enlargement of Meckel cave with petrous apex extension (*arrows*).

and dose-limiting normal structures is required (typically 3 mm clearance from the brainstem and at least 5 mm from the optic chiasm and at least one, or preferably both, optic nerves (**Fig. 11**).[27] There is radiological and histopathological overlap between skull base chondrosarcoma and chordoma, and it may be difficult to distinguish between grade 1 chondrosarcoma and chordoma.[28] Nonechoplanar diffusion-weighted imaging may help distinguish between chordoma

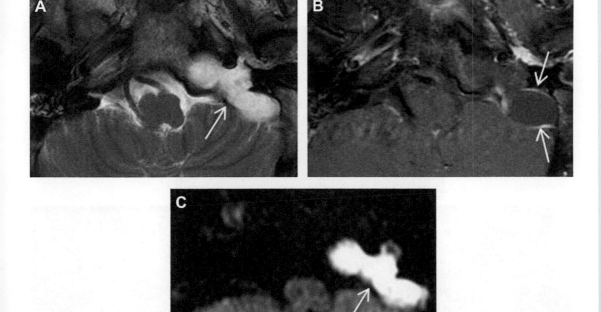

Fig. 6. Congenital cholesteatoma. (*A*) Axial T2-weighted MR image shows a hyperintense, large, well-defined, lobulated lesion in the anterior and posterior compartments of the left petrous apex (*arrow*). (*B*) Axial postcontrast T1 fat-suppressed image shows subtle thin rim enhancement only (*arrows*). (*C*) Diffusion restriction on axial DWI using non-EPI technique (*arrow*).

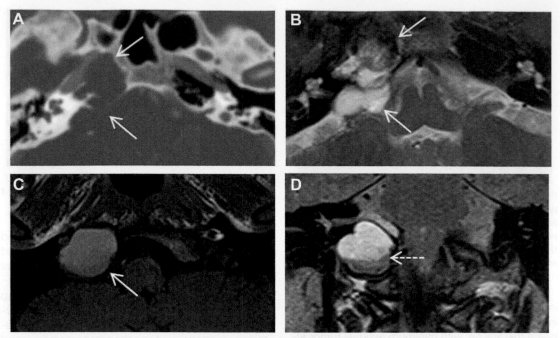

Fig. 7. Cholesterol granuloma. (*A*) Axial CT shows expansile lucent lesion in the right petrous apex (*arrows*) with erosion of the posterior petrous face and anteromedial wall of the right petrous carotid canal. (*B*) Axial T2-weighted MR image shows predominantly high signal with areas of intermediate and low signal. (*C*) Axial T1-weighted MRI shows high signal, suggesting blood products. (*D*) A fluid level on coronal T2-weighted MR image suggests recent hemorrhage (*dashed arrow*).

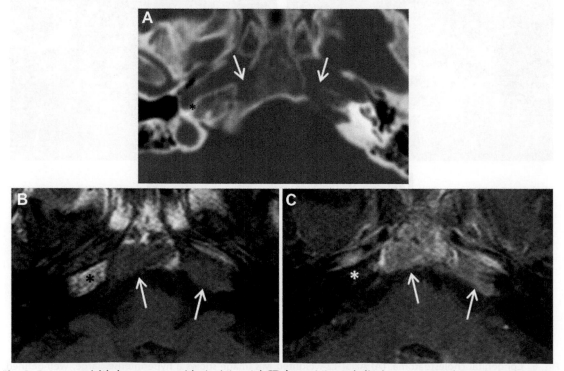

Fig. 8. Petrous apicitis in neurosarcoidosis. (*A*) Axial CT shows bilateral clival erosion, involving the right petro-occipital fissure and extending across the left petro-occipital fissure into the petrous apex (*arrows*). (*B, C*) Axial T1-weighted image shows loss of normal T1-hyperintense fatty marrow signal (*arrows*). (*C*) Postcontrast fat-suppressed T1 image shows enhancement (*arrows*). Asterisk denotes normal fat signal in the nonpneumatized right petrous apex.

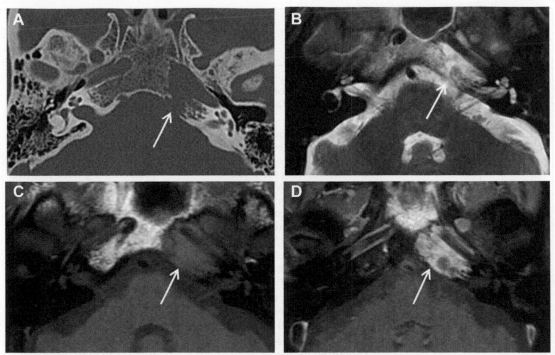

Fig. 9. Chondrosarcoma. Axial CT (*A*) shows erosion centered on the left petro-occipital fissure (*arrow*) with erosion of the adjacent wall of the left petrous ICA. (*B*) Axial T2-weighted MR image shows a predominantly hyperintense lesion (*arrow*). (*C*) Axial T1-weighted MR image shows corresponding intermediate T1 signal (*arrow*). (*D*) Enhancement on postcontrast fat-suppressed T1 image (*arrow*).

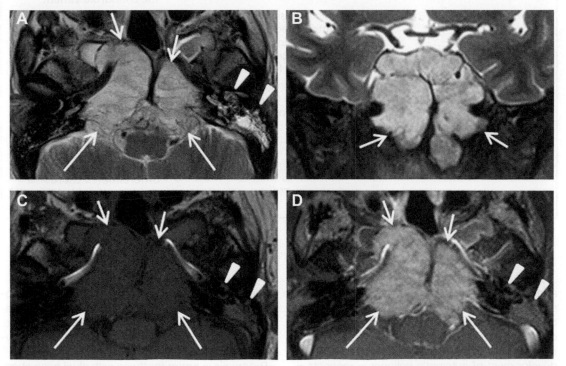

Fig. 10. Extensive clival chordoma with bilateral petrous apex extension. (*A–D*) Axial T2-weighted, coronal T2-weighted fat-suppressed, axial T1-weighted, and axial contrast-enhanced T1-weighted fat-suppressed images. There is an extensive T2-hyperintense, T1-isointense mass with enhancement centered on the clivus. The large bilateral retroclival components (*arrows* in *A, C* and *D*) displace the medulla posteriorly. Tumor extends anteriorly toward the paranasal sinuses (*short arrows* in *A, C* and *D*) and inferiorly into the prevertebral space (*short arrows* in *B*). Left otomastoiditis (*arrowheads* in *A, C* and *D*) is caused by left eustachian tube obstruction.

Table 2
Histopathological and imaging features of skull base chordoma and chondrosarcoma

	Chondrosarcoma	Chordoma
Origin	Primitive mesenchymal cells or from the embryonic rest of the cranial cartilaginous matrix	Embryonic remnants of primitive notochord
Histopathology	Four histologic subgroups: conventional, mesenchymal, clear cell, dedifferentiated; positive staining for S-100 and vimentin; 3 WHO grades, based on cellularity, mitotic activity, atypia, and nuclear size: grade I (well-differentiated), grade II (intermediately differentiated), grade III (poorly differentiated)	Three types: classical (conventional), chondroid, dedifferentiated); type predicts prognosis; positive staining for S100, vimentin and epithelial markers (epithelial membrane antigen, pan-cytokeratins); positive for Brachury,[26] a specific diagnostic marker with potential therapeutic implications
Typical location	Off midline, along skull base synchondroses (petroclival, petrosphenoidal)	Midline
CT appearances	Aggressive bony destruction; chondroid matrix mineralization; rings and arcs	Well-circumscribed; expansile soft tissue mass; normally hyperdense to brain parenchyma; lytic bone destruction; tumor calcification may be seen in the chondroid variant
MRI appearances	Low-intermediate signal on T1-weighted images, high signal on T2-weighted images; moderate to avid heterogenous enhancement	Intermediate to low signal on T1-weightedimages; very high signal on T2-weighted images; moderate to marked enhancement
Additional comments	May rarely hemorrhage, with low signal on T2-weighted images because of hemosiderin	Intratumoral hemorrhage, calcification and highly proteinaceous mucus pool may produce foci of high T1-weighted signal and more heterogeneous enhancement; poorly differentiated chordoma may show low signal on T2-weighted images

and chondrosarcoma and differentiate between different histopathological types of chordoma.[29–32] Multiparametric radiomics signatures can also help in preoperative differentiation between chondrosarcoma and chordoma.[33,34] The development of automatic volumetric reconstruction may lead to improvements in assessing growth of large, irregular, multicompartmental lesions of the skull base.[9] Elucidation of molecular events underlying the pathogenesis of chondrosarcoma and chordroma has led to the identification of several new potential therapeutic targets, especially for those with chemotherapy-refractory, inoperable or metastatic disease.[35–38] Prognosis is better for those with skull base chondrosarcoma when compared with chordoma for patients when treated with similar complex strategies.[25]

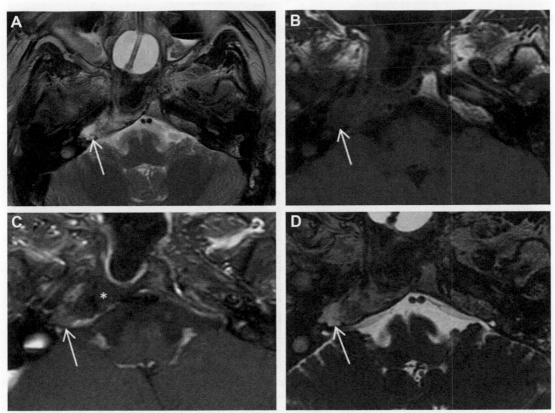

Fig. 11. Intraoperative MRI during endoscopic endonasal resection of right clival and petrous apex chondrosarcoma. (A) Axial T2-weighted MR image shows minor focal residual T2-hyperintense tumor in the right petrous apex at the posterolateral margin of the postsurgical cavity, posterior to the proximal petrous ICA (arrow). (B) On axial T1-weighted imaging, it is difficult to distinguish between tumor (arrow) and adjacent postsurgical changes. (C) Mild enhancement of residual tumor (arrow) with nonenhancement of adjacent postsurgical changes (asterisk) on postcontrast fat-suppressed T1-weighted image. (D) Axial heavily T2-weighted MR image shows relative hyperintensity of residual tumor (arrow) compared with the adjacent postsurgical cavity.

Metastases

Skull base metastases, postulated to arise because of retrograde venous seeding along the extensively interconnected midline venous system, are often asymptomatic and discovered incidentally on CT or MRI performed for other clinical reasons. The most frequently reported primary neoplasms in patients with skull base metastases are lung (Fig. 12), prostate (Fig. 13), and breast cancers.[39] Temporal bone metastases may be the first sign of cancer in approximately 28% of cases.[40] The petrous apex is the most common site of disease within the temporal bone, and patients may be asymptomatic.[39] Treatment of petrous apex and skull base metastases is primarily palliative.

Jugulotympanic Paragangliomas

Paragangliomas are rare, usually benign, tumors with an autosomal dominant inheritance.[41,42] In the head and neck, paragangliomas are described by the ganglion involved and are classified as jugulotympanic, carotid body, vagal, laryngeal, and miscellaneous, according to the World Health Organization (WHO).[43] The term glomus arose from confusion with true glomus tumors derived from thermoregulatory myoarterial structures and is no longer an accepted pathologic nomenclature. Jugulotympanic paragangliomas, arising from the jugular bulb or from Arnold or Jacobson nerves within the middle ear,[44] may extend to involve the petrous apex (Fig. 14). In patients with head and neck paragangliomas, whole-body MRI is performed on the basis of biochemical and genetic testing to identify synchronous and metachronous tumors.[41,45] Functional imaging (including fluorodeoxyglucose positron emission tomography (PET)/CT and 68-Ga DOTATATE PET/CT) may be used if specifically evaluating for metastatic disease or small multifocal lesions, with 68-Ga DOTATATE PET/CT having the highest detection rate.[46,47] [123]Iodine-labeled metaiodobenzylguanidine (MIBG) scintigraphy may be used in patients being considered for MIBG therapy. Genetic and biochemical testing are

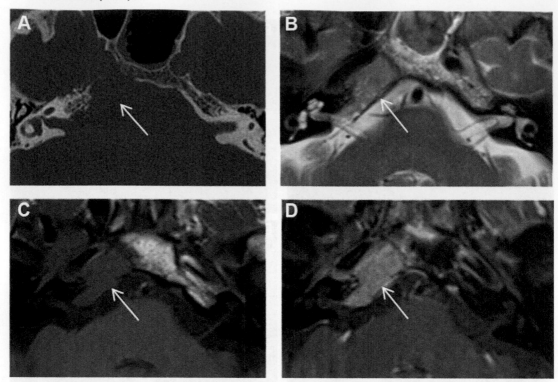

Fig. 12. Lung cancer metastasis. (*A*) Axial CT shows aggressive bony destruction of the right petrous apex, right upper clivus, and anteromedial wall of the right internal auditory canal. (*B–D*) On MRI, the lesion is T2-and T1-isointense relative to brain parenchyma (*B, C*, respectively; *arrows*), with avid enhancement on axial postcontrast T1 fat-suppressed imaging (*D, arrow*). The skull base was the only site of bony metastatic disease in this patient with nonsmall cell lung cancer (adenocarcinoma type).

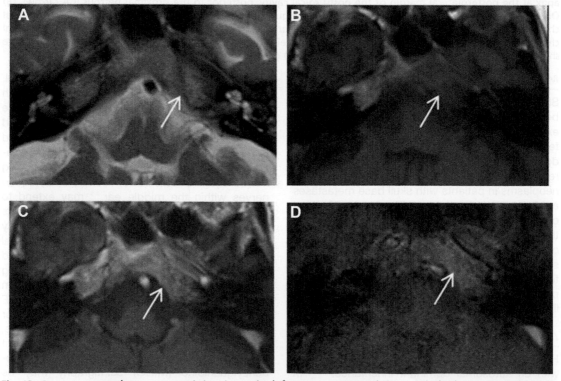

Fig. 13. Prostate cancer bony metastasis involving the left petrous apex and clivus. (*A*) The lesion (*arrow*) is difficult to appreciate on axial T2-weigted imaging, showing similar signal to normal bone marrow. (*B*) On axial T1-weighted MR image, abnormal asymmetric loss of normal high T1 marrow signal (*arrow*). (*C, D*) Axial postcontrast T1 imaging obtained without (*C*) and with (*D*) fat suppression, highlighting increased lesion conspicuity when fat suppression is applied, even in the presence of motion artifact, as in this patient.

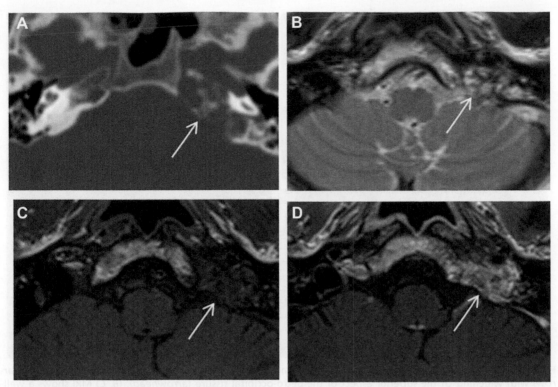

Fig. 14. Jugular paraganglioma with petrous apex extension showing a typical salt and pepper appearance on MR images (*B–D*). (*A*) Axial CT shows irregular erosion and a typical moth-eaten appearance of the left petrous apex. (*B*) On axial T2-weighted MRI, the lesion is hyperintense to brain parenchyma and contains multiple small intralesional hypointense hypervascular flow voids (pepper). (*C*) Axial T1-weighted MR image showing small intralesional foci of hemorrhage or slow flow within flow voids (salt). (*D*) Avid enhancement on postcontrast axial T1-weighted imaging. Note suboptimal delineation of the medial tumor margin on postcontrast T1-weighted imaging because fat suppression has not been applied (*D*).

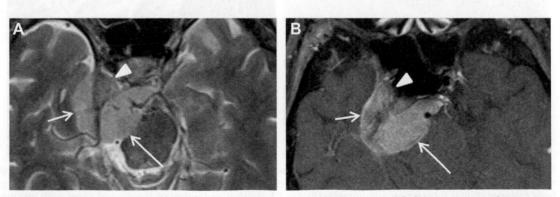

Fig. 15. Petroclival meningioma. (*A*) On axial T2-weighted MRI, the lesion is mildly hyperintense to brain parenchyma. (*B*). Axial postcontrast fat-suppressed T1-weighted image shows avid enhancement. The posterior fossa component (*long arrows*) displaces and flattens the right lower midbrain and encases the right posterior cerebral artery. There is extension into the right middle cranial fossa (*short arrows*), without adjacent temporal lobe edema, and into the superior right cavernous sinus (*arrowheads*).

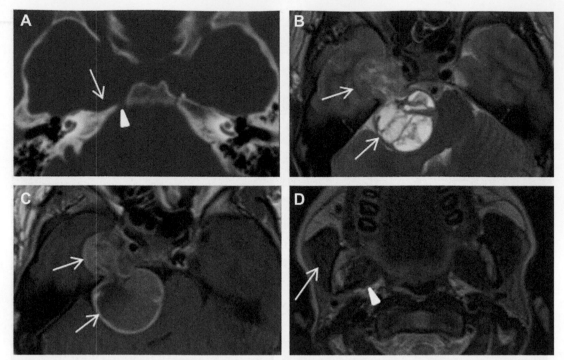

Fig. 16. Trigeminal schwannoma. (*A*) Axial CT shows smooth erosion of the right anterior petrous face (*long arrow*) with widening of the superior aspect of the petro-occipital fissure (*arrowhead*). (*B, C*) MRI shows a well-defined, dumbbell-shaped lesion in right Meckel cave and the right prepontine cistern with heterogenous signal and enhancement on T2-weighted imaging (*B*) and axial postcontrast T1 imaging (*C*) in keeping with multicystic change. The component centered in Meckel cave displaces and compresses the right temporal lobe and medially displaces the right cavernous ICA. The prepontine cistern component produces significant brainstem compression and partial effacement and displacement of the fourth ventricle. (*D*) Secondary atrophy of the right muscles of mastication (masseter, *long arrow*; medial pterygoid muscle, *arrowhead*) on axial T2-weighted imaging.

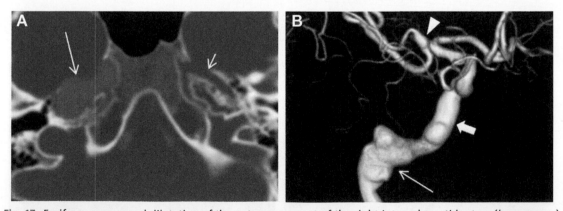

Fig. 17. Fusiform aneurysmal dilatation of the petrous segment of the right internal carotid artery (*long arrows*) on axial CT angiogram in a patient with vasculopathy of uncertain etiology (*A*) and volume-rendered imaging from catheter digital subtraction angiography (*B*). On CT, there is expansion of the carotid canal with erosion of the right petrous apex. The small-caliber left carotid canal (*A, short arrow*) related to longstanding occlusion of the left ICA (not shown). The cavernous segment of the right internal carotid artery demonstrated relative enlargement (*B, block arrow*), and the patient had previously undergone coiling of a right middle cerebral artery bifurcation aneurysm (*B, arrowhead*).

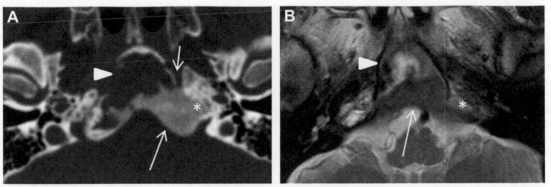

Fig. 18. Fibrous dysplasia. (*A*) Axial CT shows mixed ground glass (*arrow*) and lucency (*arrowhead*) of the inferior clivus at the level of the foramen lacerum (*short arrow*), extending across the left inferior petro-occipital fissure to the left petrous apex (*asterisk*). (*B*) Axial T2-weighted MR image shows mixed signal in the clivus. The lucent area on CT (*arrowhead*) is predominantly T2-hyperintense with areas of intermediate and low T2 signal (*arrowhead*), and the ground glass area on CT (*arrow*) is slightly hypointense to brain parenchyma (*arrow*).

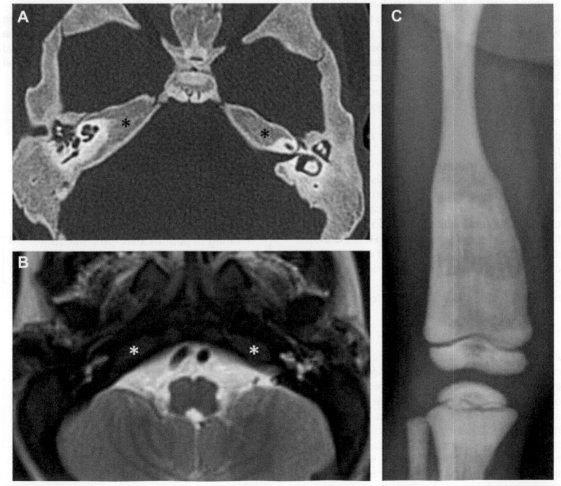

Fig. 19. Osteopetrosis. Diffuse calvarial and skull base osteosclerosis including the petrous apices (*asterisk*) on axial CT (*A*) with diffuse low signal on axial T2-weighted MR image (*B*) in a child. (*C*) Erlenmeyer flask-type deformity on an AP view of the right femur. Skeletal survey showed diffuse increased bone density (not shown).

recommended in all patients with paragangliomas.[41,48] The World Health Organization Endocrine Tumor Classification recently acknowledged metastatic potential for all paragangliomas.[49] The evaluation of radiological, pathologic, clinical, biochemical, and genetic evidence in patients with head and neck paragangliomas is optimally undertaken by a multidisciplinary team with the relevant expertise, including oncology, radiology, genetics, skull base surgery, and endocrinology.[41,48,50]

OTHER NEOPLASMS

Several other tumors, either arising within the petrous bone or extending from a closely related anatomic structure, may involve the petrous apex. Tumors such as myeloma, plasmacytoma, and lymphoma may produce aggressive bony destruction on CT with low-intermediate T1 and T2 signal (relative to brain parenchyma) and enhancement on MRI. Endolymphatic sac tumors, located along the posterior petrous face, however, with the potential for petrous apex extension, may in addition show areas of T1 hyperintensity secondary to hemorrhage. Rarer pathologies with the potential for overlapping imaging features such as fibromyxoma,[51] chondromyxoid fibroma,[52] osteosarcoma, chondroblastoma, osteoblastoma,[53] intraosseous schwannoma, granulocytic sarcoma,[54] and giant cell tumor may pose more diagnostic dilemmas, with a subsequent increased reliance on histologic analysis. In children, differential diagnosis should also include entities such as Langerhans cell histiocytosis and rhabdomyosarcoma.[55,56] More commonly seen entities with secondary involvement of the petrous apex may pose less diagnostic difficulty on account of their well-described and characteristic CT and MRI appearances, such as petroclival meningioma (Fig. 15), CN5 schwannoma (Fig. 16), and CN7 schwannoma.

VASCULAR LESIONS

Aneurysms of the petrous segment of the internal carotid artery are rare and are most often found incidentally on cross-sectional imaging; however, they may infrequently present with otologic symptoms such as hearing loss, tinnitus, and hemorrhage.[57] Their cause is unknown; however, they have been reported in the settings of trauma, infection/inflammation, radiation, and fibromuscular dysplasia.[57,58] CT bone windows are optimal for assessment of the bony carotid canal (Fig. 17). On MRI, patent aneurysms appear as flow voids on T1-and T2-weighted imaging. In thrombosed aneurysms, T2-weighted signal appears more heterogeneous. Petrous ICA aneurysms can be effectively treated by endovascular techniques.[59,60]

BONE DYSPLASIAS

The petrous apex may be involved by bone dysplasias, although rarely in isolation. These include fibrous dysplasia (Fig. 18) and osteopetrosis (Albers-Schönberg disease; Fig. 19). In Paget disease, demineralization of the petrous apex is the most common manifestation of temporal bone involvement. Diagnosis of bone dysplasias is typically made based on a combination of age, clinical features, and imaging findings using single or multiple imaging modalities, including radiographs, CT, MRI, and nuclear medicine investigations.

SUMMARY

The petrous apex may be affected by a wide range of lesions. CT and MRI are complementary in the imaging assessment of petrous apex lesions and play a key role in diagnosis, surveillance, surgical planning, and oncological contouring.

CLINICS CARE POINTS

- Radiologists should be familiar with anatomic variations in petrous apex pneumatization in order to minimize interpretative errors relating to petrous apex 'pseudolesions'.[1-4]

- Petrous apex cholesteatoma may be distinguished from cholesterol granuloma by the presence of low T1-weighted signal, and from a mucocele by the presence of restricted diffusion.[5,17]

- CT and MR imaging play a critical role in the early identification and subsequent management of petrous apicitis.[18,19]

- Evaluation of radiological, pathologic, clinical, biochemical and genetic evidence in patients with head and neck paragangliomas should optimally be undertaken by a multidisciplinary team.[41,48,50]

DISCLOSURE

The authors have nothing to disclose.

REFERENCES

1. Schmalfuss IM. Petrous apex. Neuroimaging Clin N Am 2009;19(3):367–91.
2. Isaacson B, Kutz JW, Roland PS. Lesions of the petrous apex: diagnosis and management. Otolaryngol Clin North Am 2007;40(3):479–519.
3. Razek AA, Huang BY. Lesions of the petrous apex: classification and findings at CT and MR imaging. Radiographics 2012;32(1):151–73.
4. Connor SE, Leung R, Natas S. Imaging of the petrous apex: a pictorial review. Br J Radiol 2008;81(965):427–35.
5. Chapman PR, Shah R, Curé JK, et al. Petrous apex lesions: pictorial review. AJR Am J Roentgenol 2011;196:WS26–37.
6. Li KL, Agarwal V, Moskowitz HS, et al. Surgical approaches to the petrous apex. World J Otorhinolaryngol Head Neck Surg 2020;6(2):106–14.
7. Zhang Y, Shang L, Chen C, et al. Machine-learning classifiers in discrimination of lesions located in the anterior skull base. Front Oncol 2020;10(752):1–9.
8. Rudie JD, Rauschecker AM, Bryan RN, et al. Emerging applications of artificial intelligence in neuro-oncology. Radiology 2019;290:607–18.
9. Bi WL, Hosny A, Schabath MB, et al. Artificial intelligence in cancer imaging: clinical challenges and applications. CA Cancer J Clin 2019;69(2):127–57.
10. Lingam RK, Connor SEJ, Casselman JW, et al. MRI in otology: applications in cholesteatoma and Meniere's disease. Clin Radiol 2018;73(1):35–44.
11. Boardman JF, Rothfus WE, Dulai HS. Lesions and pseudolesions of the cavernous sinus and petrous apex. Otolaryngol Clin North Am 2008;41(1):195–213.
12. Hardcastle T, McKay-Davies I, Neeff M. Petrous apex pneumatisation in children: a radiological study. J Laryngol Otol 2020;24:1–6.
13. Kwong Y, Yu D, Shah J. Fracture mimics on temporal bone CT: a guide for the radiologist. AJR Am J Roentgenol 2012;199(2):428–34.
14. Zetchi A, Labeyrie M-A, Nicolini E, et al. Empty sella is a sign of symptomatic lateral sinus stenosis and not intracranial hypertension. AJNR Am J Neuroradiol 2019;40(10):1695–700.
15. Stark TA, McKinney AM, Palmer CS, et al. Dilation of the subarachnoid spaces surrounding the cranial nerves with petrous apex cephaloceles in Usher syndrome. AJNR Am J Neuroradiol 2009;30(2):434–6.
16. Lingam RK, Bassett P. A meta-analysis on the diagnostic performance of non-echo-planar diffusion-weighted imaging in detecting middle ear cholesteatoma: 10 years on. Otol Neurotol 2017;38(4):521–8.
17. Isaacson B. Cholesterol granuloma and other petrous apex lesions. Otolaryngol Clin North Am 2015;48(2):361–73.
18. Gadre AK, Chole RA. The changing face of petrous apicitis-a 40-year experience. Laryngoscope 2017;128(1):195–201.
19. Lingam RK, Kumar R, Vaidhyanath R. Inflammation of the temporal bone. Neuroimaging Clin North Am 2018;29(1):1–17.
20. Robles LA, Matilla AF, Covarrubias MP. Sarcoidosis of the skull: a systematic review. World Neurosurg 2020;139:387–94.
21. Shah R, Roberson GH, Curé JK. Correlation of MR imaging findings and clinical manifestations in neurosarcoidosis. AJNR Am J Neuroradiol 2009;30(5):953–61.
22. Bittencourt AG, Pereira LV, Junior FC, et al. IgG4-related sclerosing disease of the temporal bone. Otol Neurotol 2013;34(3):e20–1.
23. Takanoa K, Yamamoto M, Takahashi H, et al. Recent advances in knowledge regarding the head and neck manifestations of IgG4-related disease. Auris Nasus Larynx 2017;44(1):7–17.
24. Bonhomme GR, Loevner LA, Yen DM, et al. Extensive intracranial xanthoma associated with type II hyperlipidemia. Am J Neuroradiol 2000;21(2):353–5.
25. Kremenevski N, Schlaffer S, Coras R, et al. Skull base chordomas and chondrosarcomas. Neuroendocrinology 2020;110:836–47.
26. Nibu Y, José-Edwards DS, Di Gregorio A. From notochord formation to hereditary chordoma: the many roles of Brachyury. Biomed Res Int 2013;2013:826435.
27. Mercado CE, Holtzman AL, Rotondo R, et al. Proton therapy for skull base tumors: a review of clinical outcomes for chordomas and chondrosarcomas. Head Neck 2019;41(2):536–41.
28. Coca-Pelaz A, Rodrigo JP, Triantafyllou A, et al. Chondrosarcomas of the head and neck. Eur Arch Otorhinolaryngol 2014;271(10):2601–9.
29. Yeom KW, Lober RM, Mobley BC, et al. Diffusion-weighted MRI: distinction of skull base chordoma from chondrosarcoma. Am J Neuroradiol 2013;34(5):1056–61.
30. Müller U, Kubik-Huch RA, Ares C, et al. Is there a role for conventional MRI and MR diffusion-weighted imaging for distinction of skull base chordoma and chondrosarcoma? Acta Radiol 2016;57(2):225–32.
31. Freeze BS, Glastonbury CM. Differentiation of skull base chordomas from chondrosarcomas by diffusion-weighted MRI. AJNR Am J Neuroradiol 2013;34(10):E113.
32. Guler E, Ozgen B, Mut M, et al. The added value of diffusion magnetic resonance imaging in the diagnosis and posttreatment evaluation of skull base chordomas. J Neurol Surg B Skull Base 2017;78(3):256–65.
33. Li L, Wang K, Ma X, et al. Radiomic analysis of multiparametric magnetic resonance imaging for

differentiating skull base chordoma and chondrosarcoma. Eur J Radiol 2019;118:81–7.

34. Santegoeds RGC, Temel Y, Beckervordersandforth JC, et al. State-of-the-art imaging in human chordoma of the skull base. Curr Radiol Rep 2018;6:16.

35. Yamaguchi T, Imada H, Iida S, et al. Notochordal tumors: an update on molecular pathology with therapeutic implications. Surg Pathol Clin 2017;10(3):637–56.

36. Polychronidou G, Karavasilis V, Pollack SM, et al. Novel therapeutic approaches in chondrosarcoma. Future Oncol 2017;13(7):637–48.

37. Liu C, Jia Q, Wei H, et al. Apatinib in patients with advanced chordoma: a single-arm, single-centre, phase 2 study. Lancet Oncol 2020;21:1244–52.

38. Stacchiotti S, Gronchi A, Fossati P, et al. Best practices for the management of local-regional recurrent chordoma: a position paper by the Chordoma Global Consensus Group. Ann Oncol 2017;28:1230–42.

39. Jones AJ, Tucker BJ, Novinger LJ, et al. Metastatic disease of the temporal bone: a contemporary review. Laryngoscope 2020;00:1–9.

40. Laigle-Donadey F, Taillibert S, Martin-Duverneuil N, et al. Skull-base metastases. J Neurooncol 2005;75:63–9.

41. Cass ND, Schopper MA, Lubin JA, et al. The changing paradigm of head and neck paragangliomas: what every otolaryngologist needs to know. Ann Otol Rhinol Laryngol 2020;1–9.

42. Lotti LV, Vespa S, Pantalone MR, et al. A developmental perspective on paragangliar tumorigenesis. Cancers 2019;11:273–93.

43. Williams MD, Tischler AS. Update from the 4th edition of the World Health Organization classification of head and neck tumours: paragangliomas. Head Neck Pathol 2017;11:88–95.

44. Noujaim SE, Brown KT, Walker DT, et al. Paragangliomas of the head and neck: a practical approach to diagnosis and review of detailed anatomy of sites of origin. Neurographics 2020;10(4):211–22.

45. Jasperson KW, Kohlmann W, Gammon A, et al. Role of rapid sequence whole-body MRI screening in SDH-associated hereditary paraganglioma families. Fam Cancer 2014;13(2):257–65.

46. Janssen I, Blanchet EM, Adams K, et al. Superiority of [68Ga]-DOTATATE PET/CT to other functional imaging modalities in the localization of SDHB-associated metastatic pheochromocytoma and paraganglioma. Clin Cancer Res 2015;21(17):3888–95.

47. Janssen I, Chen CC, Taieb D, et al. 68Ga-DOTATATE PET/CT in the localization of head and neck paragangliomas compared with other functional imaging modalities and CT/MRI. J Nucl Med 2016;57(2):186–91.

48. Lloyd S, Obholzer R, Tysome J, et al. British Skull Base Society clinical consensus document on management of head and neck paragangliomas. Otolaryngol Head Neck Surg 2020;163(3):400–9.

49. Kimura N, Capella C. Extraadrenal paraganglioma. In: Lloyd RV, Osamura RY, Kloppel G, editors. WHO classification of tumors of endocrine organs. 4th edition. Lyons, France: IARC Press; 2017. p. 190–5.

50. Fishbein L. Pheochromocytoma and paraganglioma: genetics, diagnosis, and treatment. Hematol Oncol Clin North Am 2016;30(1):135–50.

51. Srinivasan US. Fibromyxoma of the petrous apex. Pediatr Neurosurg 2000;32(4):209–13.

52. Wang J, Zhang Y, Li W. Chondromyxoid fibroma of the petrous apex. J Neuroradiol 2011;38(4):255–6.

53. Kraft CT, Morrison RJ, Arts HA. Malignant transformation of a high-grade osteoblastoma of the petrous apex with subcutaneous metastasis. Ear Nose Throat J 2016;95(6):230–3.

54. Lee B, Fatterpekar GM, Kim W, et al. Granulocytic sarcoma of the temporal bone. AJNR Am J Neuroradiol 2002;23(9):1497–9.

55. Touska P, Juliano AF-Y. Temporal bone tumors: an imaging update. Neuroimag Clin N Am 2019;29:145–72.

56. Chevallier KM, Wiggins RH, Quinn NA, et al. Differentiating pediatric rhabdomyosarcoma and Langerhans cell histiocytosis of the temporal bone by imaging appearance. AJNR Am J Neuroradiol 2016;37(6):1185–9.

57. Moonis G, Hwang CJ, Ahmed T, et al. Otologic manifestations of petrous carotid aneurysms. Am J Neuroradiol 2005;26(6):1324–7.

58. Bender MT, Hurtado C, Jiang B, et al. Cerebral aneurysms in patients with fibromuscular dysplasia. Intervent Neurol 2018;7:110–7.

59. Gross BA, Moon K, Ducruet AF, et al. A rare but morbid neurosurgical target: petrous aneurysms and their endovascular management in the stent/flow diverter era. J Neurointerv Surg 2017;9:381–3.

60. Deep NL, Besch-Stokes JG, Lane JI, et al. Paget's disease of the temporal bone: a single-institution contemporary review of 27 patients. Otol Neurotol 2017;38(6):907–15.

Imaging of Sella and Parasellar Region

Claudia F.E. Kirsch, MD

KEYWORDS

- Pituitary • Sellar and suprasellar region • Magnetic resonance imaging
- Computed axial tomography (CT)

KEY POINTS

- The pituitary, sellar, and suprasellar region contain unique meningeal, neural, vascular, and bony complexity; awareness of this anatomy is critical for accurate imaging interpretation.
- Magnetic resonance (MR) imaging is a primary modality for pituitary assessment; axial computed tomography (CT) may be used when MR imaging is contraindicated and provides complementary bony anatomic information.
- CT, MR angiography, or MR venography may be critical to exclude aneurysm, vascular malformations, or cavernous sinus thrombosis.

INTRODUCTION

The sellar and parasellar region is complex, with a unique meningeal, neural, vascular, and bony anatomy. Understanding the imaging anatomy is critical for accurate imaging interpretation. Magnetic resonance (MR) imaging is the primary modality for pituitary imaging; however, computed tomography (CT) may be used when MR imaging is contraindicated, and provides complementary bony anatomic information. Both CT and MR angiography and/or venography aid vascular assessment and evaluate for aneurysms, vascular malformations, or cavernous sinus thrombosis. This article reviews embryology and anatomy of the sellar and parasellar region. Imaging appearances of the more commonly identified and clinically important disorders are discussed and illustrated.

EMBRYOLOGY OF THE PITUITARY GLAND

The hypothalamic-pituitary network arises at approximately 4 4weeks' gestation. The stomodeum invaginated ectoderm forms the pituitary anterior adenohypophysis, and this eventually fuses with the posterior neurohypophysis, arising via diencephalon neuroectoderm.[1–3] The stomodeum, a primitive oral cavity lined with ectoderm and neural elements at the pharyngeal vault, arises anterior to the buccopharyngeal membrane. The anterior median primitive neural plate cells leads to Rathke pouch formation from the oral ectoderm.[4,5] The Rathke pouch is a thin-walled vesicle lined by cuboidal epithelium evaginating with a stalk attached to the stomodeal vault. It extends via a bony canal, which normally regresses, but can persist as the craniopharyngeal canal, which may be associated with developmental abnormalities or craniopharyngiomas. At the sixth to eighth weeks of development, the Rathke pouch constricts at the base and separates from the oral epithelium. As the Rathke pouch extends upward, the posterior pituitary neurohypophysis is formed by evaginating magnocellular neurons from the third ventricular floor (supraoptic and paraventricular nuclei), creating a hypothalamohypophyseal tract. In addition, mesenchyme forms the sphenoid body (**Fig. 1A**). Pituitary development is completed by the end of the first trimester. Genetic mutations can result in abnormal pituitary migration with an ectopic posterior pituitary, resulting in an autosomal dominant diabetes insipidus (as

Department of Radiology, Northwell Health, Zucker Hofstra School of Medicine at Northwell Health, Northshore University Hospital, 300 Community Drive, New York, NY 11030, USA
E-mail address: cfekirsch@gmail.com

Neuroimag Clin N Am 31 (2021) 541–552
https://doi.org/10.1016/j.nic.2021.05.010

neuroimaging.theclinics.com

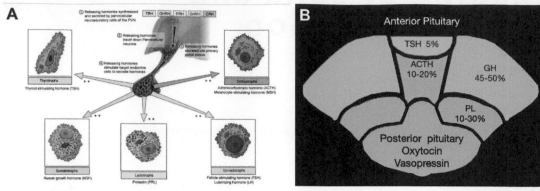

Fig. 1. (*A, B*) Pituitary adenohypophysis (anterior lobe) fuses with neurohypophysis (posterior lobe). (*A*) One trophic hormone, prolactin, acts directly on tissue to cause growth, whereas the remainder are tropic hormones stimulating organs to secrete activating hormones. (*B*) Cell type organization. ACTH, adrenocorticotropic hormone; GH, growth hormone; TSH, thyroid-stimulating hormone. ([*A*] © Informa UK Ltd (trading as Primal Pictures), 2021. Primal Pictures, an informa business www.primalpictures.com www.anatomy.tv.)

in Wolfram disease).[6] Signaling pathways allow differentiation of somatotrophs, lactotrophs and thyrotropes, corticotropes, and gonadotrophs.[7–11] The pouch of Sessel is a further invagination of the stomodeum posterior to the buccopharyngeal membrane, and this sometimes persists and becomes the source of tumors such as craniopharyngiomas.

Pituitary Anatomy and Hormonal Secretion

The anterior lobe (adenohypophysis) contains the pars distalis, which is responsible for most hormone production, and the pars tuberalis, a tubular sheath encasing the pituitary stalk (**Fig. 2**). The pars intermedia, which is located between the adenohypophysis and posterior pituitary, contains cells with a colloidal matrix, secreting melanocyte-stimulating hormone. The pituitary infundibulum or stalk also inserts between the 2 lobes. The pars tuberalis extends superiorly from the anterior

adenohypophysis, containing scant gonadotroph or corticotrophin cells, and encasing the anterior pars infundibularis. The pars infundibularis contains magnocellular supraoptic and paraventricular unmyelinated axons.

The anterior lobe (adenohypophysis) secretes a trophic hormone, prolactin (PRL), which acts directly on tissues. It also secretes 5 trophic hormones that stimulate other organs to secrete hormonal active substances: TSH (thyroid-stimulating hormone), FH and LH (follicular and luteinizing hormones), ACTH (adrenocorticotrophic hormone), and GH (growth hormone). The posterior pituitary neurohypophysis contains neurosecretory granules of antidiuretic hormone (ADH) or vasopressin, and oxytocin[12] (see **Fig. 2**B,C).

PITUITARY VASCULAR ANATOMY

The pituitary arteries comprise the superior hypophyseal artery (SHA) and inferior hypophyseal

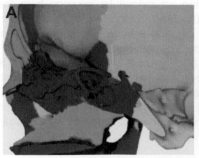
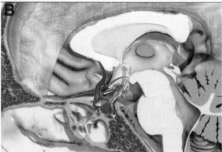
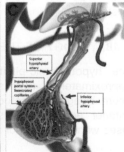

Fig. 2. (*A*) The sella turcica (*blue arrow*) with paired anterior and posterior clinoids, clivus posteriorly. Sphenoid sinus (*orange*) has variable pneumatization. (*B*) Pituitary gland (usually <1 cm in height) varies with hormonal alterations during puberty and pregnancy. (*C*) Vascular pituitary gland supplied by superior and inferior hypophyseal arteries forming anastomoses with glandular tissue adjacent to the hypophyseal portal venous fenestrated capillaries. (© Informa UK Ltd (trading as Primal Pictures), 2021. Primal Pictures, an informa business www.primalpictures.com www.anatomy.tv.)

artery (SHA) and the capsular, infundibular, pre-chiasmal, and posteroinferior hypophyseal arteries.[13]

The primary SHA (from the internal carotid artery [ICA]) branches to the superior infundibulum, optic nerves and optic chiasm, and superior adenohypophysis[13] (see Fig. 2B,C). The SHA creates a pre-infundibular anastomosis, with secondary SHAs supplying the infundibulum, tuber cinereum, optic tracts, and mamillary bodies.[13] Descending SHA branches supply the pars distalis, lower infundibulum, and posterior pituitary; however, it is controversial whether it supplies the anterior pituitary.[13,14] Descending branches also unite with infundibular and prechiasmal arteries, creating circum-infundibular anastomoses with ascending vessels to optic chiasm, tuber cinereum, and median eminence as well as descending branches to diaphragm sella and adenohypophysis.[13,14] Blood from the primary capillary network around the hypothalamus is transported via the hypophyseal portal system to the secondary capillary plexus surrounding the anterior pituitary. The pituitary cells are closely related to these hypophyseal portal fenestrated capillaries.[15–17] Animal models have shown there to be 2 portal vessel types with capillary anastomoses, allowing rapid hormone transfer into portal blood.[18,19]

The IHA supplies the posterior pituitary posterior and capsule, anastomosing with descending SHA and capsular arteries from the medial inferior cavernous ICAs.[13,14,20] Anastomoses between IHA and ICAs supply the anterior lobe and residual craniopharyngeal canal in the sphenoid sinus.[3,21,22] Posterior hypophyseal arteries anastomose with the ascending pharyngeal external carotid arteries, forming a posterior inferior hypophyseal and medial clival trunk network.[14]

Venous drainage is via hypophyseal veins that drain into the cavernous sinus.

SELLAR AND PARASELLAR ANATOMY

The midline sphenoid bone contains the sella turcica or Turkish saddle, a concavity with anterior and posterior clinoids. The tuberculum sella is anteriorly and the dorsum sella is posteriorly. Superior to the sella is the optic chiasm and the optic nerves.

Lateral to the sella is the cavernous sinus. This sinus is contained by meningeal and periosteal dura and limited laterally by the anterior petroclinoid ligament (see Fig. 2A,B; Figs. 3 and 4). The superior and lateral walls have 2 layers: a larger superficial smoother layer and an inner transparent layer, which encases the cranial nerves. The lateral, medial, and superior margins are meningeal dura, whereas the inferior margin is periorbital dura overlying the sphenoid bone.[23] The lateral wall comprises a thicker superficial layer and a thinner incomplete layer, which connects to cranial nerves III, IV, and V_1, wrapping nerves in a common meningeal sheath.[24] Cranial nerve VI is medial within the cavernous sinus. As it enters the cavernous sinus, it is fixed by endosteal dural adhesions, which sensitize the nerve to displacement by increased intracranial pressure.[25]

Posteromedial to the sella is the Meckel cave, a dural recess or pocket in the petrous apex trigeminal impression. Within the Meckel cave is the trigeminal (gasserian/semilunar) ganglion.[26]

IMAGING PROTOCOLS

MR imaging is the pituitary imaging modality of choice. If the sphenoid is well pneumatized, a

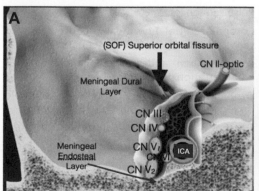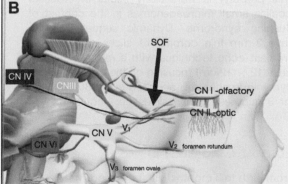

Fig. 3. The meninges, cavernous sinus cranial nerves (CNs), superior orbital fissure (SOF), and ICA. CN III, oculomotor nerve superior Edinger-Westphal nuclei controlling pupil in blue, motor portion in pink. Trochlear nerve CN IV below, CN VI medial, inferiorly first and second divisions of trigeminal nerve CN V. CN III, IV, V_1, and VI exit the superior orbital fissure (SOF), CN V_2 via foramen rotundum, CN V_3 via foramen ovale.

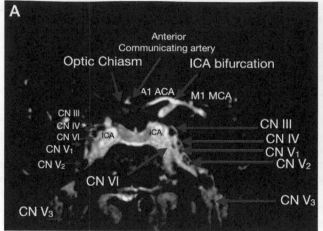
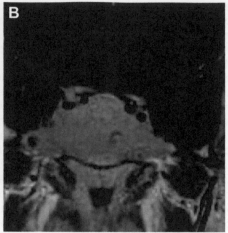

Fig. 4. (*A*, *B*) Coronal T1 gadolinium, pituitary, optic chiasm, vessel, CNs are hypointense relative to enhancing cavernous sinus. (*B*) Pituitary adenoma with cavernous sinus invasion. ACA, anterior cerebral artery; MCA, middle cerebral artery.

1.5-T system results in reduced susceptibility artifact from air-tissue interfaces. CT delineates bony structures and can be used when MR imaging is contraindicated.

Dedicated MR imaging pituitary protocols should include pre–gadolinium-enhanced and post–gadolinium-enhanced T1-weighted (T1w) sequences, with sagittal and coronal planes most beneficial, using 3-mm sections or volume sequences. To identify microadenomas, T2-weighted (T2w) coronal sequences may be useful. Fat-suppressed sequences may also be helpful in the context of adjacent fatty osseous marrow.

Because portal venous flow with fenestrated capillaries lacks a blood-brain barrier, there is rapid pituitary and infundibular enhancement.[27–29]

Dynamic imaging may increase the ability to identify microadenomas, because they enhance at slower rates than normal pituitary tissue.[27] This property is particularly useful in order to localize small microadenomas in the context of Cushing syndrome. Dynamic sequences may have 3-mm thin coronal T1 slices or a spoiled gradient echo technique with a reduced field of view (12 × 12 cm) focusing on the pituitary fossa. Dynamic images are acquired every 30 seconds for 3 minutes, with 5 slices per acquisition[27–31] (Box 1).

NORMAL IMAGING FINDINGS

From birth to 3 months, pituitary glands may measure 6 mm craniocaudally and show intrinsic T1 hyperintensity that gradually resolves.[32,33] Pituitary glands range from 5 to 9 mm in height, increasing in size during hormonal production in puberty, menarche, or pregnancy to 10 to 12 mm.[32,33] The pituitary can decrease in height in the setting of idiopathic intracranial hypertension, postpartum, pituitary apoplexy, and radiation therapy.[33–36] The anterior lobe of pituitary gland is isointense to gray matter on a T1w image, whereas the posterior pituitary shows T1w shortening and hyperintensity (likely from lipid vesicles containing ADH and oxytocin). This structure may be displaced by macroadenomas or tumors, and absence may signify diabetes insipidus.[33,36] The infundibulum can measure 3.5 mm at the median eminence, 2.8 mm at midportion, and 2 mm inferiorly. Although gadolinium contrast is used for

Box 1
Imaging protocols for the sella

Pulse sequences

Coronal, sagittal T1w ideally reduced field of view 3 mm/0 mm or volume sequence

Pregadolinium and postgadolinium contrast administration

Dynamic gadolinium-enhanced T1; multiple time points, 0, 30, 60, 90, 120, 180 seconds

Coronal T2 weighted; fat suppression helpful

Gadolinium administration: standard dose (0.1 mmol/kg body weight) for macroadenoma, reduced dose (0.05 mmol/kg body weight) for microadenoma

Brain sequences as per institutional protocol

MR or CT angiography; MR venography may be added to assess for vascular disorders

microadenoma identification, it can lead to nephrogenic systemic fibrosis and gadolinium deposition in the brain. Recent consensus guidelines in Europe suggest reducing gadolinium doses to 0.05 mmol/kg body weight and to follow up conservatively managed macroadenomas with noncontrast sequences on MR imaging.[37]

PATHOLOGIC IMAGING FINDINGS
Pituitary Adenomas

The 2 most common disorders of the sella are pituitary adenomas and Rathke cleft cysts.[38] An intrasellar adenoma smaller than 1 cm is termed a microadenoma, whereas an intrasellar tumor larger than 1 cm is referred to as a mesoadenoma. When there is extrasellar extension, an adenoma more than 1 cm is referred to as a macroadenoma, whereas the subgroup larger than 4 cm are termed giant adenomas. Hormone-producing adenomas are considered functional and endocrinologically active, whereas non–hormone-producing adenomas are nonfunctional. The most common hormone-secreting tumors are prolactinomas, occurring in approximately 30% of cases.[27,28,33,38–40]

Microadenomas are generally T1w hypointense relative to pituitary. The T1w signal may be increased because of hemorrhagic or proteinaceous products, with hemorrhage most often occurring in prolactinomas, either spontaneously or after medication treatment.

On T2w sequences, a microadenoma may be hyperintense or hypointense (**Fig. 5**). In acromegaly with excess GH, decreased T2 signal is seen in 40% to 60% of granulated GH adenomas, likely reflecting adenomas' increased density, and this may be a useful clue to diagnosis[38–41] Tumors with lower T2w signal tend to be firmer, adherent, and more difficult to surgically remove. Increased T2w signal may reflect softer cystic tumors.[7] Pituitary infundibulum is usually deviated away from the adenoma toward the residual pituitary gland.

The extrasellar extension of macroadenomas is also defined with imaging. Larger tumors often have cystic elements that are T2w hyperintense and frequently a multilobulated morphology. Approximately 80% of pituitary tumors extend superiorly through the sella into the suprasellar cistern, with confinement by the diaphragmatic sella creating a snowman shape.[38–42] Sellar and suprasellar extension compress optic nerves and

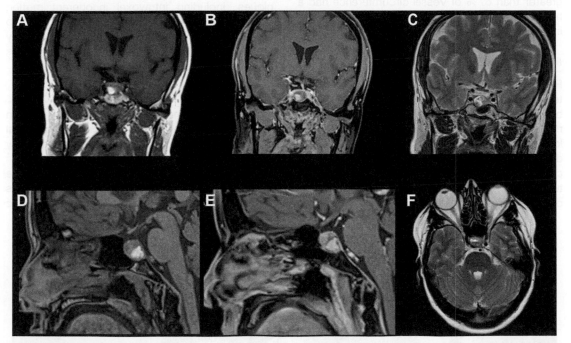

Fig. 5. (*A*) Coronal T1 MR imaging, (*B*) coronal T1 contrast fat saturation, (*C*) coronal T2 (*D*) sagittal T1 without contrast, (*E*) sagittal T1 with contrast, (*F*) axial T2. A 48-year-old woman with a hemorrhagic pituitary prolactinoma. (*A, B, C*) Intrinsic T1 hyperintensity (likely hemorrhagic), heterogenous T2w signal and additional poorly enhancing components with leftward infundibular deviation. (*D, E*) Sagittal T1 pregadolinium and postgadolinium contrast images show foci of intrinsic T1 hyperintensity and the enhancing displaced pituitary. (*F*) Axial T2 image shows a fluid-fluid level.

chiasm, causing bitemporal hemianopsia.[27,28] Up to 20% of pituitary tumors may extend into the sphenoid sinus, dorsum sella, or cavernous sinuses.[28,38–40] Imaging should identify the infundibulum, posterior pituitary, and residual pituitary preoperatively.

Lateral tumor extension can result in cavernous sinus invasion, occurring in 5% to 10% of tumors, with increasing difficulty for complete resection and with a higher likelihood of tumor residual and recurrence.[27–30,38,40–42] The delineation of meningeal layers encasing the pituitary, cavernous sinus, and cranial nerves is controversial, with research suggesting an outer dural layer with a thin inner lamina propria layer.[42–48] The determination of gland encasement may shed light on macroadenoma growth because expansion may reflect cellularity and not necessarily cavernous sinus anatomic or histologic defects.[42] It is controversial whether adenoma growth laterally is invasive, expansive, or aggressive.[42] A system describes the tumor relationship to lines along the intracavernous and supracavernous ICAs in the coronal plane, rating invasion from 0 to 4. Tumor beyond the intercarotid line (grade 2) is highly correlated with cavernous sinus invasion and tumor size at surgery[49] (see **Fig. 4**). Other investigators found that a degree of carotid encasement greater than 67% of vessel circumference had a high positive predictive value of cavernous sinus invasion of 100%.[50]

Rathke Cleft Cysts

Rathke cleft cysts (see **Fig. 7B**), sometimes termed pars intermedia cysts, were first described by Luschka in 1860.[51] They are congenital, benign, midline, unilocular cystic remnants of the embryologic Rathke pouch along the craniopharyngeal duct, developing as cystic lesions from the columnar cuboidal cells, typically between the pituitary anterior and posterior lobes. They may demonstrate an egg-in-cup configuration because

they are interposed between the 2 lobes and are hence distinguished from arachnoid cysts. They may show increased T1w signal and T2w hypointense intracystic nodules with absent or very thin wall enhancement. If there is suprasellar extension, it is usually along the ventral pituitary stalk, and the cysts are occasionally located just anterior to the infundibulum along the superior surface of the gland. Unlike craniopharyngiomas, they should not show calcification. They are asymptomatic in 17% of healthy individuals with brain imaging.[51] Clinical presentation with headaches, endocrine dysfunction, and visual disturbances are reported, with 20% recurring after resection.[39,51,52]

Meningiomas

Meningiomas are the second most common sellar and parasellar tumor and arise from arachnoid cap cells. Approximately 5% to 10% of meningiomas arise in the sellar and parasellar regions, involving either the tuberculum or diaphragma sellae, sphenoid wing, cavernous sinus, planum sphenoidale, or petroclival confluence[53–56] (**Fig. 6**). Meningiomas are usually isointense to gray matter on T1w and T2w images and markedly enhance. Associated CT features include bony hyperostosis or an enlarged sphenoid sinus, referred to as pneumosinus dilatans. Newer MR imaging techniques, including intravoxel incoherent motion and diffusion-weighted imaging (DWI), may help grade tumors.[57] Incomplete resections may require adjuvant treatments, such as Gamma Knife therapy.[58]

Craniopharyngiomas

Craniopharyngiomas are histologically benign grade I tumors, arising from craniopharyngeal duct epithelial cells. They represent approximately 2% to 5% of primary intracranial tumors.[59–61] Although their cause is unknown, theories include development from embryonic squamous cell rests along the craniopharyngeal duct, or metaplastic

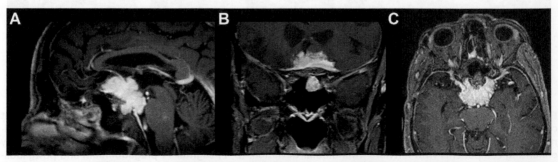

Fig. 6. (A) Sagittal, (B) coronal, (C) axial T1 postgadolinium MR imaging shows a planum sphenoidale, sellar, and suprasellar meningioma with bony hyperostosis and pneumosinus dilatans of the right sphenoid sinus.

transformation of adenohypophyseal or infundibulum cells.[62,63] The 2 major histologic subtypes are adamantinomatous craniopharyngioma (ACP) and papillary craniopharyngioma (PCP), with transitional and mixed forms occurring. Tumor chromosomal translocations and deletions, including beta-catenin gene mutations are found in the ACP variant.[64,65] Craniopharyngiomas have a bimodal distribution, with ACP presenting in pediatric patients at 5 to 16 years, whereas PCP presents in patients 45 to 60 years of age. ACP tumors are 90% to 95% suprasellar and only rarely intrasellar, but many are a large (>2 cm) and extend inferiorly to the sella. They are often cystic with solid components, with calcifications in 90%. Children with the ACP subtype may present with headache, vomiting, and papilledema, or pituitary hypofunction.[33,39,64,65] Squamous papillary tumors (which may harbor somatic $BRAF^{V600E}$ mutations) have a mixed histopathology and are more solid.[66–69] Hence the imaging appearances of the 2 subtypes can be differentiated. ACP follows the 90% rule: 90% are predominantly cystic, have notable calcifications, and have contrast enhancement of cyst margins, whereas PCPs are often solid and noncalcified.[66–69]

Arachnoid Cysts

Intra-arachnoid cysts are uncommon nonneoplastic fluid collections representing approximately 1% of intracranial masses.[70–72] The exact cause is unknown, but it is speculated that a ball valve mechanism allows cerebrospinal fluid (CSF) to enter through the diaphragma sella.[70] Surgical morbidity may be higher than with pituitary adenomas, with secondary infection, fistula formation,

and blindness.[72] On imaging, there is sella turcica expansion with CSF MR imaging signal and CT attenuation, but without enhancement or calcification (**Fig. 7**A). DWI follows CSF signal.[73] The differential diagnosis includes intrasellar arachnoid herniation (empty sella), atypical Rathke cleft cyst, cystic adenoma, or craniopharyngioma.[72] Intra-arachnoid cysts may displace the pituitary inferiorly and posteriorly, as opposed to Rathke cleft cysts, which splay the anterior and posterior lobes (**Fig. 7**B).

Aneurysms

Sellar and parasellar aneurysms can present with headache, visual defects, endocrinopathy, and cranial nerve palsies (**Fig. 8**). Sellar aneurysms are uncommon, representing 1% to 2% of intracranial aneurysms. Interestingly, intracranial aneurysm are found to coexist with pituitary adenomas in 2.3% to 6.9% of patients, a prevalence greater than in the average population.[74] Accurate preoperative delineation is critical to avoid inadvertent surgery with potential morbidity and mortality. Imaging may be altered by calcification or aneurysmal thrombus, and MR imaging appearances may be complex because of lamellated blood degradation products and flow-related signal. They are usually eccentrically located within the sella. CT angiography, MR angiography, or cerebral angiography aid the diagnosis.

Infectious and Inflammatory Lesions

Invasive fungal sinusitis may spread from the paranasal sinuses to the skull base. Angioinvasive fungal species such as *Aspergillus* produce elastase enzymes that disrupt arterial walls, leading

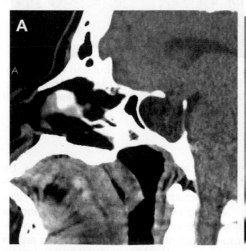
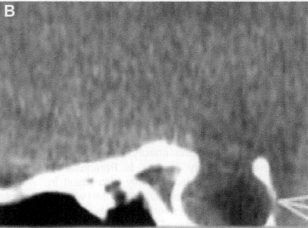

Fig. 7. (*A*) Sagittal CT scan of sellar arachnoid cyst enlarging the sella turcica and displacing pituitary posteriorly. (*B*) Rathke cleft cyst with anterior lobe of pituitary displaced anteriorly.

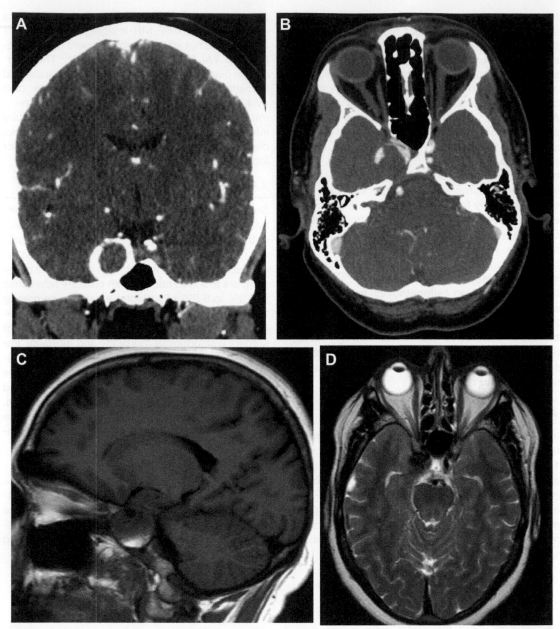

Fig. 8. (*A*) Coronal, (*B*) axial CT angiography of right cavernous ICA aneurysm with thrombus and rim calcification, right globe medial deviation, with right lateral rectus muscle denervation atrophy. (*C*) Sagittal T1 MR imaging, partially thrombosed right cavernous ICA giant aneurysm. (*D*) Axial T2 shows a right ICA giant aneurysm coil mass causing susceptibility.

to pseudoaneurysm and aneurysms, with high morbidity and mortality[75,76] (**Fig. 9**). Paranasal sinus and skull base infection may also result in cavernous sinus thrombosis, and CT or MR venography may help assess cavernous sinus enlargement with thrombosis. DWI may delineate abscesses containing diffusion-restricting pus and hyperintense DWI signal.[77]

The sellar and suprasellar region may be affected by inflammatory conditions such as neurosarcoid, immunoglobulin (Ig) G4–related disease, and granulomatosis with polyangiitis (formerly Wegener granulomatosis). These conditions more frequently involve the parasellar region and are usually of intermediate to decreased T2w signal. Although serology (eg, antineutrophil

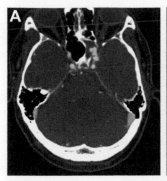 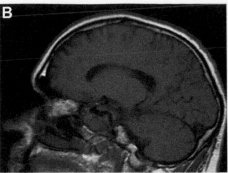 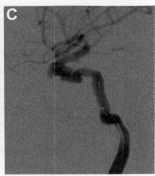

Fig. 9. (A) Axial CT angiography, (B) sagittal T1 MR imaging in a 78-year-old patient with left sphenoid sinus chronic aspergillosis infection with dehiscent left lateral sphenoid bony margin and multiple left cavernous ICA pseudoaneurysms. (C) Sagittal cerebral angiography with multiple lobulated pseudoaneurysms; during neurointerventional treatment to prevent rupture.

cytoplasmic antibodies and IgG4 levels) may be helpful for diagnosis, biopsy may be required.

Pituitary Apoplexy

Pituitary apoplexy is an uncommon clinical syndrome, secondary to infarction or hemorrhage in a pituitary adenoma, possibly caused by outgrowing of the blood supply. Although rare (2%–12% of pituitary adenomas), it may be life threatening because of corticotropic hormone deficiency if left untreated.[78] Presentation includes acute headache, visual disturbance or ocular palsies, emesis, and fatigue. On CT, there may be increased density, whereas MR imaging shows variable T1 and T2 signal depending on blood product stages.[78]

Imaging assessment of a sella and parasellar lesion.

Identify normal anatomy: pituitary anterior and posterior lobes (increased T1w signal) and midline infundibulum.

Assess adjacent structures: optic apparatus, third ventricle, cavernous sinus invasion.

Determine whether disorder arises from the pituitary gland or extrasellar location (eg, suprasellar, para sellar, clivus). Extrasellar lesions are less likely to expand the sella, and the pituitary gland may be identified separately.

Imaging characteristics: solid, cystic (fluid-fluid levels), calcification, low T2 signal, evidence of blood degradation products.

Are there anatomic variants that could affect the surgical approach?

Differential diagnosis

Congenital

Pituitary hypoplasia, Rathke cleft cysts, arachnoid cysts, pars intermedia cysts, persistent craniopharyngeal canal or skull base anomalies

Neoplastic: primary or secondary

Pituitary adenomas (microadenomas<10 mm, macroadenomas>10 mm)

Meningiomas

Craniopharyngiomas

Dermoid and epidermoid tumors

Germ cell tumors

Hypothalamic hamartomas

Pituicytoma, tancytoma, granular cell tumor

Metastases especially to infundibulum; leukemia or lymphoma

Schwannomas from cranial nerves of cavernous sinus

Optic or chiasmatic gliomas

Langerhans histiocytosis

Clival tumors, including chondromas, chondrosarcomas

Adjacent paranasal sinus tumors in the sphenoid region

Inflammatory/infectious

Infundibular neurohypophysitis

Pituitary abscess

Invasive sinus infections, including fungal

Vascular lesions

Aneurysms

Pituitary apoplexy

Cavernous sinus thrombosis

Vascular malformations

Rare intrasellar cavernous hemangioma

Pearls, pitfalls, and variants: what referring physicians need to know (clinics care points)

Use dedicated imaging protocols with reduced field of view

Sagittal and coronal T1 precontrast and postcontrast and coronal T2 sequences are useful

Pituitary adenomas and Rathke cleft cysts are the most common sellar lesions

Pediatric adamantinomatous subtype craniopharyngiomas are among the most common nonglial tumors and follow the 90% rule: suprasellar, containing calcifications, and having rim enhancement

Hemorrhagic pituitary apoplexy can be life threatening from endocrinopathy and should be treated emergently

Be wary of vascular mimics; CT angiography or MR angiography may help delineate

DISCLOSURE

C.F.E. Kirsch: consultant for Primal Pictures 3D Anatomy; royalties from Informa.

REFERENCES

1. McCabe MJ, Dattani MT. Genetic aspects of hypothalamic and pituitary gland development. Handb Clin Neurol 2014;124:3–15.

2. Bancalari RE, Gregory LC, McCabe MJ, et al. Pituitary gland development: an update. Endocr Dev 2012;23:1–15.

3. Musumeci G, Castorina S, Castrogiovanni P, et al. A journey through the pituitary gland: Development, structure and function, with emphasis on embryofoetal and later development. Acta Histochem 2015;117(4–5):355–66.

4. Bhattacharyya S, Bronner ME. Clonal analyses in the anterior pre-placodal region: implications for the early lineage bias of placodal progenitors. Int J Dev Biol 2013;57(9–10):753–7.

5. Suga H, Kadoshima T, Minaguchi M, et al. Self-formation of functional adenohypophysis in three-dimensional culture. Nature 2011;480(7375): 57–62.

6. di Iorgi N, Secco A, Napoli F, et al. Developmental abnormalities of the posterior pituitary gland. Endocr Dev 2009;14:83–94.

7. Zhang Shu, et al. Single-cell transcriptomics identifies divergent developmental lineage trajectories during human pituitary development. Nat Commun 2020;11:1–5275.

8. Andoniadou CL, et al. Sox2(+) stem/progenitor cells in the adult mouse pituitary support organ homeostasis and have tumor-inducing potential. Cell Stem Cell 2013;13:433–45.

9. Rizzoti K, Akiyama H, Lovell-Badge R. Mobilized adult pituitary stem cells contribute to endocrine regeneration in response to physiological demand. Cell Stem Cell 2013;13:419–32.

10. Amar AP, Weiss MH. Pituitary anatomy and physiology. Neurosurg Clin N Am 2003;14(1):11–23, v.

11. Baik JS, Lee MH, Ahn KJ, et al. Characteristic location and growth patterns of functioning pituitary adenomas: correlation with histological distribution of hormone-secreting cells in the pituitary gland. Clin Imaging 2015;39(5):770–4.

12. Larkin S, Ansorge O. Development And Microscopic Anatomy Of The Pituitary Gland. [Updated 2017 Feb 15]. In: Feingold KR, Anawalt B, Boyce A, et al, editors. Endotext [Internet]. South Dartmouth (MA): MDText.com, Inc.; 2000. p. 1–8.

13. Truong HQ, Najera E, Zanabria-Ortiz R, et al. Surgical anatomy of the superior hypophyseal artery and its relevance for endoscopic endonasal surgery. J Neurosurg 2018;131(1):154–62.

14. Cironi KA, Decater T, Iwanaga J, et al. Arterial Supply to the Pituitary Gland: A Comprehensive Review. World Neurosurg 2020;142:206–11.

15. Nakane PK. Classifications of anterior pituitary cell types with immunoenzyme histochemistry. J Histochem Cytochem 1970;18(1):9–20.

16. Moriarty GC. Adenohypophysis: ultrastructural cytochemistry. A review. J Histochem Cytochem 1973; 21(10):855–94.

17. Gross PM, Joneja MG, Pang JJ, et al. Topography of short portal vessels in the rat pituitary gland: a scanning electron-microscopic and morphometric study of corrosion cast replicas. Cell Tissue Res 1993; 272(1):79–88.

18. Cheng Y, Zhang H, Su L, et al. Anatomical study of cavernous segment of the internal carotid artery and its relationship to the structures in sella region. J Craniofac Surg 2013;24(2):622–5.

19. Tuccar E, Uz A, Tekdemir I, et al. Anatomical study of the lateral wall of the cavernous sinus, emphasizing dural construction and neural relations. Neurosurg Rev 2000;23(1):45–8.

20. Truong HQ, et al. Bilateral coagulation of inferior hypophyseal artery and pituitary transposition during

endoscopic endonasal interdural posterior clinoidectomy: do they affect pituitary function? J Neurosurg 2018;131(1):141–6.

21. Gorczyca W, Hardy J. Arterial supply of the human anterior pituitary gland. Neurosurgery 1987;20(3): 369–78.

22. Gibo H, Lenkey C, Rhoton AL Jr. Microsurgical anatomy of the supraclinoid portion of the internal carotid artery. J Neurosurg 1981;55(4):560–74.

23. Kawase T, van Loveren H, Keller JT, et al. Meningeal architecture of the cavernous sinus: clinical and surgical implications. Neurosurgery 1996;39(3):527–34 [discussion: 534–6].

24. Sabancı PA, Batay F, Civelek E, et al. Meckel's cave. World Neurosurg 2011;76(3–4):335–41 [discussion: 266–7].

25. Go JL, Rajamohan AG. Imaging of the Sella and Parasellar Region. Radiol Clin North Am 2017;55(1): 83–101.

26. Umansky F, Elidan J, Valarezo A. Dorello's canal: a microanatomical study. J Neurosurg 1991;75(2): 294–8.

27. Chapman PR, Singhal A, Gaddamanugu S, et al. Neuroimaging of the Pituitary Gland: Practical Anatomy and Pathology. Radiol Clin North Am 2020; 58(6):1115–33.

28. Grober Y, Grober H, Wintermark M, et al. Comparison of MRI techniques for detecting microadenomas in Cushing's disease. J Neurosurg 2018;128(4): 1051–7.

29. Bladowska J, Sasiadek M. Diagnostic imaging of the pituitary and parasellar region. In: Rahimi-Movaghar V, editor. Pituitary adenomas. Rijeka, Croatia: InTechOpen Europe; 2012. p. 1323–32.

30. Chowdhury IN, Sinaii N, Oldfield EH, et al. A change in pituitary magnetic resonance imaging protocol detects ACTH-secreting tumours in patients with previously negative results. Clin Endocrinol (Oxf) 2010;72(4):502–6.

31. Pisaneschi M, Kapoor G. Imaging the sella and parasellar region. Neuroimaging Clin N Am 2005;15(1): 203–19.

32. Lucas JW, Zada G. Imaging of the pituitary and parasellar region. Semin Neurol 2012;32(4):320–31.

33. Kirsch C. Pseudotumor cerebri syndrome (PCTS) - Losing sight in patients and doctors with regards to a growing epidemic. Clin Imaging 2018;51:vii–viii.

34. Kirsch CF, Black K. Diplopia: What to Double Check in Radiographic Imaging of Double Vision. Radiol Clin North Am 2017;55(1):69–81.

35. Rennert J, Doerfler A. Imaging of sellar and parasellar lesions. Clin Neurol Neurosurg 2007;109(2):111–24.

36. Hess CP, Dillon WP. Imaging the pituitary and parasellar region. Neurosurg Clin N Am 2012;23(4): 529–42.

37. Kucharczyk W, Truwit CL. Diseases of the Sella Turcica and Parasellar Region. 2020 Feb 15. In:

38. Hodler J, Kubik-Huch RA, von Schulthess GK, editors. Diseases of the brain, Head and Neck, spine 2020–2023: Diagnostic imaging [Internet]. Cham (CH): Springer; 2020. Chapter 1.

38. Lundin P, Nyman R, Burman P, et al. MRI of pituitary macroadenomas with reference to hormonal activity. Neuroradiology 1992;34(1):43–51.

39. Lersy F, et al. Consensus Guidelines of the French Society of Neuroradiology (SFNR) on the use of Gadolinium-Based Contrast agents (GBCAs) and related MRI protocols in Neuroradiology. J Neuroradiol 2020;47(6):441–9.

40. Hagiwara A, Inoue Y, Wakasa K, et al. Comparison of growth hormone-producing and non-growth hormone-producing pituitary adenomas: imaging characteristics and pathologic correlation. Radiology 2003;228(2):533–8.

41. Songtao Q, Yuntao L, Jun P, et al. Membranous layers of the pituitary gland: histological anatomic study and related clinical issues. Neurosurgery 2009;64(3 Suppl):ons1–9 [discussion: ons9-10].

42. Destrieux C, Kakou MK, Velut S, et al. Microanatomy of the hypophyseal fossa boundaries. J Neurosurg 1998;88(4):743–52.

43. Dolenc VV. Relation of the cavernous sinus to the sella. In: Dolenc VV, editor. Anatomy and surgery of the cavernous sinus. Vienna: Springer- Verlag; 1989. p. 118–30.

44. Yokoyama S, Hirano H, Moroki K, et al. Are nonfunctioning pituitary adenomas extending into the cavernous sinus aggressive and/or invasive? Neurosurgery 2001;49:857–63.

45. Peker S, Kurtkaya-Yapicier O, Kiliç T, et al. Microsurgical anatomy of the lateral walls of the pituitary fossa. Acta Neurochir (Wien) 2005;147:641–9.

46. Yasuda A, Campero A, Martins C, et al. The medial wall of cavernous sinus: Microsurgical anatomy. Neurosurgery 2004;55:179–90.

47. Chi JG, Lee MH. Anatomical observations of the development of the pituitary capsule. J Neurosurg 1980;52:667–70.

48. Knosp E, Steiner E, Kitz K, et al. Pituitary adenomas with invasion of the cavernous sinus space: A magnetic resonance imaging classification compared with surgical findings. Neurosurgery 1993;33:610–8.

49. Cottier JP, Destrieux CD, Brunereau L, et al. Cavernous sinus invasion by pituitary adenoma: MR imaging. Radiology 2000;215:463–9.

50. Han SJ, Rolston JD, Jahangiri A, et al. Rathke's cleft cysts: review of natural history and surgical outcomes. J Neurooncol 2014;117(2):197–203.

51. Voelker JL, Campbell RL, Muller J. Clinical, radiographic, and pathological features of symptomatic Rathke's cleft cysts. J Neurosurg 1991;74:535–44.

52. Chin BM, Orlandi RR, Wiggins RH 3rd. Evaluation of the sellar and parasellar regions. Magn Reson Imaging Clin N Am 2012;20(3):515–43.

53. Tian Z, et al. Radiomic Analysis of Craniopharyng-ioma and Meningioma in the Sellar/Parasellar Area with MR Images Features and Texture Features: A Feasible Study. Contrast media Mol Imaging 2020; 2020:4837156.

54. Kotecha RS, Pascoe EM, Rushing EJ, et al. Meningi-omas in children and adolescents: a meta-analysis of individual patient data. Lancet Oncol 2011; 12(13):1229–39.

55. Ostrom QT, Gittleman H, Liao P, et al. CBTRUS sta-tistical Report: primary brain and other central ner-vous system tumors diagnosed in the United States in 2010–2014. Neuro Oncol 2017;19(suppl_5):v1–88.

56. Yiping L, Kawai S, Jianbo W, et al. Evaluation param-eters between intra-voxel incoherent motion and diffusion-weighted imaging in grading and differen-tiating histological subtypes of meningioma: A pro-spective pilot study. J Neurol Sci 2017;372:60–9.

57. Sheehan JP, Starke RM, Kano H, et al. Gamma Knife radiosurgery for sellar and parasellar meningiomas: a multicenter study. J Neurosurg 2014;120(6): 1268–77.

58. Kleihnes P, Burger P, Scheithauer B. Histological typing of tumours of the central nervous system. WHO international histological classification of tu-mours. Springer-VerlangHeidelberg; 1993 (Germany).

59. Karavitaki N, Wass JA. Craniopharyngiomas. Endo-crinol Metab Clin North Am 2008;37(1):173–93. ix-x.

60. Parisi JE, Mena H. Nonglial tumours. In: Nelson JS, Parisi JE, Schochet SS Jr, editors. Principles and practice of neuropathology. 1st edition. St. Louis (MO): Mosby; 1993. p. 203–66.

61. Hunter IJ. Squamous metaplasia of cells of the ante-rior pituitary gland. J Pathol Bacteriol 1955;69: 141–5.

62. Asa SL, Kovacs K, Bilbao JM. The pars tuberalis of the human pituitary: a histologic, immunohistochem-ical, ultrastructural and immunoelectron microscopic analysis. Virchows Arch A Pathol Anat Histopathol 1983;399:49–59.

63. Sekine S, Shibata T, Kokubu A, et al. Craniopharyng-ioma of adamantinomatous type harbor β-catenin gene mutations. Am J Pathol 2002;161:1997–2001.

64. Eldevik OP, Blaivas M, Gabrielsen TO, et al. Cranio-pharyngioma: radiologic and histologic findings and recurrence. AJNR Am J Neuroradiol 1996;17: 1427–39.

65. Müller HL, Merchant TE, Warmuth-Metz M, et al. Cra-niopharyngioma. Nat Rev Dis Primers 2019;5(1):75.

66. Brastianos PK, et al. Exome sequencing identifies BRAF mutations in papillary craniopharyngiomas. Nat Genet 2014;46:161–5.

67. Goschzik T, et al. Genomic alterations of adamanti-nomatous and papillary craniopharyngioma. J Neuropathol Exp Neurol 2017;76:126–34.

68. Haston S, et al. MAPK pathway control of stem cell proliferation and differentiation in the embryonic pi-tuitary provides insights into the pathogenesis of papillary craniopharyngioma. Development 2017; 144:2141–52.

69. Castle-Kirszbaum MD, Uren B, King J, et al. Glimpse into Pathophysiology of Sellar Arachnoid Cysts. World Neurosurg 2018;119:381–3.

70. Cincu R, Agrawal A, Eiras J. Intracranial arachnoid cysts: current concepts and treatment alternatives. Clin Neurol Neurosurg 2007;109(10):837–43.

71. Dubuisson AS, Stevenaert A, Martin DH, et al. Intra-sellar arachnoid cysts. Neurosurgery 2007;61(3): 505–13 [discussion: 513].

72. Huo CW, Caputo C, Wang YY. Suprasellar keratinous cyst: A case report and review on its radiological features and treatment outcome. Surg Neurol Int 2018;9:15.

73. Oh MC, Kim EH, Kim SH. Coexistence of intracranial aneurysm in 800 patients with surgically confirmed pituitary adenoma. J Neurosurg 2012;116(5):942–7.

74. Horten B, Abbott G, Porro R. Fungal aneurysms of intracranial vessels. Arch Neurol 1976;33:577–9.

75. Rhodes J, Bode R, McCuan-Kirsch C. Elastase pro-duction in clinical isolates of Aspergillus. Diagn Mi-crobiol Infect Dis 1988;10:165–70.

76. Hurst RW, Judkins A, Bolger W, et al. Mycotic aneu-rysm and cerebral infarction resulting from fungal sinusitis: imaging and pathologic correlation. AJNR Am J Neuroradiol 2001;22(5):858–63.

77. Fenstermaker R, Abad A. Imaging of Pituitary and Parasellar Disorders. Continuum (Minneap Minn) 2016;22(5, Neuroimaging):1574–94.

78. Barkhoudarian G, Kelly DF. Pituitary Apoplexy. Neu-rosurg Clin N Am 2019;30(4):457–63.

Imaging Anatomy and Pathology of the Intracranial and Intratemporal Facial Nerve

Burce Ozgen Mocan, MD

KEYWORDS

- Facial nerve • Facial nerve palsy • Bell's palsy • Hemifacial spasm • Facial nerve canal

KEY POINTS

- The facial nerve has a complex course from the brainstem to the extracranial soft tissues, with a tortuous and long intratemporal segment.
- A variety of congenital, inflammatory, vascular, and neoplastic processes may affect each segment.
- Knowledge of the complex anatomy of the facial nerve is essential to localize the site of the disorder.
- Computed tomography (CT) and magnetic resonance (MR) studies are complementary but MR imaging is the modality of choice for most segments, whereas CT is reserved to assess the petrous facial nerve canal.

INTRODUCTION

The facial nerve is one of the most complex cranial nerves (CNs) and is responsible for facial expression, lacrimation, salivation, and taste. It is also one of the most commonly paralyzed nerves in the body and its palsy gets early attention because of its role in facial expression. Facial neuropathy has numerous and varied causes, including congenital, traumatic, vascular, inflammatory, and neoplastic processes. Many of those disorders can now be identified on imaging with the increased resolution of imaging studies and new magnetic resonance (MR) sequences. In addition, there are congenital anomalies and variations that may or may not be symptomatic but play a crucial role in the setting of surgical planning to avoid complications.

Appropriate imaging of the facial nerve requires detailed knowledge of its anatomy and recognition of the imaging features of the wide spectrum of pathologic processes that may affect this nerve.

NORMAL ANATOMY

The CN VII, also known as the facial nerve, is one of the most complex CNs with motor, sensory, and parasympathetic fibers (Fig. 1).[1,2]

The nerve is composed of a large motor root, containing motor fibers, and a smaller somatosensory root (containing sensory and parasympathetic fibers) called the nervus intermedius (NI).[1,3] The facial nerve has several different parts with multiple connections, but the overall course can be simplified and summarized as in Fig. 2.[4]

Intra-axial Segment

The fibers arising from 3 different nuclei, located in the pontine tegmentum, form the motor root and the NI (Fig. 3, Table 1).[1,5–8] The facial nerve fibers exit the pontomedullary sulcus at the root exit point (RExP) but they remain strongly adherent to the surface of the pons (as the attached segment), before separating from the brainstem. After this

Department of Radiology, University of Illinois at Chicago, 1740 West Taylor Street, MC 931, Chicago, IL 60612, USA
E-mail address: bozgen2@uic.edu
Twitter: @burceozgen (B.O.M.)

Neuroimag Clin N Am 31 (2021) 553–570
https://doi.org/10.1016/j.nic.2021.06.001
1052-5149/21/© 2021 Elsevier Inc. All rights reserved.

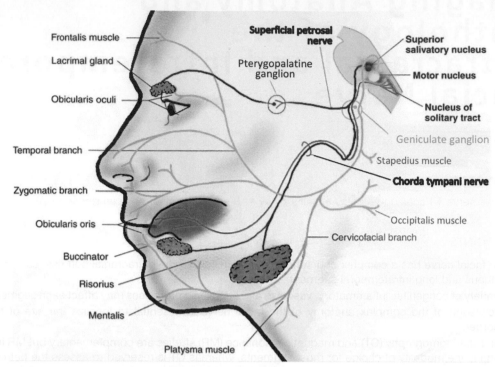

Fig. 1. The facial nerve components and its terminal branches.

root detachment point, a transition zone (TZ) is seen (where oligodendrocyte-derived central myelin is replaced by the peripheral Schwann cell–derived myelin). All the segments from the RExP to the TZ form the root exit zone (REZ) of the facial nerve.[9]

Cisternal Segment

After the REZ, the motor root (facial nerve proper) and the NI course through the cerebellopontine angle (CPA), toward the porus of the internal auditory canal (IAC) (see **Fig. 3**; **Fig. 4**). The NI (thinner than the motor part because it has fewer fibers)

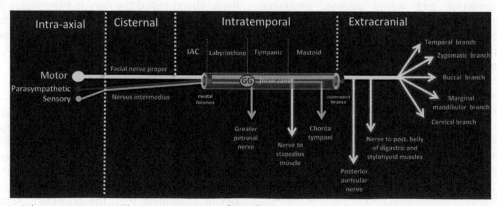

Fig. 2. Facial nerve segments. The nerve originates from the brainstem nuclei (intra-axial segment), traverses the cerebellopontine angle (cisternal segment) to enter the temporal bone (intratemporal segment). Within the temporal bone, it courses within the internal auditory canal (IAC) (canalicular/meatal segment), and then enters the facial/fallopian canal where it has a very convoluted, Z-shaped course (consisting of labyrinthine, geniculate, tympanic, and mastoid segments). It then exits through the stylomastoid foramen into the extracranial soft tissues (extracranial segment). GG, geniculate ganglion. (*Adapted from* Chung R, Dorros S, Mafee MF. Imaging of facial nerve pathology. *Operative Techniques in Otolaryngology-Head and Neck Surgery.* 2014;25(1):58-65; with permission.)

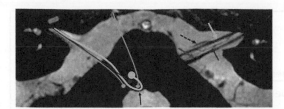

Fig. 3. The facial nuclei and components of the facial nerve in the cisternal and canalicular segments. The estimated location of the motor nucleus (*yellow*), superior salivatory nucleus (*orange*), and nucleus tractus solitarius (*green*) on the axial DRIVE (driven equilibrium radio frequency reset pulse) sequence. The facial nerve proper (*yellow arrow*) and the NI (*orange arrow*) are seen anterior to the cochleovestibular nerve (*purple arrow*). The motor fibers of facial nerve loop around the nucleus of the abducens nerve (*blue*), producing a small bulge at the floor of the fourth ventricle known as the facial colliculus (*black arrow*). An anterior and inferior cerebellar artery loop (*dashed arrow*) is seen extending into the left IAC. (*Adapted from* Harnsberger, H. R., Hudgins, P. A., Koch, B. L., Hamilton, B. E. (2016). Diagnostic Imaging: Head and Neck. United States: Elsevier Health Sciences; with permission from Elsevier.)

can be identified as it courses between the facial nerve proper and CN VIII (see **Fig. 3**).[8] The anterior and inferior cerebellar artery (AICA) usually loops more or less deeply in the CPA and can extend into the IAC (see **Fig. 3**).

Intratemporal Segment

The different segments of the intratemporal facial nerve are summarized in **Table 2**.[10]

Canalicular segment
This is the segment of the nerve within the IAC (see **Fig. 4**).[4] At the fundus of the IAC, the facial nerve enters a bony canal called the facial canal/fallopian canal. The zone of transition between the IAC and the facial canal is the narrowest part of the bony facial canal.[11] Furthermore, at this location the nerve is only covered by pial and arachnoid membranes because the dural lining terminates at the fundus of the IAC.[3] This focal narrowing and thin covering is the reason the meatal segment is the most common site of facial nerve injury when the nerve is swollen from an inflammation such as Bell's palsy (BP) or Ramsay Hunt syndrome.[3]

Labyrinthine segment
This first segment of the facial canal is the shortest and the narrowest segment of the canal (**Fig. 5A, D**).

Geniculate ganglion
The term geniculate (from the Latin meaning knee-like) refers to the abrupt posterior turn of the facial canal (**Fig. 5B**).[4] The upper bony covering of the geniculate fossa can be dehiscent in up to 15% of temporal bones, which makes the facial nerve vulnerable to injury during anterior epitympanic recess or middle cranial fossa surgeries.[3,5]

Tympanic segment
This segment descends obliquely along the medial wall of the tympanic cavity (**Fig. 5B, D**). It is located above the oval window and can be easily identified on the coronal images as a small dot, below the lateral semicircular canal (**Fig. 5E**).

Posteriorly the nerve enters the facial recess, lateral to the pyramidal eminence, where it turns

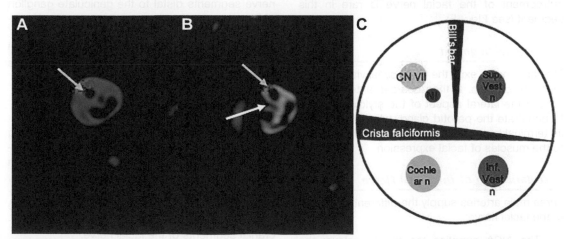

Fig. 4. The facial nerve (*yellow arrow*) is located at the anterosuperior aspect of the canal as demonstrated on the sagittal oblique DRIVE sequence (*A* and *B*) and on the diagram illustrating the IAC (*C*). Crista falciformis (*white arrow*) separates the facial nerve from inferiorly located cochlear nerve and a vertical bone crest, the Bill bar, separates it from the superior vestibular nerve, located posteriorly. n, nerve; Sup. Vest. N., superior vestibular nerve; Inf. Vest. N, inferior vestibular nerve.

Table 1
Facial nerve nuclei: locations and innervation

	Location	Nerve Fiber Type	Innervated Structures/Functions	Exit From Brainstem
Main motor nucleus	Ventrolateral pontine tegmentum, within the reticular formation	Motor fibers	• Muscles of facial expression • Stylohyoid muscle • Posterior belly of the digastric muscle • Stapedius muscle	Inferior lateral border of the pons, medial to CN VIII
Superior salivatory nucleus/lacrimal nucleus	Pontine tegmentum, posterolateral to motor nucleus	Parasympathetic secretory fibers	• Lacrimal glands • Submandibular glands • Sublingual glands	Nerve fibers join to form the nucleus intermedius, which exits the pontomedullary sulcus between the motor root and CN VII
Nucleus of tractus solitarius/gustatory nucleus	Dorsolateral medulla oblongata and lower pons, lateral to other nuclei	Special afferent sensory fibers	Taste sensation from the anterior two-thirds of the tongue	
		Somatic sensory fibers	Sensation from the pinna and external auditory canal	

inferiorly to form the second genu (**Fig. 5C**) and this part is the most susceptible portion for iatrogenic injury during surgery, especially for cholesteatoma.[10]

Mastoid segment

This segment is the longest but also the largest part of the canal; the nerve filling only half to 25% of the lumen, which is why inflammatory entrapment of the facial nerve is rare in this segment (see **Fig. 5E**).[12]

Extracranial Segment

The facial nerve exits the facial canal via the stylomastoid foramen. It then courses anterolaterally around the lateral aspect of the styloid process, to penetrate the parotid gland, where it gives off its terminal branches, providing motor innervation to the muscles of facial expression.

Vascularization of the Facial Nerve

Three main arteries supply the different segments of the facial nerve:

- The AICA supplies the facial nucleus: the cisternal, intracanalicular, and labyrinthine segments via the labyrinthine artery.
- The superficial petrosal artery (SPA), a branch of the middle meningeal artery.

- The stylomastoid artery (SMA), from the occipital artery in two-thirds of patients or from the postauricular artery.

The SMA anastomoses with the SPA at the level of the second genu and forms an arterial arcade called the facial arch, which supplies the tympanic and mastoid segments of the nerve.[13] The venous drainage parallels the arterial blood supply.[6] The nerve segments distal to the geniculate ganglion (GG) are surrounded by a venous network surrounded by a strong connective tissue sheath. The normal enhancement of the GG and distal nerve segments on postcontrast MR imaging is the result of this circumneural venous plexus.[1]

IMAGING TECHNIQUE AND PROTOCOLS

Computed tomography (CT) and MR imaging represent the primary imaging modalities for evaluating facial nerve disorder (**Table 3**). Although they may provide complementary information, MR imaging is the modality of choice in most circumstances and is preferred to evaluate the intra-axial, cisternal, canalicular, as well as extracranial segments of the facial nerve.[5,11,14,15]

Computed Tomography

CT imaging is usually performed without contrast, and, for facial nerve disorders, contrast-enhanced

Table 2
Intratemporal facial nerve segments

Segments	Location	Course	Branches	Important Imaging Points	Clinically Relevant Points
Canalicular/meatal	From porus to fundus of IAC	Anterior and laterally	—	The nerve is located in the anterosuperior quadrant of the canal	The lateral aspect is the most common site of injury from inflammatory swelling
Labyrinthine	From the meatal foramen to the GG	Anterior and laterally	—	Shortest and the narrowest segment of the facial canal	—
GG	In the geniculate fossa	Acute angled, reverse V-shaped posterior turn	GPSN • Secretory fibers to the lacrimal glands • Sensory innervation to the NC and palate mucosa	In addition to GG, it contains veins and arteries, which results in physiologic contrast enhancement	Weakest zone of canal, most common location for nerve injury in temporal bone fractures
Tympanic/horizontal/ second segment	From GG to the pyramidal eminence at the posterior wall of the middle ear cavity	Posterior and inferiorly	—	Frequently dehiscent	Most common site for congenital anomalies
Mastoid/vertical/third segment	From the posterior genu to the stylomastoid foramen inferiorly	Vertical	Nerve to the stapedius muscle, responsible for the stapedial reflex Chorda tympani nerve • Secretomotor innervation to the SM and SL glands • Sensory innervation to the anterior two-thirds of the tongue	Branching off at the level of second genu Branching off about 5–6 mm above the stylomastoid foramen	This segment is a frequent site of iatrogenic injury during posterior tympanotomy and mastoidectomy

Abbreviations: GG, geniculate ganglion; GPSN, greater superficial petrosal nerve; NC, nasal cavity; SM, submandibular; SL, sublingual.

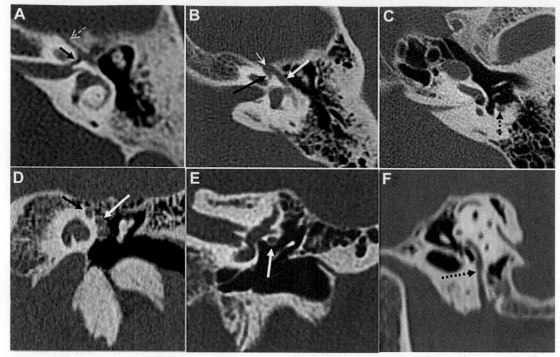

Fig. 5. Segments of the facial canal seen on axial (*A–C*), coronal (*D, E*), and Poschl (*F*) reformatted CT images. The labyrinthine segment (*black arrows*), the tympanic segment (*white arrows*), and the mastoid segments (*dotted arrow*) with the GG (*short open arrow*). Note the greater superficial petrosal nerve (GSPN) exiting anteriorly from the GG (*dashed arrow in A*).

CT should be reserved for patients who have contraindications for MR.[5] Although multidetector CT is used worldwide, cone-beam CT using flat-panel detector technology is slowly taking over for detailed evaluation of the temporal bone structures.

Magnetic Resonance Imaging

Tables 4 and 5 summarize the recommended protocol and sequences for facial nerve imaging.[2,16,17] There is building evidence that three-dimensional (3D) fluid-attenuated inversion recovery (FLAIR) MR imaging, especially after contrast, can reveal subtle changes in facial nerve disorders and should replace the standard axial contrast-enhanced T1-weighted sequences.[18,19] Similarly, balanced steady-state free precession (b-SSFP) sequences such as fast imaging employing steady-state acquisition–constructive interference (FIESTA-C) acquired after contrast can provide additional information in subtle cases.[20]

PATHOLOGY
Developmental Lesions and Variants

Aplasia/hypoplasia
Congenital facial paralysis may be seen in several syndromes, including Mobius, CHARGE

(coloboma, heart defects, atresia choanae, growth retardation, genital abnormalities, and ear abnormalities), Goldenhar, and also in brain malformations such as pontine tegmental cap dysplasia.[21]

Mobius sequence/syndrome is characterized by congenital, often bilateral, CN VII and CN VI palsies. The underlying CN VII and VI nuclei aplasia result in absence of the facial colliculus with flattening of the floor of the fourth ventricle and nonvisualization of the ipsilateral abducens and facial nerves (**Fig. 6**).[22,23]

Unilateral congenital facial nerve hypoplasia may also occur as an isolated abnormality or accompanied by inner ear anomalies.[23,24] It can be diagnosed with the imaging findings of facial canal hypoplasia on CT and small caliber of the nerve on MR (**Fig. 7**).[25]

Duplication
Duplication of the facial nerve, also called bifid facial nerve, can occur in isolation or with other ear anomalies.[23,26] Tympanic segment is the most common site, followed by the mastoid segment.[26]

Aberrant course
Abnormal course of the facial nerve can be seen in isolation but is usually seen in 3 conditions:

Table 3
Imaging techniques and suggested clinical indications with their corresponding imaging recommendations

Imaging Modality	Indications	Study Selection	Advantages	Disadvantages	
CT	• Initial evaluation after trauma • Presurgical assessment of osseous anatomy	MDCT	Widely available	Higher radiation dose compared with CBCT	HR bone algorithm with st ≤0.6 mm. MPR in the axial, coronal, Poschl and Stenvers planes
—	• Assessment of bone erosion in inflammation and neoplasia	CBCT	Higher resolution of small or thin structures, such as lateral wall of tympanic segment, with a lower dose	• Longer acquisition • Increased motion artifact • Requires GA in children	—
MR imaging	Nontraumatic facial palsy	Dedicated MR imaging of the temporal bones with contrast	Ability to evaluate the nerve and the brainstem in the setting of inflammation, neoplasia, or vascular lesion	• Longer acquisition • Prone to artifact	—

Abbreviations: CBCT, cone-beam CT; GA, general anesthesia; HR, high-resolution; MDCT, multidetector CT; MPR, multiplanar reconstruction; st, slice thickness.

Table 4
Sequences used for facial imaging and the corresponding abbreviations

Fluid-attenuated inversion recovery	FLAIR
Balanced steady-state free precession	b-SSFP
Fast spin echo	FSE
Constructive interference into steady state	CISS
Fast imaging employing steady-state acquisition	FIESTA
Fast imaging employing steady-state acquisition–constructive interference	FIESTA-C
Driven equilibrium radiofrequency reset pulse	DRIVE
Sampling perfection with application optimized contrasts using different flip angle evolution	SPACE
Spoiled gradient recalled acquisition in the steady state	SPGR
Volumetric interpolated breath-hold examination	VIBE
Magnetization prepared rapid gradient echo	MPRAGE
Brain volume imaging	BRAVO

- Congenital aural dysplasia: the tympanic and mastoid segments are most commonly affected.[21,23]
- Congenital middle ear and ossicular anomalies (because of common origin of the ossicles and facial nerve from second branchial arch). There is usually inferomedial displacement of the tympanic segment (**Fig. 8**A, B).[27]
- Congenital inner ear anomalies (IEAs).[28,29] The direction of abnormal displacement depends on the severity and type of underlying IEA.[29] IP-III results in superior dislocation of the labyrinthine segment, whereas cochlear aplasia/hypoplasia and common cavity anomaly usually result in anterior displacement of labyrinthine segment and inferior dislocation of the tympanic segment.

On coronal reformatted CT images, the absence of the dot beneath the lateral semicircular canal should raise suspicion of the abnormal course of the facial nerve (see **Fig. 8**A, B). Preoperative identification of such an anomalous course is crucial to surgeons and can help avoid an inadvertent iatrogenic facial nerve paralysis.[23]

Dehiscence
The facial canal dehiscence has been reported in more than half the cases histopathologically,

Table 5
Recommended magnetic resonance imaging sequences and parameters for facial neuropathy and for hemifacial spasm

Sequence	ST (mm/Gap)	FOV (cm)	Imaging Details
Limited Brain			
Sagittal T1	5/1	23–24	Entire brain
Axial FLAIR	5/1	22	Entire brain
Axial T2 brain stem	3/1	22	Include parotids
DWI	5/1	22	—
High-resolution IAC			
Axial 3D T2 b-SSFP or 3D FSE (CISS/FIESTA/DRIVE/SPACE…)	0.6	16–18	—
Precontrast and postcontrast T1WI	—	—	—
Axial 3D T1 (T1-SPACE/3D-SPGR/VIBE)	1	20–22	Preferred
Axial and coronal T1 TSE	2	16–18	≤2 mm, if 3D unavailable
Add-ons			
Postcontrast axial 3D FLAIR	1.2	22	In suspected inflammation
3D TOF MRA	—	—	For hemifacial spasm

Abbreviations: 3D, three-dimensional; DWI, diffusion-weighted imaging; FLAIR, fluid-attenuated inversion recovery; FOV, field of view; MRA, magnetic resonance angiography; TOF, time-of-flight; TSE, turbo spin echo.

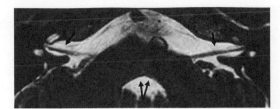

Fig. 6. Mobius sequence. Axial constructive interference into steady state (CISS) image performed on a 10-year-old boy with facial paralysis and abnormal gaze since birth, shows bilateral absence of the facial colliculi (*double arrows*) and flattening of the fourth ventricle with absence of the bilateral CN VII (*black arrows*) and CN VI. (*Courtesy of* K. K.Oguz, MD, Ankara, Turkey.)

most common in the tympanic portion, mastoid segment, and near the GG (**Fig. 8C, D**).[30] At the tympanic segment, the facial nerve may prolapse inferiorly from the dehiscence and lie in close contact with the stapes. Again, because of the embryonic association of facial nerve with other second arch derivatives, a dehiscence of the facial canal can be associated with additional middle ear or ossicular anomalies.[1,23] Although most patients with dehiscence are asymptomatic, conductive hearing loss may be the presenting symptom. In addition, a dehiscence may predispose the nerve to injury during a middle ear surgery.

Epineurial pseudocysts

An epineurial pseudocyst of the intratemporal facial nerve is a developmental lesion, located

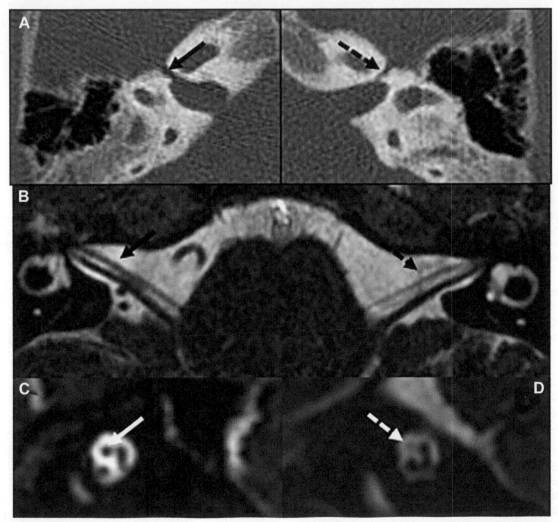

Fig. 7. Facial canal and facial nerve hypoplasia. Axial CT (*A*), axial (*B*) and bilateral sagittal oblique CISS from right (*C*) and left (*D*) IACs, showing left facial canal and facial nerve hypoplasia (*dotted arrows*) compared with the normal-sized canal and nerve (*straight arrows*) on the right.

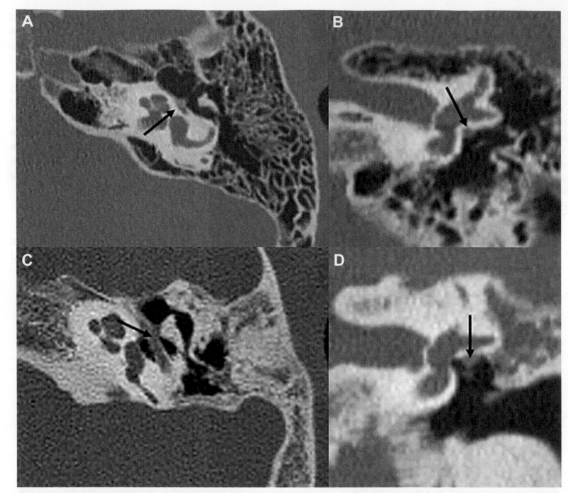

Fig. 8. Axial (*A*) and coronal (*B*) reformatted images of temporal bone CT of a 8-year-old boy showing aberrant course of the left facial nerve (*arrow*) with inferomedial displacement of the tympanic facial canal and accompanying oval window atresia (*A and B*). Axial (*C*) and coronal (*D*) reformatted images of temporal bone CT scans in another adult patient showing dehiscent facial canal (*arrow*).

adjacent to the mastoid segment of the facial nerve (**Fig. 9**). The lesions consist of dense fibroadipose tissue without a true wall and are probably an incidental imaging finding.[31]

Inflammatory/Infectious Disorders

Studies have shown that infection/inflammation accounts for more than 70% of cases presenting with facial palsy.[11]

Bell palsy
BP, also called idiopathic facial palsy, is the most common cause of facial paralysis.[32,33] It is characterized by a rapid unilateral facial nerve paresis or paralysis of unknown cause. Although a viral cause (herpes simplex virus reactivation) is suspected, the exact mechanism of BP is currently unknown.[34] The BP is thought to result from

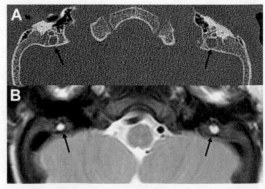

Fig. 9. Epineurial pseudocysts seen as bilateral cystic lesions (*arrows*) along the course of the mastoid facial segment on axial CT (*A*) and T2 turbo spin-echo MR image (*B*).

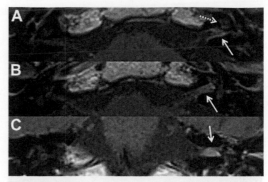

Fig. 11. Ramsey-Hunt disease. Axial (*A* and *B*) and coronal (*C*) postcontrast T1WI images of a 34-year-old woman presenting with 1-month history of left facial paralysis and vertigo. There is abnormal thickening and enhancement involving both the facial and vestibulocochlear nerves (*straight arrows*) with subtle enhancement of the cochlea (*dashed arrow*). The patient had history of vesicular rash in her pinna at the onset, confirming the diagnosis.

inflammatory edema of the facial nerve, with resultant compression of the vascular supply within the narrow facial canal.[34] The narrowest regions of the canal, the labyrinthine segment and especially the meatal foramen, are thus the most susceptible areas to injury from ischemia. Furthermore, those areas constitute a watershed zone between the vertebral and carotid artery systems, which makes them susceptible to ischemic injury.[11] The disease is usually self-limiting, with improving weakness in all cases, and complete recovery in up to 80% of patients at 6 months. The diagnosis of BP is one of exclusion, where history and physical

examination are crucial in making the diagnosis. The latest guidelines do not consider imaging to be contributive in BP, unless the symptoms are atypical (**Box 1**).[32]

When imaging is needed, dedicated contrast-enhanced MR imaging of the temporal bone should be performed, covering the entire course of the facial nerve, including the parotid glands, to rule out other conditions that could present with facial paralysis.

The characteristic imaging finding of BP is linear intense contrast enhancement along the distal canalicular and labyrinthine segments of the nerve (**Fig. 10**A). Although any enhancement in the canalicular segment is considered abnormal for routine turbo spin-echo (TSE) imaging, faint focal enhancement can occasionally be seen at the IAC fundus in normal individuals, on 3D sequences such as spoiled gradient recalled acquisition in the steady state (SPGR) and fast spin-echo (FSE).[35,36] Furthermore, physiologic enhancement is usually seen in the geniculate, tympanic, and mastoid segments caused by previously described vascular plexus. In addition, compared with routine T1 spin-echo sequences, increased signal can be observed both before and after contrast and in all facial nerve segments on 3D inversion recovery–prepared fast spoiled gradient echo sequences (such as magnetization prepared rapid gradient echo [MPRAGE] and brain volume imaging [BRAVO]) (**Fig. 10**B, C).[37] Determination of pathologic facial nerve enhancement on these sequences must thus be made with caution, because the apparent enhancement may instead

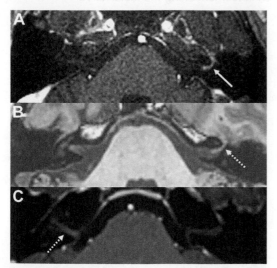

Fig. 10. BP in a 49-year-old woman presenting with left-sided facial paralysis that had started 6 weeks ago, seen as abnormal enhancement along the labyrinthine segment (*arrow*) on postcontrast 3D T1-weighted imaging (T1WI) (*A*). On different patients without any facial symptoms, increased signal along the normal nerve (*dotted arrows*) on precontrast brain volume imaging (BRAVO) sequence (*B*) and on postcontrast magnetization prepared rapid gradient echo (MPRAGE) sequence (*C*).

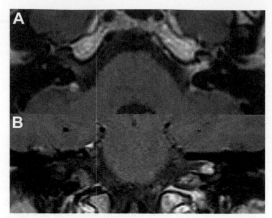

Fig. 12. Neurosarcoidosis patient with contrast enhancement at the fundus of IAC on axial (*A*) and coronal (*B*) postcontrast BRAVO.

reflect the increased visualization of the nerve on this sequence.[37] The postcontrast 3D-FLAIR images can improve the specificity and overall accuracy of MR imaging in patients with BP.[19]

Herpes zoster oticus

Herpes zoster oticus (HZO), also called Ramsay Hunt syndrome, is the second most common inflammation of the facial nerve and results from reactivation of latent varicella zoster virus in the GG.[6,11,38] It is characterized by acute facial palsy and facial pain, accompanied by CN VIII symptoms (including sensorineural hearing loss and vertigo) and also by vesicular rash in the periauricular region and external auditory canal. The characteristic imaging findings are thickening and enhancement along the involved nerves, CN VII and CN VII, a distinguishing feature from BP (**Fig. 11**).[18,39,40] The presence of associated increased signal and enhancement of the

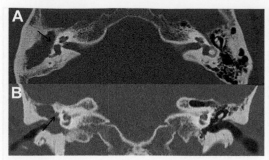

Fig. 14. Large middle ear cholesteatoma with facial canal erosion (*arrows*) on axial (*A*) and coronal (*B*) reformatted images of temporal bone CT.

labyrinth, best seen on the 3D-FLAIR sequences, was also found to be useful in distinguishing HZO from BP.[18,40]

Lyme disease

Lyme disease is caused by the infection by the spirochete *Borrelia burgdorferi* and is a common cause of facial paralysis is children. The central nervous system (CNS) involvement can cause meningitis and cranial neuropathies, facial palsy being the most common.[41] The facial paralysis can be present bilaterally in up to 25% of cases.[41] The imaging findings are nonspecific, with linear enhancement along the facial nerve.[41]

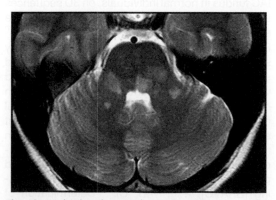

Fig. 13. Multiple sclerosis in 28-year-old woman with multiple demyelinating plaques at the brain stem, also involving the regions of the facial nerve and facial colliculus.

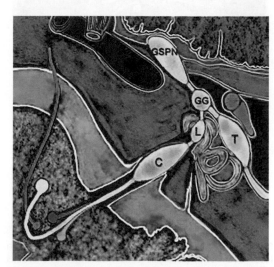

Fig. 15. The most common locations for facial schwannoma: the canalicular segment (C), the labyrinthine segment (L), the GG, the GSPN, and the tympanic segment (T). (*Adapted from* Mundada P, Purohit BS, Kumar TS, Tan TY. Imaging of facial nerve schwannomas: diagnostic pearls and potential pitfalls. *Diagnostic and interventional radiology.* 2016;22(1):40-46.)

Sarcoidosis

Sarcoidosis is a noncaseating granulomatous inflammation that can affect the CNS. Facial nerve palsy is the most commonly seen CN disorder.[42] Neurosarcoidosis manifests as leptomeningeal enhancement, typically involving the basal surfaces of the brain, and enhancing dural masses/diffuse dural thickening. The facial nerve, when involved, shows focal nodular or linear enhancement (Fig. 12).[42]

Other inflammatory conditions affecting the facial nerve/nucleus

Demyelinating diseases such as multiple sclerosis may involve the facial nerve nucleus, but the facial palsy is rarely isolated and is rarely the presenting symptom (Fig. 13).[11]

Autoimmune disorders such as chronic inflammatory demyelinating polyneuropathy or Sjögren syndrome can also present with facial nerve palsy, and enhancement along the involved nerve can be seen on postcontrast images.[43]

Secondary involvement from acute/chronic middle ear and skull base infections

Acute and chronic infections of the middle ear including cholesteatoma can result in facial palsy.[11] Facial palsy is seen in 1% of cases with cholesteatoma, and the tympanic segment of the nerve is the most frequently affected site (Fig. 14).[44] Similarly, facial palsy is seen in more than one-third of patients with skull base osteomyelitis and is also a sign of poor prognosis.[11,45]

Tumoral Lesions

Several benign and malignant tumors can occur along the facial nerve but the primary tumors of CN VII are rare and the nerve is more frequently affected by lesions arising in the adjacent structures (such as vestibular schwannoma) or is secondarily involved by metastatic disease and perineural tumor spread.

Facial schwannoma

Facial nerve schwannoma (FNS) is a rare benign neoplasm but it represents the most common

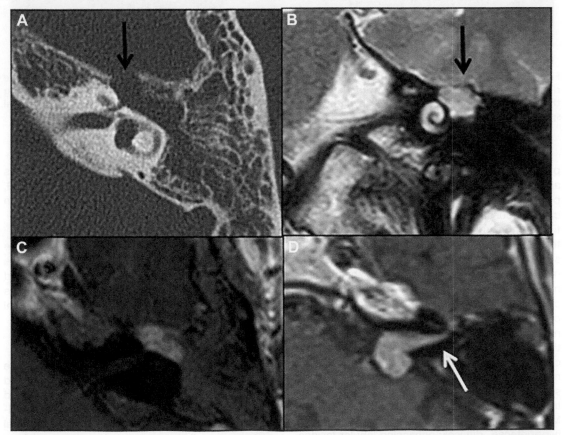

Fig. 16. Facial schwannoma (*arrow*) with widening of the GG and extension into the middle ear (*A*). The coronal T2-weighted imaging (WI) (*B*) and the axial postcontrast T1WI (*C*) show expansile, homogeneous, and avidly enhancing lesion centered at the GG. In another patient (*D*), an IAC mass extending to the facial canal (*arrow*), suggestive of a facial schwannoma.

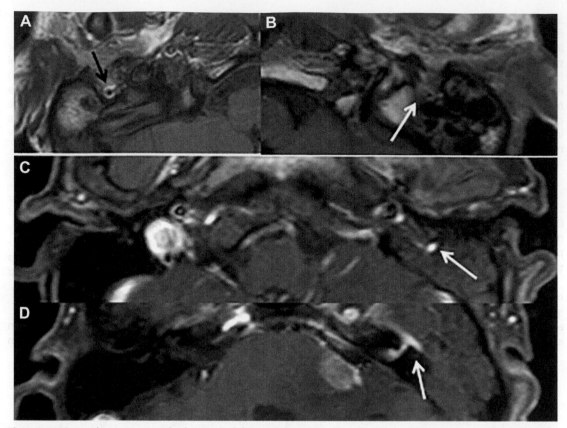

Fig. 17. Perineural tumor spread. The normal fat signal surrounding the nerve (*black arrow*) preserved on the right (*A*), decreased (*white arrow*) on the left on T1WI (*B*). Asymmetric increased enhancement (*arrow*) along the mastoid (*C*) tympanic, geniculate, labyrinthine, and cisternal segments (*D*) on the left suggestive of perineural spread.

primary neoplasm of the facial nerve. It can involve any segment, but most lesions are centered at the perigeniculate area (**Fig. 15**).[16,46] Although most cases occur sporadically, it can also be seen in patients with neurofibromatosis type 2 or after radiotherapy.[47] Facial palsy is the most frequent symptom but is not always present (because the motor nerves have thicker myelin sheaths and may be more resistant to slowly increasing compression) and the patients may present from compressive symptoms to the adjacent cochlear nerve.[2,47] FNSs are typically small fusiform tumors that grow along the path of least resistance and can involve multiple contiguous segments of the nerve.[16,46] On CT, the lesions typically cause smooth expansion of the canal, but they can protrude into the middle ear cavity (**Fig. 16**A). On MR imaging, they are usually homogeneous, T2-hyperintense, diffusely enhancing lobular lesions, although cystic degeneration may result in heterogeneous enhancement (**Fig. 16**B, C).[16] At the CPA or IAC, FNS cannot be differentiated from a

vestibular schwannoma unless the tumor extends to the labyrinthine segment (**Fig. 16**D). At the GG, the lesion can enlarge superiorly and present as an extra-axial middle cranial fossa mass.

Other benign lesions affecting the facial nerve
Primary meningiomas of the facial nerve canal are very rare (they are mostly centered at the GG), and the facial nerve is mostly affected by meningiomas originating from the CPA/IAC and middle cranial fossa regions.[2,5,11]

Perineural spread of tumor
Several head and neck malignancies can involve the facial nerve as perineural tumor spread (PNTS).[48] The most common primaries are parotid gland malignancies (adenoid cystic and mucoepidermoid carcinomas), but external auditory canal squamous cell carcinoma, melanoma, and lymphoma can also spread through the nerve. The PNTS might cause gradual facial palsy but is often asymptomatic and can only be detected on

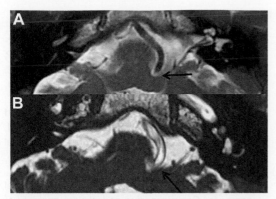

Fig. 18. In a 45-year-old male patient presenting with hemifacial spasm, the T2WI (*A*) and the FIESTA sequence (*B*) show a tortuous vertebrobasilar artery causing compression of the facial nerve at REZ (*arrows*), with indentation in the ventrolateral aspect of the brainstem.

imaging. The tumor spread typically occurs centripetally, from the extracranial nerve or greater superficial petrosal nerve toward the brain stem, but so-called skip lesions are common. Furthermore, the spread may also extend in the reverse direction from a branching point of the main nerve trunk. PNTS is seen as asymmetric and thickened enhancement along the involved nerve and can even be seen as enhancement extending all the way to the brain stem (**Fig. 17**).[49] Obliteration of the fat signal at the level of the stylomastoid foramen on T1-weighted imaging (T1WI) is an important finding suggestive of PNTS (see **Fig. 17**A, B).

Metastases to the surrounding bones as well as leptomeningeal metastases along the cisternal and canalicular segments of the nerve can also result in facial palsy. In adult patients, the most common primaries are breast and lung.[5] In addition, lymphoma and leukemia can also cause CN infiltration that usually involves multiple CNs.

Vascular Lesions

Hemifacial spasm

Hemifacial spasm is a complex symptom that consists of involuntary, painless spasms of the facial muscles, most commonly seen in middle-aged women.[9] The spasm can be secondary to the facial nerve/nucleus irritation (from tumors, demyelinating disorders, trauma, and infections) but is most frequently primary and caused by a neurovascular conflict, from a vascular structure that causes facial nerve compression.[50,51] The previously described REZ, especially the centrally myelinated axons from the RExP to TZ, are the most vulnerable for focal injury and demyelination from repeated vascular pulsations.[9] The most commonly implicated vessels are AICA, PICA, and vertebral artery (**Fig. 18**).[9,50] However, it is important to remember that numerous vessels course in the CPA and cross the facial nerve but most are not symptomatic; therefore, the radiological diagnosis or suggestion should only be used in patients who are symptomatic and who have objective distortion of the facial nerve on imaging.[51]

Venous vascular malformation of the facial nerve

Venous vascular malformation (VVM) of the facial nerve is a vascular lesion that was historically referred to as facial hemangioma or ossifying hemangioma.[52] It is most frequently seen in the GG with extension to the labyrinthine segment (usually presenting with facial nerve symptoms) or at the IAC (presenting with gradually progressive sensorineural hearing loss).[4,53] On MR, VVMs are seen as expansile, heterogenous, and avidly enhancing masses that may be difficult to differentiate from schwannomas (**Fig. 19**). However, the CT findings showing characteristic honeycomb appearance with internal bony spicules and poorly defined

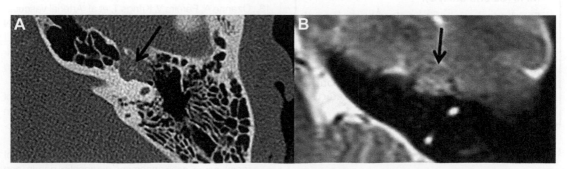

Fig. 19. VVM of the facial nerve seen as expansile mass, centered at the GG, with internal trabecular calcifications (*arrow*) on axial CT (*A*) and heterogenous appearance on T2WI (*B*).

margins allow the differential diagnosis from FNS (see **Fig. 19**).[2,11,15]

The facial nerve can also be involved in temporal trauma and can be secondarily affected by skull base tumors and tumors arising from adjacent structures, but these entities are discussed separately elsewhere in this issue.

SUMMARY

The facial nerve is a complex structure, affected by a wide spectrum of disorders. The appropriate radiological assessment of a patient presenting with facial neuropathy requires a thorough knowledge of its anatomy, of the normal imaging appearance of the nerve/canal both on CT and MR, and characteristic and atypical imaging features of different affecting disorders for an accurate differential diagnosis.

CLINICS CARE POINTS

- Abnormal course of the facial nerve can be seen in isolation but is usually seen in the setting of congenital aural dysplasia, congenital middle ear and ossicular anomalies or with congenital inner ear anomalies. It is thus crucial to assess the course of the nerve in those cases to help surgical planning and prevent iatrogenic injury.

- In routine TSE imaging any enhancement in the canalicular segment of the facial nerve is considered abnormal. However, faint enhancement can occasionally be seen at the IAC fundus in normal individuals, on 3D sequences such as SPGR and FSE. Additionally, increased signal can be observed both before and after contrast and in all facial nerve segments on 3D inversion recovery-prepared fast spoiled gradient-echo sequences (such as MPRAGE and BRAVO).

- Facial nerve might be involved by perineural tumor spread (PNTS) in several head and neck malignancies including parotid gland malignancies, external auditory canal squamous cell carcinoma and melanoma. The PNTS might cause gradual facial palsy but is often asymptomatic and can only be detected on imaging.

DISCLOSURE

The author has nothing to disclose.

REFERENCES

1. Curtin H, Gupta R, Bergeron R. Embryology, anatomy, and imaging of the temporal bone. In: Som P, Curtin H, editors. Head and neck imaging, vol. 2, 5th edition. Philadelphia: Elsevier Mosby; 2011. p. 1053–96.
2. Phillips C, Hashisaki G, Vellion F. Anatomy and development of the facial nerve. In: Swartz J, Harnsberger H, editors. Imaging of the temporal bone. 4th edition. New York: Thieme; 2009. p. 444–79.
3. Mansour S, Magnan J, Ahmad HH, et al. Facial nerve. In: Comprehensive and clinical anatomy of the middle ear. Cham: Springer International Publishing; 2019. p. 175–96.
4. Chung R, Dorros S, Mafee MF. Imaging of facial nerve pathology. Oper Tech Otolaryngol Head Neck Surg 2014;25(1):58–65.
5. Veillon F, Ramos-Taboada L, Abu-Eid M, et al. Imaging of the facial nerve. Eur J Radiol 2010;74(2): 341–8.
6. Raghavan P, Mukherjee S, Phillips CD. Imaging of the facial nerve. Neuroimaging Clin N Am 2009; 19(3):407–25.
7. Kouo T, Morales RE, Raghavan P. Imaging of the facial nerve. In: Chong V, editor. Skull Base Imaging. Elsevier; 2018. p. 197–213.
8. Burmeister HP, Baltzer PA, Dietzel M, et al. Identification of the nervus intermedius using 3T MR imaging. AJNR Am J Neuroradiol 2011;32(3):460–4.
9. Campos-Benitez M, Kaufmann AM. Neurovascular compression findings in hemifacial spasm. J Neurosurg 2008;109(3):416.
10. Ozgirgin ON, Cenjor C, Filipo R, et al. Consensus on treatment algorithms for traumatic and iatrogenic facial paralysis. Mediterr J Otol 2007;3:150–8.
11. Borges A. Pathology of the facial nerve. In: Lemmerling M, De Foer B, editors. Temporal bone imaging. Berlin, Heidelberg: Springer Berlin Heidelberg; 2015. p. 257–306.
12. Lindeman H. The fallopian canal: an anatomical study of its distal part. Acta Otolaryngol 1960; 52(sup158):204–11.
13. Ozanne A, Pereira V, Krings T, et al. Arterial vascularization of the cranial nerves. Neuroimaging Clin N Am 2008;18(2):431–9, xii.
14. Policeni B, Corey AS, Burns J, et al. ACR Appropriateness Criteria(®) cranial neuropathy. J Am Coll Radiol 2017;14(11s):S406–20.
15. Park SU, Kim HJ, Cho YK, et al. The usefulness of MR imaging of the temporal bone in the evaluation of patients with facial and audiovestibular dysfunction. Korean J Radiol 2002;3(1):16–23.
16. Mundada P, Purohit BS, Kumar TS, et al. Imaging of facial nerve schwannomas: diagnostic pearls and

potential pitfalls. Diagn Interv Radiol 2016;22(1): 40–6.

17. Veillon F, Taboada LR, Eid MA, et al. Pathology of the facial nerve. Neuroimaging Clin N Am 2008;18(2): 309–20.

18. Chung MS, Lee JH, Kim DY, et al. The clinical significance of findings obtained on 3D-FLAIR MR imaging in patients with Ramsay-Hunt syndrome. Laryngoscope 2015;125(4):950–5.

19. Lim HK, Lee JH, Hyun D, et al. MR diagnosis of facial neuritis: diagnostic performance of contrast-enhanced 3D-FLAIR technique compared with contrast-enhanced 3D-T1-fast-field echo with fat suppression. Am J Neuroradiol 2012;33(4):779–83.

20. Hector M, Alnadji A, Veillon F, et al. Imaging of facial neuritis using T2-weighted gradient-echo fast imaging employing steady-state acquisition after gadolinium injection. Eur Arch Otorhinolaryngol 2020; 278(7):2501–9.

21. Robson CD, Robertson RL, Barnes PD. Imaging of pediatric temporal bone abnormalities. Neuroimaging Clin N Am 1999;9(1):133–55.

22. Herrera DA, Ruge NO, Florez MM, et al. Neuroimaging findings in moebius sequence. AJNR Am J Neuroradiol 2019;40(5):862–5.

23. Romo LV, Casselman JW, Robson CD. Congenital anomalies of the temporal bone. In: Som P, Curtin H, editors. Head and neck imaging, vol. 2, 5th edition. Philadelphia: Elsevier Mosby; 2011. p. 1097–165.

24. Mohammad SA, Abdelaziz TT, Gadelhak MI, et al. Magnetic resonance imaging of developmental facial paresis: a spectrum of complex anomalies. Neuroradiology 2018;60(10):1053–61.

25. Ramanathan S, Al Heidous M, Kumar D, et al. Three-dimensional constructive interference in steady-state magnetic resonance imaging diagnosis of isolated unilateral facial nerve hypoplasia. Neurol India 2016; 64(2):358–9.

26. Glastonbury CM, Fischbein NJ, Harnsberger HR, et al. Congenital bifurcation of the intratemporal facial nerve. AJNR Am J Neuroradiol 2003;24(7):1334–7.

27. Jahrsdoerfer RA. The facial nerve in congenital middle ear malformations. Laryngoscope 1981;91(8): 1217–25.

28. Romo LV, Curtin HD. Anomalous facial nerve canal with cochlear malformations. AJNR Am J Neuroradiol 2001;22(5):838–44.

29. Sennaroğlu L, Tahir E. A novel classification: anomalous routes of the facial nerve in relation to inner ear malformations. Laryngoscope 2020;130(11): E696–703.

30. Baxter A. Dehiscence of the Fallopian canal. An anatomical study. J Laryngol Otol 1971;85(6): 587–94.

31. Delrue S, Cammaert T, Heylbroeck P, et al. Epineurial pseudocyst of the intratemporal facial nerve: a case series study. J Int Adv Otol 2020;16(2):266–70.

32. Baugh RF, Basura GJ, Ishii LE, et al. Clinical practice guideline: Bell's Palsy. Otolaryngol Head Neck Surg 2013;149(3_suppl):S1–27.

33. Borges A, Casselman J. Imaging the cranial nerves: Part I: methodology, infectious and inflammatory, traumatic and congenital lesions. Eur Radiol 2007; 17(8):2112–25.

34. Eviston TJ, Croxson GR, Kennedy PG, et al. Bell's palsy: aetiology, clinical features and multidisciplinary care. J Neurol Neurosurg Psychiatry 2015; 86(12):1356–61.

35. Radhakrishnan R, Ahmed S, Tilden JC, et al. Comparison of normal facial nerve enhancement at 3T MRI using gadobutrol and gadopentetate dimeglumine. Neuroradiol J 2017;30(6):554–60.

36. Warne R, Carney OM, Wang G, et al. Enhancement patterns of the normal facial nerve on three-dimensional T1W fast spin echo MRI. Br J Radiol 2021;94(1122):20201025.

37. Dehkharghani S, Lubarsky M, Aiken AH, et al. Redefining normal facial nerve enhancement: healthy subject comparison of typical enhancement patterns–unenhanced and contrast-enhanced spin-echo versus 3D inversion recovery-prepared fast spoiled gradient-echo imaging. AJR Am J Roentgenol 2014;202(5):1108–13.

38. Zimmermann J, Jesse S, Kassubek J, et al. Differential diagnosis of peripheral facial nerve palsy: a retrospective clinical, MRI and CSF-based study. J Neurol 2019;266(10):2488–94.

39. Iwasaki H, Toda N, Takahashi M, et al. Vestibular and cochlear neuritis in patients with Ramsay Hunt syndrome: a Gd-enhanced MRI study. Acta Otolaryngol 2013;133(4):373–7.

40. Kuya J, Kuya K, Shinohara Y, et al. Usefulness of high-resolution 3D multi-sequences for peripheral facial palsy: differentiation between Bell's Palsy and Ramsay Hunt Syndrome. Otol Neurotol 2017; 38(10):1523–7.

41. Lindland ES, Solheim AM, Andreassen S, et al. Imaging in Lyme neuroborreliosis. Insights Imaging 2018;9(5):833–44.

42. Nowak DA, Widenka DC. Neurosarcoidosis: a review of its intracranial manifestation. J Neurol 2001; 248(5):363–72.

43. Shibuya K, Tsuneyama A, Misawa S, et al. Cranial nerve involvement in typical and atypical chronic inflammatory demyelinating polyneuropathies. Eur J Neurol 2020;27(12):2658–61.

44. Irving R. Facial palsy in cholesteatoma: presenting author: richard irving. J Laryngol Otol 2016; 130(S3):S126–7.

45. Dabiri S, Karrabi N, Yazdani N, et al. Facial nerve paralysis in malignant otitis externa: comparison of

the clinical and paraclinical findings. Acta Otolaryngol 2020;140(12):1056–60.

46. Wiggins RH III, Harnsberger HR, Salzman KL, et al. The many faces of facial nerve schwannoma. AJNR Am J Neuroradiol 2006;27(3):694–9.

47. Carlson ML, Deep NL, Patel NS, et al. Facial nerve schwannomas: review of 80 cases over 25 years at mayo clinic. Mayo Clin Proc 2016;91(11):1563–76.

48. Badger DMD, Aygun NMD. Imaging of perineural spread in head and neck cancer. Radiol Clin North Am 2016;55(1):139–49.

49. Ginsberg LE. MR imaging of perineural tumor spread. Magn Reson Imaging Clin North Am 2002; 10(3):511–25.

50. Donahue JHMD, Ornan DAMD, Mukherjee SMD. Imaging of vascular compression syndromes. Radiol Clin North Am 2016;55(1):123–38.

51. Haller S, Etienne L, Kövari E, et al. Imaging of neurovascular compression syndromes: trigeminal neuralgia, hemifacial spasm, vestibular paroxysmia, and glossopharyngeal neuralgia. AJNR Am J Neuroradiol 2016;37(8):1384–92.

52. Benoit MM, North PE, McKenna MJ, et al. Facial nerve hemangiomas: vascular tumors or malformations? Otolaryngol Head Neck Surg 2010;142(1):108–14.

53. Yue Y, Jin Y, Yang B, et al. Retrospective case series of the imaging findings of facial nerve hemangioma. Eur Arch Otorhinolaryngol 2015;272(9):2497–503.

Imaging of Acute and Chronic Skull Base Infection

Sriram Vaidyanathan, MD, FRCR[a],*,
Ravi Kumar Lingam, MB BCh, MRCP, FRCR, EDiHNR[b]

KEYWORDS

- Skull base infection • Osteomyelitis • MR imaging • CT • Gallium 67 • FDG-PET/CT
- Necrotizing otitis externa • Malignant otitis externa

KEY POINTS

- The commonest cause of skull base infection is necrotizing otitis externa, followed by complicated sinusitis.
- Multimodality imaging using high-resolution CT and multiparametric magnetic resonance imaging are the cornerstones for diagnosing and estimating disease extent.
- Transspatial spread crossing the midline in the subtemporal neck, and involvement of lower cranial nerves, meninges, or brain, are adverse prognostic signs.
- Response assessment is challenging but critical in identifying treatment end point, and imaging plays a key role alongside clinical assessment.

INTRODUCTION

Skull base infections are uncommon but can have a devastating impact on patient survival without timely recognition and treatment.[1] The skull base is a unique structure between the intracranial and extracranial environments that functions both as a rampart and a fenestrated interface, the latter making it susceptible to adjacent disorders. Skull base sepsis is usually a worsening consequence of otologic or sinogenic infection and can have an intractable and recurrent course. It is often termed skull base osteomyelitis (SBO) and even used interchangeably with necrotizing otitis externa (NOE), a testament to it being the predominant cause of SBO. However, there are other causes of SBO, albeit less common, which merit mention and are discussed in this review.[2]

Imaging has a crucial role in establishing diagnosis because of limitations of clinical assessment posed by nonspecific symptoms and inaccessibility for tissue sampling. A multimodality imaging approach can help in characterizing extent, evaluating for complications, and in assessing treatment response.

CAUSES AND PATHOPHYSIOLOGY

There are no population-based studies to estimate the incidence and prevalence of SBO. A retrospective analysis of patients on the National Inpatient Sample database with NOE, the commonest

---

[a] Department of Radiology and Nuclear Medicine, St James's University Hospital, Leeds Teaching Hospitals NHS Trust, Beckett Street, Leeds LS9 7TF, UK; [b] Department of Radiology, Northwick Park & Central Middlesex Hospitals, London North West University Healthcare NHS Trust, Imperial College London, Watford Road, London HA1 3UJ, UK

* Corresponding author.

E-mail address: svaidyanathan@nhs.net

Neuroimag Clin N Am 31 (2021) 571–598
https://doi.org/10.1016/j.nic.2021.06.002

cause of SBO, yielded an approximate incidence of 11 cases per million.[3]

The population at risk for NOE-related SBO are the elderly with diabetes, which not only causes a reduction in host immune response and impairment of T-cell function but also alters the local microenvironment by causing microangiopathy and a increased pH of cerumen.[3] SBO can also occur with other causes of systemic immunosuppression, such as chemotherapy, neutropenia, end-stage renal failure, human immunodeficiency virus/acquired immunodeficiency syndrome, alcoholism, and corticosteroid therapy. Other factors, such as radiation therapy, cause susceptibility to osteomyelitis by damaging the external ear epithelium, reducing cerumen production, and altering the vascularity of bone.[4]

Complicated rhinosinusitis is the second commonest cause of SBO. Bacterial sinusitis can affect children and adults, including those with intact immune systems. In contrast, angioinvasive fungal sinusitis is almost exclusively a condition of the severely immunosuppressed. Table 1 enumerates common and rare causes of SBO.

IMAGING TECHNIQUES/PROTOCOLS

SBO is difficult to diagnose and may remain clinically occult until serious sequelae, such as cranial neuropathy, declare themselves. Even when symptoms are present at the outset, they are nonspecific and may not indicate the site of origin.

This diagnostic delay can be compounded by an inability in elderly or immunocompromised patients to mount a robust inflammatory response. Optimized imaging therefore has a crucial role to play in making a timely diagnosis and in estimating disease severity. A variety of structural and functional imaging techniques have been used in SBO, but most of the data are from small series or single-patient case studies because of the uncommonness of the disease. The relative merits and weaknesses of imaging modalities are summarized in Table 2.

High-resolution computed tomography (CT) and multiparametric magnetic resonance (MR) imaging are the workhorses in assessing the skull base and are complementary to each other.[5] MR imaging is superior to CT for depicting disease extent (and hence pretreatment assessment) by virtue of its ability to assess marrow infiltration of the skull base (notably the basiocciput/clivus and petrous apex), soft tissues of the subtemporal region, intracranial and extracranial vessels, and intracranial contents (dura, leptomeninges, ventricles, and brain) (Fig. 1).

Conventional nuclear medicine techniques have been used for decades in SBO and can be advantageous for problem solving in complex cases (Table 2). These techniques are being supplanted by higher-resolution techniques such as ^{18}F-fluorodeoxyglucose (FDG)-PET/CT.[6] Using dedicated skull base protocols, FDG-PET/CT can be acquired in less time than MR imaging. In a recent

Table 1 Causes of skull base infection	
Anterior Skull Base	Complicated sinusitis: frontal and ethmoid[a] Orbital cellulitis[a]
Central Skull Base	Otologic (NOE and otomastoiditis)[a] Complicated sinusitis: sphenoid[a] Cavernous sinus thrombosis Retropharyngeal/perivertebral space infection (rare) Masticator space/temporomandibular joint infection Extension of craniofacial actinomycosis (rare)
Posterior Skull Base	Otologic (NOE and otomastoiditis)[a] Craniocervical junction osteomyelitis
Any Site: Local Causes	Trauma Postsurgical Chemoradiation
Systemic Conditions (Rare)	Destructive nasopharyngeal granulomatosis with polyangiitis with superinfection[39] Hematogenous seeding; eg, atypical mycobacterial infections, cryptococcal sepsis in liver transplant patients, bony vaso-occlusive episodes with superimposed infection in sickle-cell disease[40–42]

[a] Denotes common causes of SBO.

Table 2
Imaging modalities in skull base osteomyelitis

Modality/ Technique	Recommended Protocol/Mechanism of Action	Advantages	Disadvantages	Key Imaging Features	Response Assessment
CT	• Bone-weighted volumetric multiplanar high-resolution CT with 0.625–1 mm slice thickness • Soft tissue weighted with or without iodinated contrast	• Rapid acquisition, which is well tolerated in elderly and infirm • Ease of availability and interpretation • High spatial resolution • Iodinated contrast helpful in soft tissue, vascular and intracranial assessment • Alternative in those with contraindication to MR imaging • For problem-solving incidental findings seen on MR imaging in the petrous apex and for foraminal assessment	• Low sensitivity for early disease • Underestimates central skull base marrow involvement compared with MR imaging as reliant on indirect signs of infection; eg, trabecular demineralization	• Site of origin of infection; eg, external auditory canal swelling and erosion, sinus opacification, and osteitis • Regional skull base changes such as asymmetric demineralization, bone erosion (eg, around the eustachian tube and carotid canal) • Chronic changes of infection; eg, osseous sclerosis, especially in treated bone, osteoneogenesis, and sinus formation[15,43] • Intracranial, vascular, and sub-temporal neck space assessment (less accurate than MR imaging)	• CT can show ongoing lucent and sclerotic bone changes for months to years that may never completely resolve (Fig. 21)[15,34]

(continued on next page)

Table 2
(continued)

Modality/ Technique	Recommended Protocol/Mechanism of Action	Advantages	Disadvantages	Key Imaging Features	Response Assessment
MR imaging	• At least 2 orthogonal planes using spin-echo (conventional or fast) T1-weighted precontrast, a fluid-sensitive sequence such as T2 with fat suppression or STIR, and gadolinium-enhanced T1-weighted images with fat suppression • 512 matrix for high resolution, slice thickness of 3–4 mm without gap especially for T1-weighted precontrast images.[44] Parallel imaging techniques may reduce acquisition time for high-resolution sequences[44,45]	• High contrast resolution • Superior to CT for early disease and marrow involvement • No ionizing radiation advantageous especially when serial imaging required	• Patient tolerance and suitability can be an issue; eg, pacemakers, coils • Prolonged acquisition time • Gadolinium may be contraindicated because of renal impairment, especially in elderly patients with diabetes • Fat suppression with the use of frequency-selective fat-suppression pulses is prone to inhomogeneity artifacts in the skull base, and in such cases STIR imaging can be helpful[30]	• Spin-echo T1-weighted pregadolinium MR imaging is the sequence par excellence for assessment of involvement of bone marrow and the subtemporal deep neck fascial spaces, which is indicated by intermediate-signal inflammatory soft tissue replacing normal fat signal (see **Fig. 1**) • T2-weighted sequences show high signal change in the bone but may show a slightly more intermediate signal in the subjacent soft tissue because of active inflammation occurring on a background of	• Signal changes in the skull-base on T1, STIR, and postgadolinium sequences are more responsive to treatment than CT but can still lag behind clinical improvement • Echoplanar DWI with ADC map has been shown to add value to MR imaging in assessing SBO as a novel technique for monitoring therapy response[35]

Technique			
	• DWI MR imaging to differentiate infection from malignancy, detect abscess formation, and monitoring therapy response[35]	fibrosis and granulation tissue[17,46] • Fat suppression pregadolinium can enhance the conspicuity of inflammation by improving the contrast compared with background fatty marrow without use of contrast • Fat suppression postgadolinium sequences can emphasize infected areas, highlight abscess formation and intracranial extension of disease	Focal moderate to intense tracer activity at the site of active infection with supportive features on the concomitant CT component if SPECT-CT performed
			—
Conventional nuclear medicine imaging (bone scan, white cell scintigraphy, gallium-67 scintigraphy)	—	• Low specificity • Poor resolution (improves with SPECT-CT) • Difficult anatomic localization unless SPECT-CT is used • Ionizing radiation • Longer acquisition times compared with CT and MR imaging	• Well-established experience with use in diagnosis and response assessment in SBO[47] • Useful in patients with renal failure, when MR imaging is contraindicated, or in iodinated contrast allergy • Functional changes on nuclear medicine imaging tend to precede changes on structural scans[6]

(continued on next page)

Table 2
(continued)

Modality/ Technique	Recommended Protocol/Mechanism of Action	Advantages	Disadvantages	Key Imaging Features	Response Assessment
		• Role for a 1-stop hybrid scan combining functional and morphologic information, especially if performed as contrast-enhanced SPECT-CT			
99mTc hydroxymethylene diphosphonate or methylene diphosphonate (99mTc-HDP/MDP) bone scintigraphy	• Analogue of inorganic pyrophosphate that binds avidly to hydroxyapatite crystals and incorporates into sites of active bone turnover; ie, osteoblastic activity such as in osteomyelitis or malignancy[48] • At least 2 phases: blood-pool at 5 min and delayed at 2–4 h after tracer injection	• High sensitivity and negative predictive value for SBO, so good for ruling out SBO (Fig. 22)	—	—	• Residual tracer activity can be present for an extended length of time because of ongoing osteoblastic activity, making it a poor choice for response assessment
99mTc99m-HMPAO or 111In-oxyquinolone white blood cell scintigraphy	• Uses radiolabeled autologous white blood cells with serial image acquisition after tracer injection at multiple time points up to 24–30 h	• Established use in acute infection	• Long acquisition time, labor intensive • Up to 30 h between injection and imaging	—	• Inaccurate for monitoring because of a high false-negative rate

Technique	Mechanism	Advantages	Disadvantages		Comments
[67]Gallium-citrate scintigraphy	• Tracer accumulates in areas of infection by binding to leukocytes, forming a complex with lactoferrin and by direct bacterial uptake[47] • Imaging performed 18–72 h after injection	• Decades of experience with tracer use in infection and inflammation imaging[47,49] • Demonstrated role in response assessment[50]	• Technical challenges eg, degree of labeling • Blood-product handling • Low sensitivity in chronic osteomyelitis, which is a *sine qua non of SBO* (Fig. 23)[6] • Needs adequate circulating white cell count so may be false-negative in neutropenia[47] • Poor spatial and contrast resolution • 48–72 h before tracer distribution normalizes to allow imaging so impractical in the infirm or obtunded patient • Limited availability	—	• Has been successfully used in clinical practice for response assessment and SPECT-CT hybrid imaging may improve diagnostic accuracy (Fig. 24)[50]
FDG-PET/CT	• FDG is a biomarker of glycolytic metabolism and accumulates in infection because of a differential increase in tissue glycolysis in inflamed tissue[6]	• Highly sensitive and specific for the diagnosis of chronic osteomyelitis in the axial and appendicular skeleton[51] • High resolution compared with traditional nuclear medicine techniques	• May show only low-grade FDG uptake in fungal SBO where MR imaging may be superior[7] • Expensive • Limited availability • Risk of nondiagnostic scans in the context of uncontrolled diabetes in SBO	—	Emerging role in response assessment but more data needed

(continued on next page)

Table 2
(continued)

Modality/Technique	Recommended Protocol/Mechanism of Action	Advantages	Disadvantages	Key Imaging Features	Response Assessment
		• Shorter acquisition times compared with traditional nuclear medicine imaging • Hybrid imaging combining functional and structural information • Allows for semiquantitative analysis	• Ionizing radiation		

Abbreviations: ADC, apparent diffusion coefficient; CT, computed tomography; DWI, diffusion-weighted imaging; HDP, hydroxymethylene diphosphonate; MDP, methylene diphosphonate; MR, magnetic resonance; SPECT, single-photon emission computed tomography; STIR, short-tau inversion recovery.

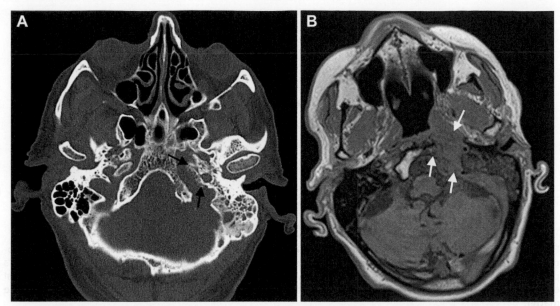

Fig. 1. Role of CT and MR imaging in assessing extent of SBO. (*A*) Axial bone-weighted CT. Subtle bone erosion in left petrous apex (*black arrows*). (*B*) Axial T1-weighted (T1W) MR. Extensive marrow signal change in the clivus and petrous bone with cellulitis in left perivertebral and poststyloid parapharyngeal spaces (*white arrows*).

study, the sensitivity, specificity, positive predictive value, negative predictive value, and accuracy of FDG-PET/CT in diagnosing SBO were 96.7%, 93.3%, 98.3%, 87.5%, and 96.1%, respectively, and had comparable accuracy with MR imaging.[7]

ANTERIOR SKULL BASE INFECTION
Relevant Anatomy

The anterior skull base (ASB) forms the border between the anterior cranial fossa superiorly from the frontal and ethmoid sinuses, and the orbits, making them leading causes of ASB osteomyelitis.

Causes

Although uncommon in the postantibiotic era, up to 3% to 5% of patients with acute rhinosinusitis experience significant orbital or intracranial complications.[8] The putative mechanism for spread of infection is transmission through a valveless emissary vein network connecting the sinus mucosa to the diploic veins and dura. Infection can transit across the sinus without discernible bony erosion on CT. These emissary veins are most abundant in the frontal sinuses, especially during adolescence, when there is active sinus growth.[9] Consequently, bacterial frontal sinusitis is the commonest cause of ASB osteomyelitis.

Frontal Sinusitis

Complicated frontal sinusitis can lead to extracranial complications such as subgaleal abscess

formation (Pott's puffy tumor) and intracranial complications, such as epidural/subdural empyema, meningitis, cortical vein thrombosis, and intraparenchymal abscess (**Fig. 2**). Pott's puffy tumor is associated with intracranial complications in up to 85% of cases and the presence clinically of a boggy forehead swelling in acute sinusitis should necessitate both sinus and intracranial imaging.[10]

Ethmoid Sinusitis

Ethmoid sinusitis initially involves the adjacent orbit through the thin fenestrated lamina papyracea rather than the skull base directly. Contrast-enhanced CT is the imaging modality of choice, with findings including erosion of the lamina papyracea, corruption of orbital fat in the medial postseptal space, and subsequent progression to a lentiform rim-enhancing subperiosteal abscess (**Fig. 3**). The abscess commonly occupies the superomedial quadrant where the periosteum is most slack. Rarely, orbital cellulitis can lead on to SBO, frontal lobe cerebritis, and brain abscess (see **Fig. 3**). An uncommon complication is cavernous sinus thrombosis (CST), which occurs because of septic thrombophlebitis spreading through superior ophthalmic veins. Direct signs of CST include asymmetric enlargement, convex configuration of the lateral wall, and filling defects within the sinus, whereas indirect signs include an engorged or thrombosed superior ophthalmic vein, stranding of orbital fat, and proptosis.[11]

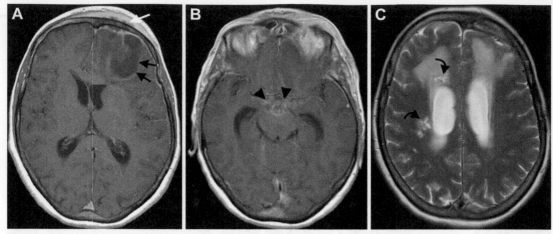

Fig. 2. Complicated acute frontal sinusitis in a 50-year-old woman. (*A* and *B*) Axial T1W postcontrast MR. Heterogeneous signal change left frontal bone in keeping with osteomyelitis, subgaleal cellulitis, and abscess; ie, Pott's puffy tumor (*white arrow*), left frontal intraparenchymal abscess (*black arrows*), and suprasellar leptomeningeal enhancement (*black arrowheads*). (*C*) Axial T2-weighted MR. Multifocal infarcts in the right cerebral deep white matter.

Fungal Sinusitis

Rarely, sinusitis may be fungal, and the most fulminant phenotype is acute angioinvasive sinusitis (**Fig. 4**). This rapidly progressing infection is seen in severely immunocompromised patients and has a high mortality of 50% to 80%.[12] There may be little bony skull base involvement because rampant disease extension occurs along vascular channels with widespread tissue necrosis.[12] The infection commences in the nasal cavity and quickly progresses to involve the sinuses, infratemporal fossa, orbit, skull base, and brain. Noncontrast CT shows hypodense sinus opacification, in contrast with chronic allergic fungal sinusitis where the sinus mucosa is hyperdense, although the presence of blood products can cause dependent layering in sinus cavities. A characteristic feature of invasive fungal sinusitis is soft tissue stranding across bony walls with minimal or no bone destruction (eg, involving periantral fat in the infratemporal fossa or along the orbital floor in maxillary sinusitis, which should immediately raise suspicion in an immunocompromised patient; see **Fig. 4**). Necrotic regions show marked hypointense T2 signal, nonenhancement, and a lack of restricted diffusion in contrast with pyogenic abscess.[9] However, these patients usually succumb to vascular and brain complications before significant SBO can set in.

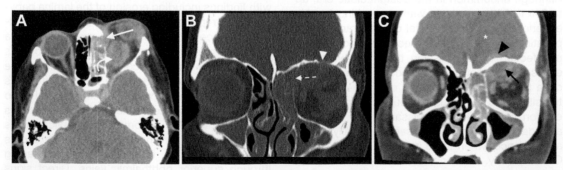

Fig. 3. Orbital cellulitis with epidural abscess and cerebritis. (*A*) Axial contrast-enhanced CT. Acute ethmoid sinusitis with periosteal elevation (*white arrow*), postseptal collection displacing the medial rectus (*curved white arrow*), with severe proptosis. (*B*) Coronal bone-weighted CT. Erosion of left lamina papyracea (*dashed arrow*) and osteomyelitis left orbital roof (*white arrowhead*). (*C*) Coronal contrast-enhanced CT. Subperiosteal abscess in superomedial orbit (*black arrow*), left frontal epidural abscess (*black arrowhead*), and low-density change left frontal lobe (*white asterisk*) in keeping with cerebritis.

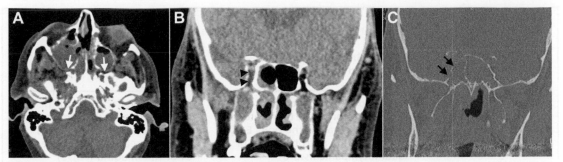

Fig. 4. Acute angioinvasive fungal sinusitis. (*A* and *B*) Contrast-enhanced CT. Severe maxillary sinusitis, inflammatory stranding right pterygopalatine fossa compared with the left without bone erosion (*white arrows*), and cellulitis extending to the inferior orbital fissure (*black arrowheads*). (*C*) Bone-weighted CT: permeative erosion right sphenoid sinus. (*Courtesy of* Dr Ashok Adams (Consultant Neuroradiologist, Barts Health NHS Trust).)

CENTRAL AND POSTERIOR SKULL BASE INFECTION
Relevant Anatomy

A unique feature of the clivus and petrous apex is their embryologic formation through endochondral ossification, in contrast with the flat bones of the skull, which form by intramembranous ossification. This feature informs their architecture by imparting a generous fatty marrow space. There are numerous venous channels traversing the length of the petrous bone. In addition to the large petrosal sinuses, there are also small venules within the anterior petrous apex, which provide an alternative route for the passage of venous blood from the cavernous to the inferior petrosal sinus or jugular bulb.[13] Moreover, the cavernous sinus, with its unique osteo-dural-meningeal structure, communicates with the orbit, pterygopalatine fossa, masticator space, and the posterior fossa.[14] These venous channels provide a route for the spread of infection along the skull base and possibly the neck.

Necrotizing Otitis Externa

Background
NOE, or malignant otitis externa, is the commonest cause of SBO. It starts as a severe erosive infection, typically at the osseous-cartilaginous junction of the external auditory canal (EAC), because this is where granulation tissue is usually found clinically. The archetypal patient is an elderly, poorly controlled diabetic with unremitting otalgia and otorrhea refractory to topical treatment with/without a facial palsy. *Pseudomonas aeruginosa* is the most common implicated organism, although isolating the bacteria may be difficult if antibiotics have been commenced before culture.[1] Because *Pseudomonas* is not a normal commensal of the EAC, it is postulated that moisture contamination with local trauma (eg, ear canal

irrigation) may be the primary insult initiating NOE. Other pathogens, including gram-positive bacteria and *Aspergillus fumigatus*, have also been incriminated.[15]

Pathophysiology
A crucial distinction from otomastoiditis and petrous apicitis is the mechanism of disease spread. NOE is not solely an osteitis. Histopathologic studies have shown that it primarily spreads along vascular channels (lateral venous sinus, petrosal sinuses, and submucosal venules), unlike the coalescent destruction of pneumatic spaces seen in otomastoiditis. This proposed pathologic mechanism is consistent with a predilection for *Pseudomonas* to spread along vessels in experimental pathologic models.[16] In SBO there is a concurrence of active osteomyelitis, new bone formation, and fibrosis at the disease front with relative sparing of the pneumatized portions of the temporal bone.[17] The disease thus behaves as a combination of an osteomyelitis, vasculitis, and fasciitis, with fasciitis also facilitating its progression in the subtemporal region.

Pattern of spread
Certain patterns of disease spread can be observed in NOE-related SBO, but there is no predictable order of events, and these patterns may occur on their own or in combination (Table 3).

Other Otologic Causes

Although uncommon in the postantibiotic era, coalescent otomastoiditis remains the commonest cause of lateral compartment central SBO. *Streptococcus pneumoniae*, *Hemophilus influenzae*, and *Staphylococcus aureus* are the most common causal organisms. Unlike NOE, it is a disease of the pneumatic spaces, characterized by a progressive bony resorption and destruction of mastoid septae with abscess formation (Fig. 11). This

Table 3
Patterns of spread in necrotizing otitis externa–related skull base osteomyelitis

Direction of Spread	Structures Breached, Spaces Involved, and Key Neurovascular Anatomy	Imaging Tips
Anterior	• Spread to the retrocondylar region by erosion of the thin plate of the anterior wall of the bony EAC or through the petrotympanic or squamotympanic fissure • If EAC wall is intact, the bone adjacent to the eustachian tube should be scrutinized for erosion on CT • A variant anatomic structure known as a persistent foramen of Huschke (foramen tympanicum) anteroinferior to the EAC has been described as an alternative route of spread of infection to and from the temporomandibular region[52] • In severe infection, temporomandibular joint osteomyelitis and masticator space abscess may be seen	• Medial condylar space of the temporomandibular region is said to be one of the earliest sites of disease spread and can be seen on CT or MR imaging (**Fig. 5**)[5]
Inferior	• Spread through the fissures of Santorini in the floor of the cartilaginous EAC to the subtemporal region • From here, the stylomastoid and submastoid region may be involved (**Fig. 6**) and result in facial nerve paralysis, which is said to be the commonest and first neurologic abnormality to develop[53] • Mastoid tip and styloid process may also show erosion on CT	• Facial nerve involvement in SBO tends to be reversible and is not a poor prognostic sign
Medial	• Cellulitis spreads from the subtemporal region to the poststyloid parapharyngeal space enveloping the internal carotid artery and internal jugular vein (see **Fig. 7**) • Vascular complications, such as marked narrowing of the internal carotid artery, and occlusion or thrombosis of the internal jugular vein can develop • The disease can extend more medially, with involvement of the adjacent perivertebral region and the area medial to the eustachian tube and deep to the nasopharynx (see **Fig. 7**) • The clivus is involved eventually from its anterior aspect once the prevertebral fascia is breached	• The prestyloid parapharyngeal space and masticator space are not commonly involved because of the strong tensor-vascular-styloid and pterygoid fasciae and this is observed as a sparing of the prestyloid parapharyngeal space best appreciated on MR imaging (see **Fig. 7**) • The mucosa of the nasopharynx is typically spared because of the protection of the robust pharyngobasilar fascia and this helps to differentiate SBO from nasopharyngeal cancer. In addition, unlike nasopharyngeal carcinoma, the soft tissue shows free diffusivity on the DWI imaging (see **Fig. 7**)

(continued on next page)

Table 3
(continued)

Direction of Spread	Structures Breached, Spaces Involved, and Key Neurovascular Anatomy	Imaging Tips
Transspatial	• In severe cases there is transspatial involvement spanning the pericondylar, poststyloid parapharyngeal, perivertebral space and retropharyngeal spaces deep to the nasopharynx mucosa (Fig. 8) • Focal abscess formation is particularly common in the perivertebral space and petroclival region and this can extend down to the cervical spine causing osteomyelitis (see Fig. 8)	• Transspatial involvement crossing the midline has been shown to confer a poor prognosis[54] • DWI MR imaging is useful for demonstrating abscess formation within an area of cellulitis and is seen as a low ADC focus
Posterior	• Uncommon pattern seen as bone destruction and enhancement in the region of the jugular foramen and sigmoid sinus (Fig. 9). Can occur with concurrent involvement of the otomastoid complex in NOE. • This presents as glossopharyngeal, vagus, or accessory nerve palsy • Rarely, hypoglossal, trigeminal, and abducens nerve involvement have also been described[1]	• Lower cranial nerve involvement is an adverse prognostic sign in NOE, likely caused by it being a surrogate marker of advanced disease[55,56]
Superior	• Can occur with both midline and paramidline SBO; eg, when the tegmen is breached or through the petroclival synchondrosis, and results in meningeal and brain parenchymal infection (Fig. 10) • Typically, the abscess is located in the temporal lobe but may also occur in the cerebellum when there is a posterior pattern of spread • Superior extension can also occur extracranially with abscess formation in the periauricular area or temporal fossa as a variant	• MR imaging is the test of choice for meningeal or intracranial involvement

condition can result in dehiscence of the lateral mastoid cortex and abscess formation in the postauricular region. The bone can also erode internally, resulting in subdural empyema and brain abscess in the posterior cranial fossa. A common complication is sigmoid sinus thrombosis caused by a thin sigmoid plate and thrombophlebitis of valveless emissary veins (see Fig. 11).

Petrous apicitis is a similar pathologic process to coalescent mastoiditis and is caused by medial extension of otomastoiditis through the pneumatized spaces of the petrous temporal bone. Patients with petrous apicitis are usually febrile and

systemically unwell with some or all of the symptoms of the Gradenigo triad of ipsilateral abducens palsy, severe facial pain in distribution of V1, and otalgia.[18] Typically, there is focal bone destruction, which can progress to abscess formation with a high incidence of intracranial complications.

Sphenoid Sinusitis

Sphenoid sinusitis is an uncommon cause of SBO caused by a robust unfenestrated bony covering unlike the ethmoid sinuses and a lack of a prominent emissary venous network like the frontal sinus. Complicated sphenoid sinusitis involves the

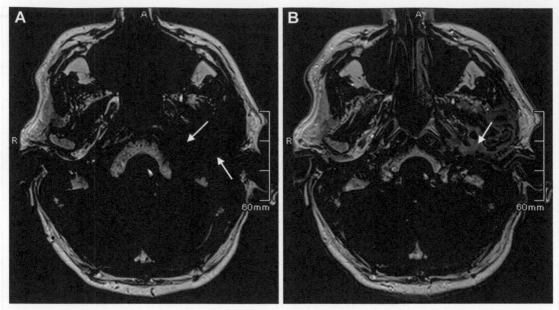

Fig. 5. Anterior-pattern NOE. (*A*) T1W precontrast MR. Intermediate-signal cellulitis in the left medial pericondy-lar space and left mandible condyle (*white arrows*). (*B*) T1W postcontrast MR shows enhancement in these areas (*white arrow*).

adjacent planum sphenoidale, clivus, and cavernous sinus, and is often associated with smooth dural enhancement in the middle cranial fossa (**Fig. 12**).

Atypical CSB Osteomyelitis

Central skull base (CSB) osteomyelitis can also occur without an obvious otologic or sinogenic source, and is termed atypical or idiopathic in such cases.[19,20] This cause is the third most common after NOE and sinus disease. The patient demographic and clinical course are the same as for NOE and imaging features are indistinguishable from a medial disease pattern with the exception of ear canal involvement (see **Table 3, Fig. 7**). Some cases of atypical SBO are probably

secondary to partly treated NOE and sparing of the nasopharyngeal mucosa with a persisting tongue of cellulitis in the retrocondylar region can be useful imaging observations to point to a cause and help distinguish this from cancer. However, when imaging findings are not conclusive, a deep prevertebral space biopsy accessed through the nasopharynx may be required to ascertain a microbiologic diagnosis.

Miscellaneous Causes of CSB and Posterior Skull Base Infection

Temporal bone osteoradionecrosis is a rare but serious late-onset complication of radiation therapy in head and neck cancer that is prone to superimposed bacterial and fungal infections and

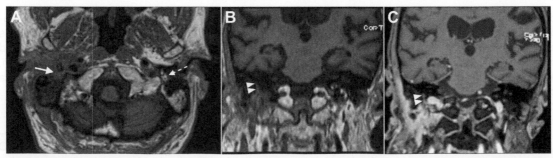

Fig. 6. Inferior pattern NOE in patient with right facial palsy. (*A*) Axial T1W MR. Intermediate-signal inflammation right stylomastoid region (*white arrow*) with loss of the perineural fat compared with left (*dashed white arrow*). (*B*) Coronal T1W MR. Thickening of the mastoid portion of the right facial nerve, which shows avid enhancement on postgadolinium MR (*C*).

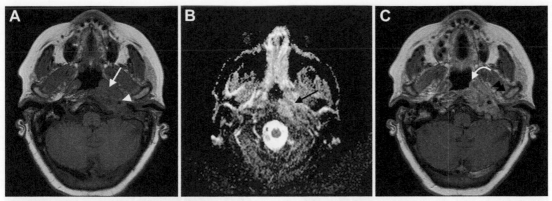

Fig. 7. Medial pattern NOE. (*A*) T1W precontrast MR. Intermediate-signal inflammation left perivertebral and retropharyngeal space deep to the nasopharynx mucosa (*white arrow*), narrowing left internal carotid artery (ICA) indicating inflammation is under pressure (*white arrowhead*). (*B*) apparent diffusion coefficient (ADC) map shows free diffusivity in the inflammation, differentiating it from nasopharyngeal carcinoma and ruling out abscess. (*C*) T1W postcontrast MR. Enhancement in the deep space cellulitis, sparing of the nasopharyngeal mucosa (*curved white arrow*), and prestyloid parapharyngeal space (*black arrowhead*).

can result in severe SBO and fatal intracranial complications (**Fig. 13**).[21] The temporal bone is considered susceptible given its thin skin covering, communication with the upper airway via the eustachian tube, and resident flora in the EAC.[21] There are also rare reports of craniocervical junction osteomyelitis involving the posterior skull base (PSB) after radiation therapy for oropharyngeal and nasopharyngeal cancer.[22] **Fig. 14** shows a patient with craniocervical junction osteomyelitis in an intravenous drug user, with involvement of the posterior skull base and resulting in a pseudoaneurysm of the vertebral artery.

Masticator space infections including mandible osteomyelitis and temporomandibular joint septic arthritis tend to remain intraspatial because of the presence of strong fascial barriers and spreads toward the suprazygomatic region laterally, rather than toward the CSB.[23] There is 1 case report of refractory craniofacial actinomycosis spreading from the masticator space to the skull base in an otherwise healthy individual.[24] **Fig. 15** shows an unusual example of masticator space infection involving the CSB in a patient with a history of immunosuppression. Rarely, temporomandibular joint septic arthritis and osteomyelitis may involve the mandibular fossa and the lateral CSB (**Fig. 16**).

It is exceptional for pharyngitis to involve the skull base because of the barrier posed by the strong pharyngobasilar fascia and the prevertebral

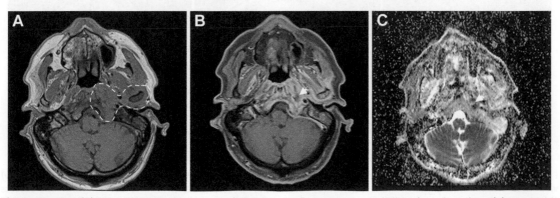

Fig. 8. Transspatial NOE. (*A*) T1W MR. Intermediate-signal inflammatory cellulitis in the left pericondylar, poststyloid parapharyngeal, perivertebral, and retropharyngeal spaces deep to the nasopharynx mucosa, left mandible condyle, and clivus (*dashed line*). (*B*) T1W postcontrast MR shows heterogeneous enhancement with a small unenhancing area (*short white arrow*) with restricted diffusivity on ADC map indicating abscess formation (*C, short white arrow*). There is also reactive pachymeningeal enhancement in the posterior fossa along the clivus.

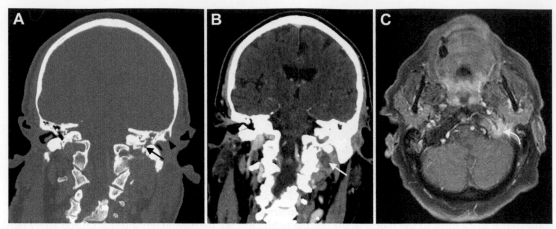

Fig. 9. Posterior pattern NOE. (*A*) Coronal bone-weighted CT. Soft tissue thickening in the left external auditory canal and middle ear. Bone erosion left hypotympanum into left jugular foramen (*black arrow*) and into mastoid (*black arrowhead*). (*B*) Coronal contrast-enhanced CT. Abscess around the left internal jugular vein. (*C*) T1W postcontrast MR. Avid enhancement left jugular foramen and skull base.

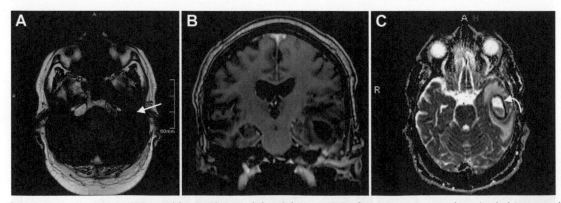

Fig. 10. Superior pattern NOE and brain abscess. (*A*) Axial T1W MR. Left otitis externa and media (*white arrow*) with mild intermediate signal in the left clivus. (*B*) Coronal T1W postcontrast MR shows left temporal lobe abscess (*black arrow*) and extensive enhancing osteomyelitis in the lateral skull base. High-resolution CT showed a tegmen defect (not shown). (*C*) ADC map shows rim-pattern restricted diffusion in the abscess without dual-rim sign and diffusion restriction of the abscess contents (*curved white arrow*), raising the possibility of a fungal rather than a bacterial pathogen on imaging appearance. However, pus cultures grew *Streptococcus pneumoniae*.

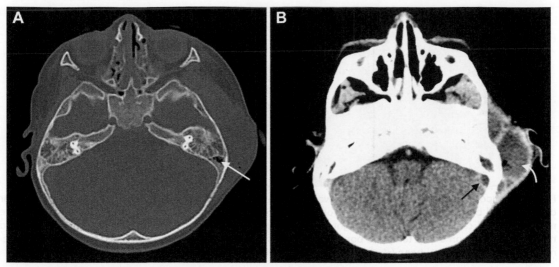

Fig. 11. Coalescent mastoiditis with subperiosteal abscess. (*A*) Bone-weighted CT. Opacified mastoid air cells with gas in the bone (*white arrow*) pathognomonic of osteomyelitis. (*B*) Contrast CT shows a multiloculated subperiosteal abscess (*curved white arrow*) and left sigmoid sinus thrombus (*black arrow*).

fascia. Even when retropharyngeal abscesses reach up to the base of the skull, it is uncommon for disease to traverse these fascial barriers. There are a few case reports in the pediatric literature of severe pharyngitis caused by *Fusobacterium necrophorum* infection causing clival osteomyelitis and intracranial complications, including septic thrombophlebitis (ie, a form of Lemierre syndrome).[25] Some cases of pediatric clival osteomyelitis are postulated to be caused by spread of pharyngeal infection through an anatomic variant, persistent fossa navicularis.[26] **Fig. 17** shows an unusual example of CSB osteomyelitis caused

by severe pharyngitis in an adult on immunotherapy for psoriatic arthropathy.

Some investigators have reported skull base infection after direct inoculation from penetrating trauma, including an unusual case report of a human bite causing SBO, surgical site infections, and scalp monitoring lead infection.[27–29] **Fig 18** shows an example of anterior SBO occurring as a complication of functional endoscopic sinus surgery. Interestingly, blunt cranial trauma can also predispose to infection when complex fracture lines breach the mastoid or sinus cavities resulting in spillover of secretions with consequent

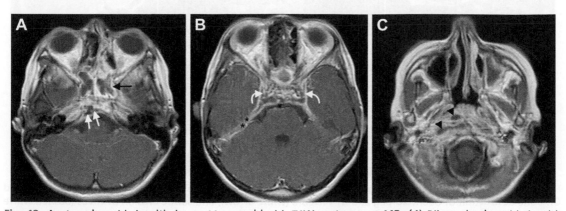

Fig. 12. Acute sphenoid sinusitis in an 11-year-old girl. T1W postcontrast MR. (*A*) Bilateral sphenoid sinusitis (*black arrow*), heterogeneous enhancement of the central skull base with epidural abscess (*white arrows*). (*B*) Bilateral nonocclusive CST (*curved white arrows*) and pachymeningeal enhancement (*asterisks*). (*C*) Abscess in perivertebral space (*black arrowheads*) tracking to C2 vertebra (not shown).

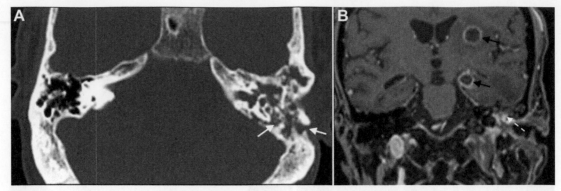

Fig. 13. Temporal bone osteoradionecrosis with SBO and brain abscesses. A 60-year-old man with left ear discharge and bleeding, history of osteoradionecrosis following chemoradiation for Epstein-Barr virus–positive nasopharyngeal carcinoma. (*A*) Bone-weighted CT. Permeative sclerotic and lucent bone texture, erosion, and mastoid opacification of left temporal bone (*white arrows*). (*B*) T1W postcontrast MR shows abnormal enhancement of the left temporal bone (*dashed white arrow*) and ring-enhancing cerebral abscesses (*black arrows*).

meningitis and cerebritis (**Fig. 19**). **Table 4** summarizes potential complications of SBO.

INITIAL IMAGING APPROACH AND RESPONSE ASSESSMENT

No single imaging test is comprehensive in evaluating SBO, and factors such as patient tolerance, contraindications, and local availability/expertise may alter the initial imaging approach.

Although CT can be performed as a quick rule-out test for excluding SBO when clinical suspicion is low, it underestimates the extent of skull base marrow involvement because it relies primarily on indirect signs such as trabecular demineralization and erosion.[30] When there is a strong clinical suspicion for SBO, MR imaging provides the most comprehensive and accurate assessment. In case MR imaging is contraindicated, or patient tolerance is an issue, a high-

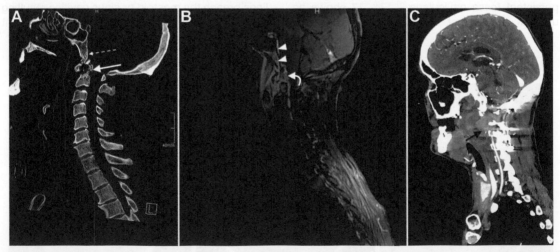

Fig. 14. Craniocervical junction spinal osteomyelitis in 50-year-old male intravenous drug user. (*A*) Bone-weighted CT. Bone destruction of odontoid peg and C1 vertebra (*white arrow*), and subtle erosion of clivus (*dashed white arrow*). (*B*) T1W postcontrast MR shows epidural and prevertebral abscess (*curved white arrow*), extensive prevertebral cellulitis, clivus osteomyelitis, and pachymeningeal enhancement (*white arrowheads*). (*C*) CT angiogram performed after surgical fixation shows truncated upper V2 segment right vertebral artery and hematoma in keeping with a mycotic pseudoaneurysm (*black arrow*).

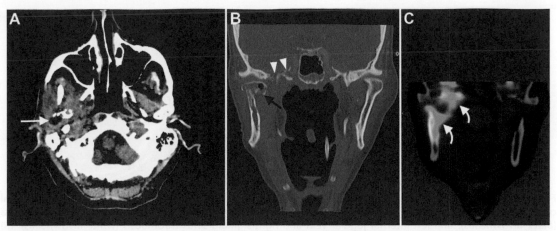

Fig. 15. Right mandible osteomyelitis with SBO in insulin-dependent diabetic and prior chemotherapy for lymphoma. (*A*) Axial contrast CT. Bone destruction and abscess around the right mandible condyle. (*B*) Coronal bone-weighted CT. Permeative destruction of the right hemimandible with gas in bone (*black arrow*), erosion right central skull base (*white arrowheads*). (*C*) FDG-PET/CT. Intense tracer uptake in right hemimandible and central skull base.

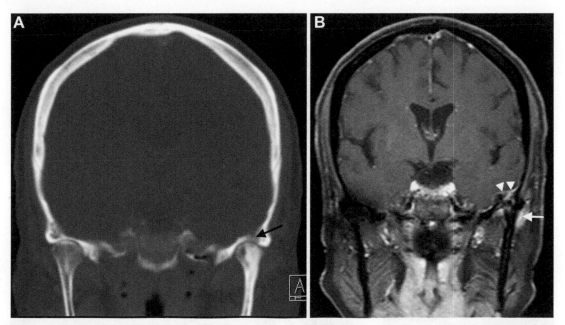

Fig. 16. Left temporomandibular joint (TMJ) septic arthritis with SBO and epidural abscess. (*A*) Contrast CT shows erosion and osteitis (indicating chronicity) in left mandibular fossa, loss of joint space, and subchondral cyst formation in the left mandible condyle head. (*B*) T1W postcontrast MR. Enhancing synovial thickening left TMJ (*white arrow*) and shallow left temporal fossa subdural collection (*white arrowheads*). The patient did not have any neurologic symptoms and was treated conservatively with antibiotics.

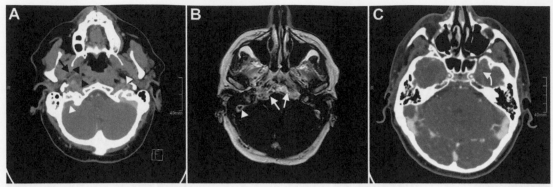

Fig. 17. Severe pharyngitis with SBO in 58-year-old man on immunotherapy for psoriatic arthritis. (*A*) Axial contrast-enhanced CT shows right parapharyngeal inflammation (*black arrow*), right retropharyngeal abscess (*black arrowheads*), and left internal jugular vein and right sigmoid sinus thrombosis (*white arrowheads*). (*B*) T1W postcontrast MR. Heterogenous enhancement of clivus in keeping with osteomyelitis (*white arrows*) and right sigmoid sinus thrombosis (*white arrowhead*). (*C*) CTV shows nonfilling expansion of left cavernous sinus compatible with thrombosis (*curved white arrow*).

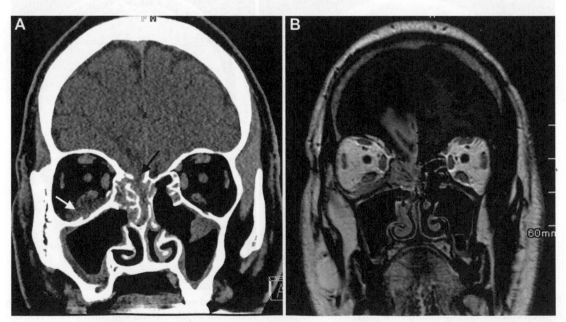

Fig. 18. Functional endoscopic sinus surgery complication. (*A*) Coronal CT shows dehiscent right cribriform plate (*black arrow*) and cellulitis in the inferior extraconal right orbit (*white arrow*). (*B*) T1W postcontrast MR shows a right frontal lobe abscess (*black arrows*).

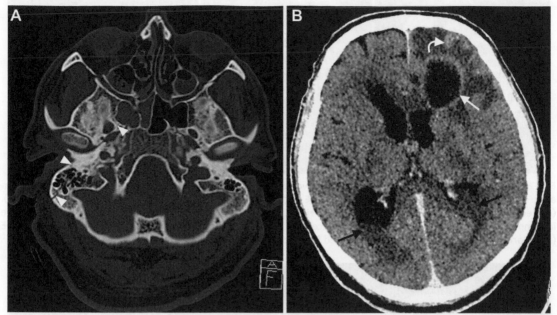

Fig. 19. Brain abscess and ventriculitis as sequelae of skull base fracture. (*A*) Bone-weighted CT shows a fracture through the right mastoid and sphenoid bone involving the right sphenoid sinus (*white arrowheads*). There were contrecoup left frontal lobe contusions. The patient presented a month later with altered sensorium. (*B*) Contrast CT shows ventricular debris (*black arrows*), left frontal lobe abscess (*white arrow*), and resolving left frontal contusions (*curved white arrow*).

Table 4 Complications of skull base infection	
Nerve	Subtemporal spread of infection and involvement of the facial nerve at stylomastoid foramen
	Jugular foramen (glossopharyngeal nerve, vagus nerve, and accessory nerve: Vernet syndrome)
	Hypoglossal canal (Collete-Sicard syndrome)
	Gradenigo syndrome: petrous apicitis, abducens nerve palsy and retro-orbital/facial pain
	Optic neuropathy
Brain	Meningitis, cerebritis, abscess formation: subdural empyema, intraparenchymal abscess, ventriculitis, hydrocephalus
	Cerebral infarction
	Brainstem involvement; eg, lateral medullary syndrome
Vascular	Occlusion
	Thrombosis
	Mycotic pseudoaneurysm
Abscess Formation	Subperiosteal and deep neck space collections
Secondary Involvement	Temporomandibular joint septic arthritis, mandible osteomyelitis
	Cervical spine osteomyelitis
	Septic pulmonary emboli

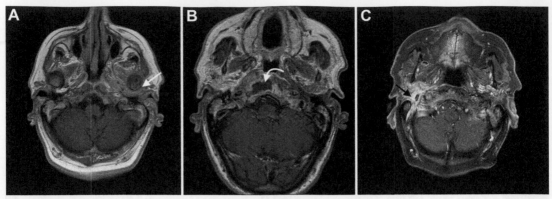

Fig. 20. Recrudescence of central SBO in 80-year-woman with uncontrolled diabetes. T1W postcontrast MR images. (*A*) Index episode with anterior-pattern NOE with inflammation in left pericondylar space (*white arrow*). (*B*) Recurrent infection a few months later with right perivertebral abscess (*curved white arrow*) and extensive inflammatory change in clivus and petrous apices. (*C*) MR a few months after. Right stylomastoid-pattern NOE (*black arrow*). These episodes are likely caused by residual unresolved infection.

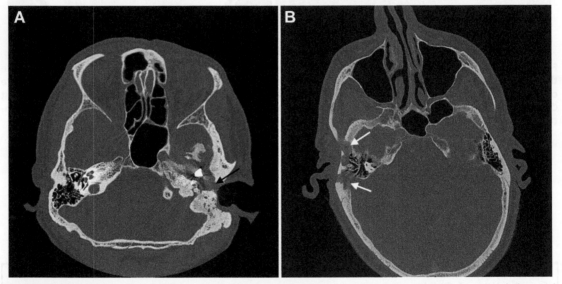

Fig. 21. Chronic SBO in different patients. Bone-weighted CT. (*A*) Central SBO caused by retained shrapnel. Despite mastoidectomy and debriding surgery, there is chronically discharging cavity with recurrent infections (*black arrow*). (*B*) Multiple sinuses (*white arrows*) in right temporal bone with osteoneogenesis indicating chronic osteomyelitis.

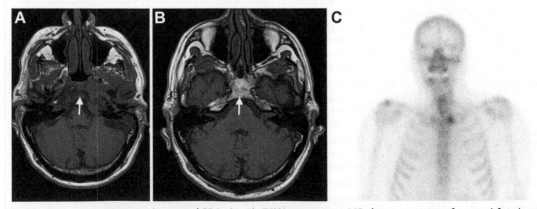

Fig. 22. Response assessment in central SBO. (*A, B*). T1W precontrast MR shows a return of normal fat signal (*arrows*) in clivus after successful treatment. ^{99m}Tc-hydroxymethylene diphosphonate bone scan anterior view (*C*). Normal tracer uptake in skull base indicating complete response to treatment.

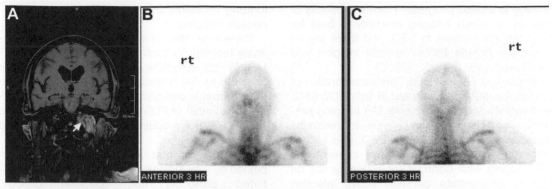

Fig. 23. False-negative ¹¹¹In-oxine leukocyte scintigraphy in central SBO. (*A*) T1W postcontrast MR shows active left-sided SBO (*white arrow*). ¹¹¹In-oxine–labeled leukocyte scintigraphy 3-hour anterior (*B*) and posterior (*C*) images do not show corresponding tracer uptake.

resolution CT scan with contrast using both bone and soft tissue algorithms is a good alternative.

Treatment of SBO understandably depends on the underlying cause but is largely medical. NOE-related SBO is associated with significant morbidity and often requires long-term antimicrobial management, regular aural toilet, and close surveillance for secondary complications.[31] Surgery is of little proven benefit in NOE-related SBO and is mainly performed for obtaining specimens for culture and to exclude malignancy.[32]

However, long-term antibiotics involve toxicity and can result in antibiotic resistance, so should not be given for longer than necessary. The principal challenge in SBO is to know when treatment

can be stopped. Undertreatment is the commonest cause of resurgence of infection and results in a recalcitrant fluctuating clinical course. SBO can recur in other sites following apparent resolution at the primary site of disease, but this is usually caused by recrudescence from residual foci of infection as opposed to true reoccurrence (**Fig. 20**). In particular, the subtemporal soft tissues can act as a sump of residual infection that can reactivate illness.

Response assessment is based on a combination of the clinical picture, serum inflammatory markers, and imaging findings.[33] Performing response assessment scans along with a comprehensive clinical assessment 8 to 10 weeks after instituting appropriate treatment is a useful

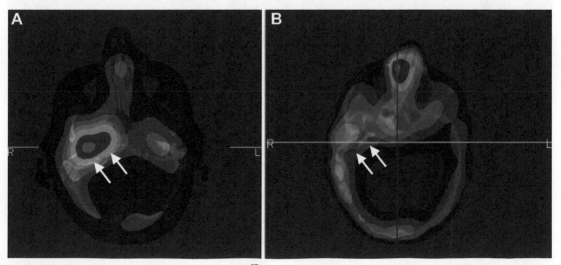

Fig. 24. Response assessment in central SBO using ⁶⁷Ga-citrate in 87-year-old woman with chronic kidney disease. Axial fused single-photon emission computed tomography (SPECT)–CT images. (*A*) Baseline showing increased tracer activity (*arrows*) in right petrous temporal bone and clivus corresponding with the osteomyelitis. (*B*) The 12-week posttreatment scan shows complete response. (*Courtesy of* Dr Lynne Armstrong and Dr Julian Kabala, Consultant Radiologists University Hospitals Bristol and Weston NHS Foundation Trust, United Kingdom.)

strategy to assess progress. There is a paucity of data as to which imaging modality is best for response assessment in SBO, and there are no consensus criteria for an optimal imaging end point (see **Table 2**).[34]

Recently, in a small study, the incorporation of echoplanar diffusion-weighted imaging (DWI) MR sequences into a conventional MR imaging protocol was shown to add value to response assessment in NOE-related SBO (**Fig. 25**).[35] DWI may especially help where conventional MR imaging with contrast (or CT) may not be able to differentiate between active infection and postinflammatory fibrosis and granulation tissue, which can persist for more than a year after the initial insult.[15,34] The other advantages of using DWI for initial staging and response assessment is that it can provide added MR assessment in patients who are not able to have intravenous contrast and does not involve

ionizing radiation, as opposed to CT and radionuclide imaging.[35]

There is an also an emerging role for hybrid imaging techniques such as FDG-PET/CT and PET-MR in osteomyelitis (**Fig. 26**).[6,36] It may be possible to use software-based techniques such as deformable coregistration to harness the synergistic potential of FDG-PET and MR imaging and perform a multimodality assessment in selected patients.[37]

It is important that treatment of SBO is underpinned by a multidisciplinary approach using dedicated protocols and specialist otology, microbiology, head and neck radiology (and nuclear medicine), and nursing input to improve patient outcomes and experience. It has been shown that such a coordinated interdisciplinary approach to management results in a decreased hospital stay and length of treatment.[38]

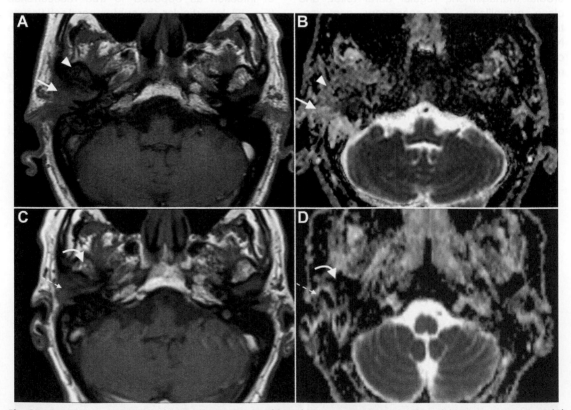

Fig. 25. Response assessment in SBO using DWI MR. (*A* and *C*) T1W precontrast MR and (*B* and *D*) ADC map. (*A*) Intermediate signal in the right retrocondylar space (*white arrow*) and articular eminence of the temporal bone (*white arrowhead*) with corresponding high ADC values (*B*) caused by right-sided NOE extending anteriorly. (*C*) and (D) are 3 months after antibiotic treatment and show near-complete resolution of infection in the retrocondylar region (*dashed white arrow*) and articular eminence (*curved white arrow*), seen as a restoration of normal fat signal on T1WI (*C*) and corresponding reduction in ADC values (*D*).

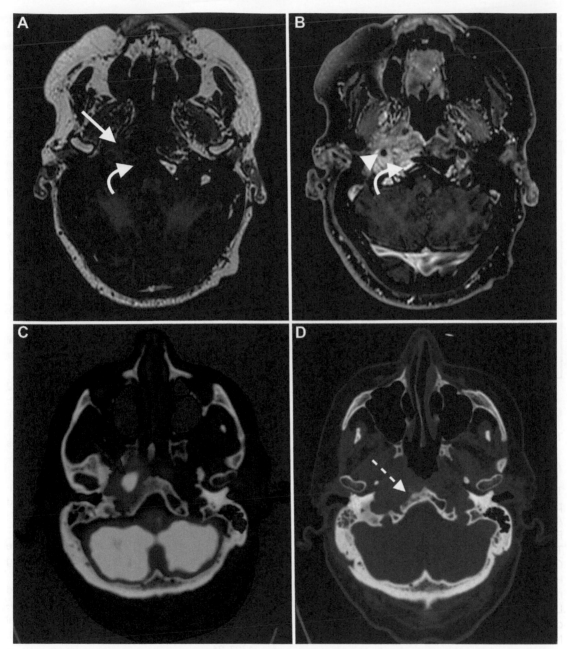

Fig. 26. Response assessment in central SBO using FDG-PET/CT. (*A*) T1W precontrast MR. Cellulitis in right deep neck space (*white arrow*) with intermediate signal in the right side of clivus (*curved white arrow*). (*B*) T1W post-contrast MR shows enhancement in this region (*curved white arrow*) and narrowing of the right ICA (*white arrowhead*). (*C*) Fused PET/CT shows intense tracer uptake in the soft tissue component, indicating residual disease at this site but complete response in the bone despite ongoing bony changes on CT (*D*).

SUMMARY

Imaging plays a critical role in aiding the diagnosis of SBO because of nonspecific symptoms and inaccessibility for tissue diagnosis. The commonest causes of SBO are (in order) NOE, complicated sinusitis, and idiopathic causes; other causes are

rare. Although no single imaging test is comprehensive in evaluating SBO, the initial assessment is best performed by a combination of high-resolution CT and multiparametric MR imaging, the latter providing a superior and more comprehensive evaluation. A multimodality and multidisciplinary approach using a dedicated protocol can help improve patient outcomes. Monitoring treatment response is a fundamental part of the imaging contribution and can be challenging; however, there are emerging promising imaging tools such as DWI MR and FDG-PET/CT.

CLINICS CARE POINTS

- MRI is superior to CT in assessing skull-base marrow involvement and T1 pre-contrast sequence is the most sensitive.
- Infection crossing the midline in the neck and involving cranial nerves portends a poor prognosis.
- Imaging features can lag behind symptoms and serum inflammatory markers during recovery and should be interpreted in the appropriate clinical context.
- A multidisciplinary approach to treatment using dedicated protocols and specialist input can improve patient outcomes and experience.

DISCLOSURE

The authors have nothing to disclose.

ACKNOWLEDGMENTS

The authors would like to thank our colleagues for providing some clinical cases and images: Mr. Amit Prasai and Mr. Justin Murphy (consultant ENT surgeons, Leeds Teaching Hospitals NHS Trust); Drs Stuart Currie, Mark Igra, and Harun Gupta (consultant radiologists, Leeds Teaching Hospitals NHS Trust); Dr Ashok Adams (consultant neuroradiologist, Barts Health NHS Trust); and Drs Lynne Armstrong and Julian Kabala (consultant radiologists, University Hospitals Bristol and Weston NHS Foundation Trust).

REFERENCES

1. Grandis JR, Branstetter BF, Yu VL. The changing face of malignant (necrotising) external otitis: clinical, radiological, and anatomic correlations. Lancet Infect Dis 2004;4(1):34–9.
2. Koch BL, Hamilton BE, Hudgins PA, et al. Diagnostic imaging: head and neck. Third edition. Salt Lake City (UT): Elsevier, Inc.; 2016.
3. Durand ML, Deschler DG. Durand, ML [Internet]. In: Infections of the ears, nose, throat, and sinuses. 2018. 115–30. Available at: https://doi.org/10.1007/978-3-319-74835-1. Accessed December 25, 2020.
4. Jereczek-Fossa BA, Zarowski A, Milani F, et al. Radiotherapy-induced ear toxicity. Cancer Treat Rev 2003;29(5):417–30.
5. Lingam RK, Kumar R, Vaidhyanath R. Inflammation of the Temporal Bone. Neuroimaging Clin N Am 2019;29(1):1–17.
6. Vaidyanathan S, Patel CN, Scarsbrook AF, et al. FDG PET/CT in infection and inflammation—current and emerging clinical applications. Clin Radiol 2015; 70(7):787–800.
7. Kulkarni SC, Padma S, Shanmuga Sundaram P. In the evaluation of patients with skull base osteomyelitis, does 18F-FDG PET CT have a role? Nucl Med Commun 2020;41(6):550–9.
8. Schupper AJ, Jiang W, Coulter MJ, et al. Intracranial complications of pediatric sinusitis: Identifying risk factors associated with prolonged clinical course. Int J Pediatr Otorhinolaryngol 2018;112:10–5.
9. Vilanilam GK, Gopal N, Gupta V, et al. A comprehensive review of the imaging of skull base infections – Part I. Radiol Infect Dis 2019; 6(3):87–94.
10. Ziegler A, Patadia M, Stankiewicz J. Neurological complications of acute and chronic sinusitis. Curr Neurol Neurosci Rep 2018;18(2):5.
11. Mahalingam HV, Mani SE, Patel B, et al. Imaging spectrum of cavernous sinus lesions with histopathologic correlation. RadioGraphics 2019;39(3): 795–819.
12. Aribandi M, McCoy VA, Bazan C. Imaging Features of Invasive and Noninvasive Fungal Sinusitis: A Review. RadioGraphics 2007;27(5):1283–96.
13. Gadre A, Brodie H, Fayad J, et al. Venous channels of the petrous apex: Their presence and clinical. Otolaryngol Head Neck Surg 1997; 116(2):168–74.
14. Charbonneau F, Williams M, Lafitte F, et al. No more fear of the cavernous sinuses! Diagn Interv Imaging 2013;94(10):1003–16.
15. Al-Noury K, Lotfy A. Computed tomography and magnetic resonance imaging findings before and after treatment of patients with malignant external otitis. Eur Arch Otorhinolaryngol 2011;268(12): 1727–34.
16. Nadol JB. Histopathology of pseudomonas osteomyelitis of the temporal bone starting as malignant external otitis. Am J Otolaryngol 1980;1(5):359–71.
17. Kohut RI, Lindsay JR. Necrotizing ("Malignant") External Otitis Histopathologic Processes. Ann Otol Rhinol Laryngol 1979;88(5):714–20.
18. Schmalfuss IM. Petrous Apex. Neuroimaging Clin N Am 2009;19(3):367–91.
19. Chang PC, Fischbein NJ, Holliday RA. Central Skull Base Osteomyelitis in Patients without Otitis Externa: Imaging Findings. AJNR Am J Neuroradiol 2003; 24(7):1310–6.

20. Clark M, Pretorius P, Byren I, et al. Central or Atypical Skull Base Osteomyelitis: Diagnosis and Treatment. Skull Base 2009;19(04):247–54.

21. Sharon JD, Khwaja SS, Drescher A, et al. Osteoradionecrosis of the temporal bone: a case series. Otol Neurotol 2014;35(7):1207–17.

22. Lalani N, Huang SH, Rotstein C, et al. Skull base or cervical vertebral osteomyelitis following chemoradiotherapy for pharyngeal carcinoma: A serious but treatable complication. Clin Transl Radiat Oncol 2018;8:40–4.

23. Schuknecht B, Stergiou G, Graetz K. Masticator space abscess derived from odontogenic infection: imaging manifestation and pathways of extension depicted by CT and MR in 30 patients. Eur Radiol 2008;18(9):1972–9.

24. McCann A, Alvi SA, Newman J, et al. Atypical Form of Cervicofacial Actinomycosis Involving the Skull Base and Temporal Bone. Ann Otol Rhinol Laryngol 2019;128(2):152–6.

25. Severino M, Liyanage S, Novelli V, et al. Skull base osteomyelitis and potential cerebrovascular complications in children. Pediatr Radiol 2012;42(7):867–74.

26. Prabhu SP, Zinkus T, Cheng AG, et al. Clival osteomyelitis resulting from spread of infection through the fossa navicularis magna in a child. Pediatr Radiol 2009;39(9):995–8.

27. Phillips I, Robertson N IJA. Osteomyelitis of the skull vault from a human bite. Br J Neurosurg 1997;11(2):168–9.

28. Mortazavi MM, Khan MA, Quadri SA, et al. Cranial Osteomyelitis: A Comprehensive Review of Modern Therapies. World Neurosurg 2018;111:142–53.

29. McGregor JA, McFarren T. Neonatal cranial osteomyelitis: a complication of fetal monitoring. Obstet Gynecol 1989;73(3 Pt 2):490–2.

30. Borges A. Imaging of the Central Skull Base. Neuroimaging Clin N Am 2009;19(3):441–68.

31. Evans IT, Richards SH. Malignant (necrotising) otitis externa. J Laryngol Otol 1973;87(1):13–20.

32. Spielmann PM, Yu R, Neeff M. Skull base osteomyelitis: current microbiology and management. J Laryngol Otol 2013;127(S1):S8–12.

33. Mahdyoun P, Pulcini C, Gahide I, et al. Necrotizing otitis externa: a systematic review. Otol Neurotol 2013;34(4):620–9.

34. Courson AM, Vikram HR, Barrs DM. What are the criteria for terminating treatment for necrotizing (malignant) otitis externa?: Necrotizing Otitis Externa: Ending Treatment. Laryngoscope 2014;124(2):361–2.

35. Cherko M, Nash R, Singh A, et al. Diffusion-weighted Magnetic Resonance Imaging as a Novel Imaging Modality in Assessing Treatment Response in Necrotizing Otitis Externa. Otol Neurotol 2016;37(6):704–7.

36. van Kroonenburgh AMJL, van der Meer WL, Bothof RJP, et al. Advanced imaging techniques in skull base osteomyelitis due to malignant otitis externa. Curr Radiol Rep 2018;6(1):3.

37. Bhatnagar P, Subesinghe M, Patel C, et al. Functional imaging for radiation treatment planning, response assessment, and adaptive therapy in head and neck cancer. RadioGraphics 2013;33(7):1909–29.

38. Sharma S, Corrah T, Singh A. Management of necrotizing otitis externa: our experience with forty-three patients. J Int Adv Otol 2017;13(3):394–8.

39. von Itzstein MS, Abeykoon JP, Summerfield DD, et al. Severe destructive nasopharyngeal granulomatosis with polyangiitis with superimposed skull base *Pseudomonas aeruginosa* osteomyelitis. BMJ Case Rep 2017. https://doi.org/10.1136/bcr-2017-220135. bcr-2017-220135.

40. Xu X, Lao X, Zhang C, et al. Chronic Mycobacterium avium skin and soft tissue infection complicated with scalp osteomyelitis possibly secondary to anti-interferon-γ autoantibody formation. BMC Infect Dis 2019;19(1):203.

41. Pudipeddi AV, Liu K, Watson GF, et al. Cryptococcal osteomyelitis of the skull in a liver transplant patient. Transpl Infect Dis 2016;18(6):954–6.

42. Saito N, Nadgir RN, Flower EN, et al. Clinical and Radiologic Manifestations of Sickle Cell Disease in the Head and Neck. RadioGraphics 2010;30(4):1021–34.

43. Adams A, Offiah C. Central skull base osteomyelitis as a complication of necrotizing otitis externa: Imaging findings, complications, and challenges of diagnosis. Clin Radiol 2012;67(10):e7–16.

44. Casselman JW. The skull base: tumoral lesions. Eur Radiol 2005;15(3):534–42.

45. Parmar H, Gujar S, Shah G, et al. Imaging of the Anterior Skull Base. Neuroimaging Clin N Am 2009;19(3):427–39.

46. Sreepada GS, Kwartler JA. Skull base osteomyelitis secondary to malignant otitis externa. Curr Opin Otolaryngol Head Neck Surg 2003;11(5):316–23.

47. Palestro CJ. Radionuclide Imaging of Osteomyelitis. Semin Nucl Med 2015;45(1):32–46.

48. Waller ML, Chowdhury FU. The basic science of nuclear medicine. Orthop Trauma 2016;30(3):201–22.

49. Garty I, Rosen G, Holdstein Y. The radionuclide diagnosis, evaluation, and follow-up of malignant external otitis (MEO): The value of immediate blood pool scanning. J Laryngol Otol 1985;99(2):109–15.

50. Stokkel MPM, Takes RP, van Eck-Smit BLF, et al. The value of quantitative gallium-67 single-photon emission tomography in the clinical management of malignant external otitis. Eur J Nucl Med Mol Imaging 1997;24(11):1429–32.

51. Basu S, Chryssikos T, Moghadam-Kia S, et al. Positron Emission Tomography as a Diagnostic Tool in

Infection: Present Role and Future Possibilities. Semin Nucl Med 2009;39(1):36–51.

52. van der Meer WL, van Tilburg M, Mitea C, et al. A persistent foramen of huschke: a small road to misery in necrotizing external otitis. AJNR Am J Neuroradiol 2019;40(9):1552–6.

53. Mehrotra P, Elbadawey MR, Zammit-Maempel I. Spectrum of radiological appearances of necrotising external otitis: a pictorial review. J Laryngol Otol 2011;125(11):1109–15.

54. Lee S, Hooper R, Fuller A, et al. Otogenic cranial base osteomyelitis: a proposed prognosis-based system for disease classification. Otol Neurotol 2008;29(5):666–72.

55. Pincus D, Armstrong M, Thaller S. Osteomyelitis of the craniofacial skeleton. Semin Plast Surg 2009; 23(02):073–9.

56. Rubin J, Yu VL. Malignant external otitis: Insights into pathogenesis, clinical manifestations, diagnosis, and therapy. Am J Med 1988;85(3):391–8.

Imaging of Skull Base Trauma
Fracture Patterns and Soft Tissue Injuries

Ashok Adams, MBBS, EDiNR, MRCP, FRCR

KEYWORDS

- Anterior • Central and posterior skull base • Cerebrospinal fluid leak • Vascular injury
- Cranial nerve deficit

KEY POINTS

- The different patterns of skull base trauma can help predict the severity of associated injuries and anticipate subsequent complications.
- Significant complications of skull base trauma include vascular and cranial nerve injuries, cerebrospinal fluid leaks, and intracranial sepsis.
- Knowledge of skull base anatomy and anatomical variants is key to identifying pseudofracture.

INTRODUCTION

Traumatic brain injury is a major cause of mortality and morbidity, and in England and Wales approximately 1.4 million patients per year are admitted to the hospital following a head injury.[1] In the authors' institution at a level I trauma unit, there are approximately 3000 trauma cases per year with an incidence of skull base fractures of approximately 5%.[2] Skull base fractures are more common in nonpenetrating versus penetrating head injuries and are most often related to high-energy trauma, particularly road traffic accidents.[3]

The skull base is uniquely placed to absorb force imparted to both the facial skeleton and/or cranial vault during trauma.[4] Clinical signs of suspected skull base fracture include the presence of cerebrospinal fluid (CSF) otorrhea/rhinorrhea, hemotympanum, and periorbital ("raccoon eyes") and retroauricular ("Battle" sign) ecchymoses; however, they correlate poorly with imaging findings.[5] Detection of basilar skull fractures assists acute patient management, particularly anterior skull base (ASB) fractures that have implications for airway management and passage of nasoenteric tubes. Identification of potential vascular injuries is essential to prevent secondary complications, whereas treatment decisions in the patients with polytrauma, particularly with regard to anticoagulation and neurointervention, are guided by the severity of coexistent traumatic injuries that may be more life threatening.

Identification of skull base fractures prompts assessment for coexistent intracranial injuries that may require surgical intervention given their strong association with skull base fractures.[6] Skull base fractures, including subtle nondisplaced fractures, can be associated with complications that include CSF leaks that may also necessitate further surgical intervention.[7]

OSSEOUS SKULL BASE ANATOMY

The skull base is composed of the unpaired ethmoid, sphenoid, and occipital bones with paired frontal and temporal bones. The skull base is subdivided into the anterior, central, and posterior skull base with the anatomic landmarks summarized in **Table 1**.

PEARLS, PITFALLS, AND VARIANTS

It is important to be aware of normal anatomic variants that can be misinterpreted as linear undisplaced fractures of the skull base, the so-called

No commercial or financial disclosures.
BartsHealth NHS Trust, Queen Mary University of London, Neuroradiology Department, Royal London Hospital, Whitechapel Rd, London E1 1BB, UK
E-mail address: Ashok.adams@nhs.net

Table 1
Anatomic divisions of the anterior, central, and posterior skull base

Skull Base Subdivsion	Anatomical Landmarks
Anterior skull base (ASB)	The ASB is formed by the frontal and ethmoid bones, and the border between the anterior and central skull base is delineated by the lesser wing of the sphenoid bone, anterior clinoid process, and planum sphenoidale[8]
	The floor of the anterior cranial fossa is composed of the orbital part of the frontal bones, and between them is the ethmoid bone with its cribriform plate
	The olfactory grooves are located lateral to the midline crista galli and the floor of the olfactory groove is formed by the thin cribriform plates (Fig. 1)
CSB	The CSB is formed by the sphenoid and paired temporal bones.[9] The anterior border is delineated by the posterior margin of the lesser wing of the sphenoid bone, anterior clinoid processes and tuberculum sella.
	Posteriorly, the border between the central and posterior skull base is formed centrally by the dorsum sella and basisphenoid portion of the clivus and laterally by the petrous ridges of the temporal bones. The lesser wings of the sphenoid bone extend horizontally toward the lateral cranial fossa and between the lesser and greater wings of the sphenoid bone is the superior orbital fissure (Fig. 2).
	The middle cranial fossa floor is partially formed by the petrous and tympanic components of the temporal bone and both the roof of the tympanic cavity and antrum separate the middle cranial fossa structures from the middle ear and mastoid cavity.
PSB	The PSB is formed by the temporal and occipital bones, and the border between the central and posterior skull base is formed by the dorsum sella, basisphenoid portion of the clivus, and by the petrous ridges of the temporal bones[3]
	The inferior border of the posterior fossa is formed by basioccipital portion of the clivus, occipital condyles, mastoid segment of the temporal bone, and squamous portion of the occipital bone
	The inferior border outlines the foramen magnum, whereas the jugular foramen is divided into a pars nervosa and pars vascularis by the jugular spine (Fig. 3)
	The hypoglossal canal is located inferior and medial to the jugular foramen. and the hypoglossal nerve passes through the canal

Abbreviations: CSB, central skull base; PSB, posterior skull base.

pseudofractures.[10] These variants include a variety of accessory skull base foramina, synchondroses, fissures, and sutures (Table 2). The combination of multiplanar reconstructed computed tomographic (CT) imaging, correlation with the mechanism of injury, and presence of associated injuries aids differentiation between traumatic fractures from normal variants (Fig. 4).

IMAGING MODALITIES

The imaging modalities and techniques available for skull base imaging are outlined in Table 3. CT remains the first-line imaging modality in the acute trauma setting given its availability, scanning speed, and efficiency. In patients with polytrauma, the brain, spine, and body can be imaged within a

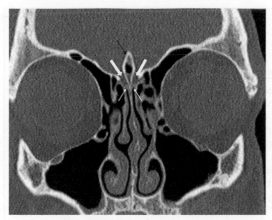

Fig. 1. Coronal CT image of the ASB demonstrating the olfactory grooves (*thick white arrows*) located lateral to the midline crista galli (*black arrow*); the floor of the olfactory groove is formed by the thin cribriform plates (*thin white arrows*).

short time interval, and in the author's institution, initial imaging of the brain and cervical spine is performed without intravenous contrast.[2] Additional imaging of vascular injuries is performed with a CT angiogram and/or venogram. MR imaging of the brain is performed to assess the extent of primary injuries and for secondary complications, providing important prognostic information. MR imaging of the orbits and neck soft tissues is included in the presence of visual symptoms and new-onset cranial nerve palsies. If there is a suspected CSF leak, cisternography is undertaken if it is difficult to identify the source of a CSF leak

on the initial trauma imaging.[3] The preferred technique in the author's institution is CT given the logistical considerations of imaging the patients with polytrauma, although MR cisternography is an alternative.

ANTERIOR SKULL BASE TRAUMA
Trauma Mechanisms and Anatomic Considerations

Frontobasal fractures are typically observed in the setting of severe head trauma, most commonly blunt trauma.[13] Penetrating trauma can also result in frontobasal fractures with the penetrating object or projectile traversing the orbits and/or sinonasal compartment to access the ASB. Anatomically, the frontal component relates to the upper face including the frontal bone, frontal sinus, and superior orbital rim, whereas the basal component relates to the ASB including the cribriform plate, ethmoidal roof, and planum sphenoidale.

The ASB can be subdivided into central and lateral compartments. The medial central compartment is composed of interorbital structures including the frontal sinuses, ethmoidal labyrinths, nasal cavity, and sphenoid sinuses. These structures are weaker than the lateral compartment, and thus the midfacial structures act as a "crumple zone." This crumple zone acts to protect both the contents of the orbit and the intracranial contents by dissipating traumatic forces before they reach these structures. The lateral compartment relates to the lateral aspect of the frontal

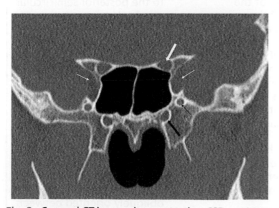

Fig. 2. Coronal CT image demonstrating CSB anatomy. The superior orbital fissures (*thin white arrows*) are located between the lesser and greater wings of the sphenoid bone through which pass the oculomotor, trochlear, abducens, and trigeminal nerve ophthalmic division. The left optic nerve canal (*thick white arrow*), foramen rotundum (*thin black arrow*), and vidian nerve canal (*thick black arrow*) are highlighted.

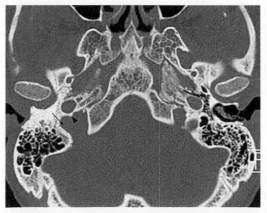

Fig. 3. The jugular foramen is divided into a pars nervosa (*thin white arrow*) and pars vascularis (*thin black arrow*) by the jugular spine (*thick black arrowhead*). The glossopharyngeal nerve, Jacobson nerve and inferior petrosal sinus pass through the anterior pars nervosa, whereas the vagus nerve, accessory nerve, Arnold nerve, and jugular bulb pass through the pars vascularis.

Table 2
Normal anatomic variant vascular channels, fissures, synchondroses, and foramina within the skull base

Anterior Skull Base	Central Skull Base	Posterior Skull Base
Anterior ethmoidal canal that transmits the anterior ethmoidal artery branch of the ophthalmic artery and associated nerve. It passes from the orbit and via the nasal cavity to access the anterior skull base *Posterior ethmoidal canal* that transmits the posterior ethmoidal artery branch of the ophthalmic artery and associated nerve. It passes from the orbit and via the nasal cavity to access the anterior skull base *Supraorbital foramen or notch* transmits the supraorbital nerve branch of the ophthalmic division of the trigeminal nerve and associated artery and nerve. It is located at the medial aspect of the superior orbital margin of the frontal bone *Sphenofrontal suture* within the roof of the orbit represents the articulation between the frontal bone and the greater wing of the sphenoid bone.	*Foramen meningo-orbitale* extends from the middle cranial fossa to the superolateral orbit and is an embryonic remnant *Foramen Vesalius* located between the foramen ovale and rotundum transmits a venous emissary between the pterygoid plexus and cavernous sinus *Canaliculus innominatus* is a small channel connecting the foramen spinosum and foramen ovale and transmits branches of the lesser petrosal nerve *Palatovaginal canal* is inferomedial to the vidian nerve canal and extends from the pterygopalatine fossa to the nasopharyngeal roof *Craniopharyngeal canal* is a congenital remnant canal that extends from the sellar base to the nasopharynx *Petroclival/petro-occipital fissure* between the basiocciput and apex of the petrous temporal bone *Sphenopetrosal suture* is located between the posterior aspect of the greater wing of the sphenoid bone and petrous apex *Sphenosquamosal suture* is a vertical suture between the sphenoid and temporal bone that fuses during childhood, located lateral to the foramen spinosum *Spheno-occipital synchondrosis* that fuses during adolescence and is located between the basisphenoid and basioccipit	*Canalis basilaris medianus* is located in the midline and extends from the pharynx to the basioccipital location and can be associated with recurrent meningitis. It is considered a notochord remnant *Petromastoid canal* transmits the subarcuate artery and vein and extends from the subarcuate fossa and passes between the limbs of the superior semicircular canal to open in the mastoid cavity *Inferior tympanic canaliculus* transmits the tympanic branch of the glossopharyngeal nerve (Jacobson nerve). It extends from the jugular foramen superiorly to the middle ear *Mastoid canaliculus* transmits the auricular branch of the vagus nerve (Arnold nerve). It extends from the jugular foramen to the descending mastoid segment of the facial nerve. It emerges from the tympanomastoid suture *Singular canal* extends from the internal auditory canal to the posterior semicircular canal and transmits the posterior ampullary/singular nerve *Tympanomastoid fissure* divides the tympanic part of the temporal bone and mastoid process *Tympanosquamous fissure* is located anterior to the bony external auditory canal and continues medially to the petrosquamous and petrotympanic fissure *Petrosquamous fissure* is obliquely oriented between the medial petrous and lateral squamous temporal bone *(continued on next page)*

Table 2 (continued)		
Anterior Skull Base	**Central Skull Base**	**Posterior Skull Base**
		Petrotympanic fissure is a fissure that connects the glenoid fossa and the tympanic cavity and transmits the chorda tympani
		Occipitomastoid suture located posterior to the mastoid process
		Posterior condylar canal extends between the jugular foramen and condylar fossa and contains an emissary vein

Data from Baugnon KL, Hudgins PA. Skull Base Fractures and Their Complications. Neuroimaging Clin N Am. 2014;24(3):439-465 and Connor SE, Tan G, Fernando R, Chaudhury N. Computed tomography pseudofractures of the mid face and skull base. Clin Radiol. 2005;60(12):1268-79.

sinus, orbital roof, and supraorbital rim, and the lack of collapsible interface results in an increased energy transfer to the intracranial contents during trauma. Thus, if the direction of force applied to the ASB is more lateral, the severity of injury is greater.[4]

Although frontobasal fractures can occur in isolation, they are typically associated with other osseous and soft tissue injuries given the relationship of the ASB to the midface naso-orbito-ethmoidal (NOE) complex, orbits, paranasal sinuses, and central skull base.[14]

NOE fractures in particular are associated with ASB and frontal bone fractures with possibility of posterior frontal sinus wall disruption. Posterior sinus wall fractures results in increased risk of

intracranial hemorrhage, CSF leak, pneumocephalus, contusion, or laceration of the brain parenchyma.

Proposed Classification Systems

There are classification systems proposed to categorize ASB fracture patterns with consideration of anatomic factors, mechanism of injury, potential complications, and surgical management.[15–17] In the classification system proposed by Madhusudan and colleagues,[17] patients who sustained frontobasal fractures with concomitant involvement of the midfacial skeleton ("impure" fractures) demonstrated a reduced incidence of brain contusion compared with those with frontobasal

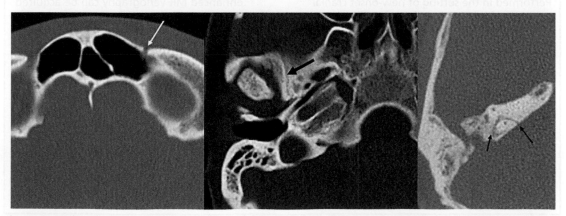

Fig. 4. Examples of anatomic variants and pseudofractures of the skull base. In the left-hand image there is a soft tissue injury overlying the left orbit; however, the white arrow indicates the normal supraorbital foramen/notch (*white arrow*). In the central image the linear lucency represents the normal sphenosquamosal suture (*thick black arrow*). In the right-hand temporal bone image there is a conspicuous subarcuate/petromastoid canal running in between the crura of the superior semicircular canal that should not be mistaken for a fracture line (*thin black arrow*).

Table 3
Imaging modalities and techniques available for imaging skull base trauma

Modality	Technique
CT head	Supine position, scanning from C2 to vertex
Performed in initial trauma imaging	0.75–1 mm slice thickness enables multiplanar reconstruction
Noncontrast study	
CT angiogram	Dedicated bone algorithm for skull base anatomy
Performed in suspected arterial vascular injury in penetrating trauma. In blunt trauma this can be based on modified Memphis criteria or Denver criteria[11,12] (Table 3)	Supine position, arms adducted
	Scanning from aortic arch to vertex
	0.75 mm slice thickness. Approximately 150 mL nonionic iodinated contrast with flow rate of approximately 6 mL/s
CT venogram	Supine position, arms adducted
Performed in skull base fractures that involve the transverse sinus, sigmoid sinus, or jugular foramen. Presence of extra-axial collection in the posterior fossa.	Scanning from C2 to vertex
	0.75 mm slice thickness.
CT cisternography	Approximately 75–100 mL nonionic iodinated contrast with flow rate of approximately 4 mL/s. Scanned at 45 s delay
Performed in setting of suspected skull base CSF leak to confirm both a leak and site of leak to guide surgical intervention	Precontrast CT image acquired. Lumbar puncture performed with 3–10 mL nonionic iodinated contrast injected into the theca. Patient rotated on table and head tilted down. Postcontrast imaging acquired
MR brain imaging	Routine sequences including T1, T2, FLAIR, DWI, and gradient recall echo or susceptibility-weighted imaging.
Assess for primary injuries and secondary complications due to skull base fractures and associated vascular injury	High-resolution CISS sequences and combination of volumetric T1- and T2-weighted sequences of the intracranial compartment skull base to assess for meningoencephaloceles
MR angiography	Time-of-flight or contrast-enhanced MR angiography of the intracranial and extracranial vessels supplemented by axial T1 and T2 fat-suppressed neck imaging dissection protocol
Same criteria applied as for CT angiography	
MR venography	
Same criteria applied as for CT venography	Time of flight, phase contrast, or contrast-enhanced MR venography can be acquired to assess patency and flow. In the trauma setting this can be impaired by the presence of blood products in addition to the flow-related artifacts that can affect the TOF and phase contrast imaging in particular
MR orbits and neck soft tissues	
Performed in cases of suspected traumatic optic neuropathy based on mechanism of injury or pattern of craniofacial fracture with involvement of orbital apex/optic nerve canal	Coronal T2 and fat-suppressed T2-weighted sequences of the orbits to assess the optic nerve
Performed in the setting of new-onset cranial nerve palsies and speech and swallowing difficulties	DWI sequences can accentuate any changes within the optic nerve and there may be a role for diffusion tensor imaging
	Conventional T2, STIR, T1, and T1 postcontrast imaging acquired to assess extracranial pathway of the cranial nerves and target organs

Abbreviations: CISS, constructive interference in steady state; DWI, diffusion-weighted imaging, FLAIR, fluid-attenuated inversion recovery; STIR, short tau inversion recovery; TOF, time of flight.

fractures that resulted from direct trauma to the frontobasal region ("pure" fracture); this is confirmed in cadaveric studies and in the study by Manson and colleagues[16] subdividing frontobasal fractures into types I to III (Table 4).

Complications and Soft Tissue Injuries

The dura within the floor of the anterior cranial fossa is adherent to the ASB that predisposes to laceration during trauma with subsequent risk of CSF leak, pneumocephalus, and orbitofrontal brain parenchymal contusion/laceration.[18]

Trauma is the most common cause for a CSF leak, and patients most commonly present with rhinorrhea. In combination with the CSF leak, the direct communication between the intracranial compartment and sinonasal cavity results in an increase of meningitis and potential complications, including extradural/subdural empyema, cerebritis, and parenchymal abscess formation (Fig. 8). Rarely, CSF oculorrhea has been reported in the setting of severe orbital trauma.[19] Intraorbital traumatic pseudomeningoceles can also complicate orbital trauma; this occurs due to an extradural collection of CSF that can extend into the orbit if the orbital fracture resulted in a dural tear. Intraorbital traumatic pseudomeningoceles can present both acutely and as a delayed complication.[20] Clinically this may be difficult to distinguish from a caroticocavernous fistula because orbital pseudomeningoceles may also be pulsatile in nature secondary to CSF pulsations.

Most CSF leaks present during the acute setting, but delayed presentations can occur years after the acute traumatic episode. A low threshold for imaging in patients with recurrent meningitis with a history of prior skull base trauma is required because this may portend an underlying CSF leak. The presence of CSF within nasal discharge can be confirmed with testing for β2 transferrin or β trace protein.[21] In the acute setting, CSF leaks can resolve with conservative management techniques, but if persistent, CSF diversion procedures and surgical intervention may be required.

Pneumocephalus or pneumatocele is an abnormal collection of air in the cranial cavity that can complicate traumatic head injuries. The accumulation of intracranial air can be acute or delayed, and in most circumstances it is benign and asymptomatic. When intracranial air causes intracranial hypertension and has a mass effect with neurologic deterioration, it is called *tension pneumocephalus,* which may necessitate neurosurgical decompression.[7]

Traumatic fracture disruption of the cribriform plate and fovea ethmoidalis with potential traumatic contusions of the orbitofrontal and temporal

Table 4
Classification of frontobasal fractures

Fracture Type	Fracture Pattern
Type I fractures Type I frontobasal fractures were less frequently associated with complications[13]	Linear fractures located parallel to the cribriform plate extending posteriorly along the sella and petrous ridge separating the anterior and middle cranial fossa from the posterior cranial fossa (Fig. 5)
Type II fractures Type II fractures were associated with more severe intracranial injuries and higher risk of CSF leak[15,16]	Vertical linear fractures of the frontal bone and anterior skull base extending to the lateral supraorbital rim, orbital roof, lateral orbital wall, and orbital apex (Fig. 6)
Type III fracture Type III fractures were associated with the most severe intracranial injuries and higher risk of CSF leak[15,16]	Most severe and classified as comminuted fractures involving the central and lateral frontobasilar compartments (Fig. 7)

Data from Manson PN, Stanwix MG, Yaremchuk MJ et al. Frontobasal Fractures: Anatomical Classification and Clinical Significance: Plast Reconstr Surg. 2009;124(6):2096-2106 and Madhusudan G, Sharma RK, Khandelwal N et al. Nomenclature of Frontobasal Trauma: A New Clinicoradiographic Classification: Plast Reconstr Surg. 2006;117(7):2382-2388.

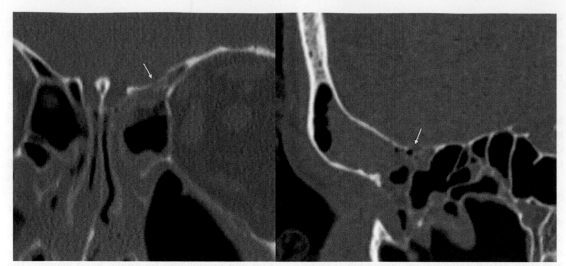

Fig. 5. Coronal and sagittal CT images in a patient who fell with direct impact to the frontal area. Type 1 frontobasal fracture; there is a linear minimally displaced fracture (*thin white arrows*) traversing the left fovea ethmoidalis, with the fracture line orientated parallel to the cribriform plate.

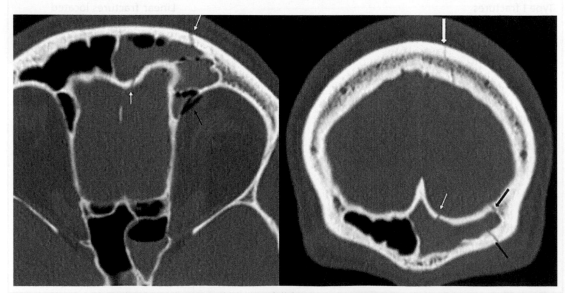

Fig. 6. Axial and coronal CT images in a patient who fell from height. Type II frontobasal fracture with a vertical linear fracture of the frontal bone (*thick white arrow*) extending inferiorly to traverse the left frontal sinus, extending to the lateral supraorbital rim (*thick black arrow*) and orbital roof (*thin black arrow arrows*).

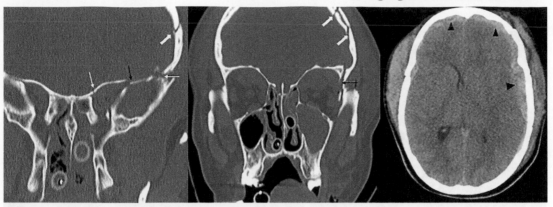

Fig. 7. Coronal and axial CT images in a patient who fell from height sustaining comminuted fractures involving the lateral frontobasilar compartment. Type III frontobasal fracture with comminuted and displaced fractures of the left frontal bone (*thick white arrows*), anterior skull base (*thin white arrows*), and superior/lateral orbital walls (*thin black arrows*). Significant intracranial injuries included subdural hematomata (*black arrowheads*) and cerebral swelling affecting the left hemisphere with right-sided midline shift.

lobe parenchyma can result in olfactory pathway trauma.[22] Disruption of the olfactory pathways can also occur in the absence of skull base fracture with shear-type injuries that can disrupt the olfactory nerves. Posttraumatic disruption of the olfactory pathways is typically irreversible, but potential for any potential rehabilitation can be expedited by predicting these injuries on initial imaging (Fig. 9).

In the presence of ASB fractures, assessment of the integrity of the orbital walls and posterior extension toward the orbital apex with involvement of the optic nerve canal is required to assess the risk of traumatic optic neuropathy.

Orbital blow-in fractures may occur as part of the NOE fracture complex, and in this setting, assessment of the orbits requires specific evaluation of the medial canthal tendon (MCT) attachment site given the implications for subsequent surgical management. The MCT inserts by 2 fascicles, an anterior fascicle in the anterior lacrimal crest of the maxillary frontal process and a posterior fascicle in the posterior lacrimal crest of the lacrimal bone. The MCT represents the medial insertion of the eyelids, and the lacrimal sac is present between the 2 crests, thus it plays a role in lacrimal sac drainage. The classification system by Markowitz and colleagues[23] subdivides the fracture patterns into 3 different types (Table 5).

Assessment of the paranasal sinuses requires assessment of both frontal sinuses and integrity of the anterior and posterior walls. The degree of pneumatization of the paranasal sinuses is important, particularly in the pediatric population where the frontal sinuses have not developed with higher rate of orbital rim fractures. Important considerations include the presence of pneumocephalus, possibility of a CSF leak and risk of meningitis if the posterior wall is fractured. Involvement of the

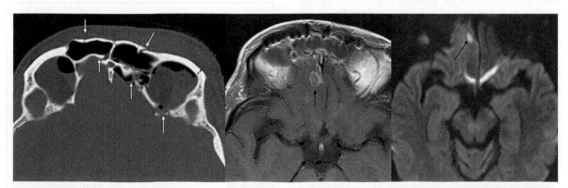

Fig. 8. Axial noncontrast CT image and MR images including axial T1 postcontrast, axial b1000 diffusion-weighted image (apparent diffusion coefficient [ADC] map not shown). This patient was involved in an road traffic accident (RTA) and sustained facial, orbital, and anterior skull base fractures (*white arrows*). The patient underwent obliteration of the frontal sinuses but developed a combination of a subdural empyema (not shown) and a parenchymal abscess (*black arrows*).

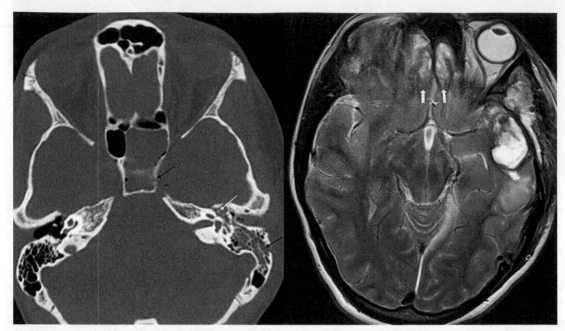

Fig. 9. Axial CT image and axial T2-weighted MR image in a cyclist hit by a truck. There are skull base fractures involving the left temporal bone (*thin black arrows*). There are parenchymal contusions and disruption of the gyrus rectuses (*thick white arrows*) that resulted in disruption of the olfactory pathways. The fracture complex traversed the geniculate ganglion (*thin white arrow*) and proximal tympanic segment of the facial nerve canal resulting in facial nerve paralysis.

frontal sinus drainage pathway and nasofrontal duct also has the potential to cause subsequent mucocele formation that is best assessed on sagittal reformats. Persistent opacification and enlargement of the frontal sinus on follow-up imaging may prompt surgical intervention and irrigation with methylene blue for further evaluation. Surgical intervention is considered for frontal sinus fracture involvement, and strategies include frontal sinus obliteration or cranialization with flap reconstruction.[7,8] Patients with severe trauma that results in disruption of greater than 25% of the posterior table should be considered for frontal sinus cranialization, which involves exposure of the entire sinus, removal of all sinus mucosa, and removal of the posterior table bone. Isolated fractures of the anterior wall may also be managed surgically with consideration of the degree of comminution and potential cosmetic deformity.

CENTRAL SKULL BASE TRAUMA
Trauma Mechanisms and Anatomic Considerations

Central skull base fractures are observed in the setting of high-energy blunt trauma. The fracture patterns relate to areas of weakness in relation to the central skull base with the anterior and posterior walls of the sphenoid sinus considered as

points of transition.[11] Anteriorly there is a transition between the posterior ethmoidal labyrinth with the relatively unsupported lateral walls of the sphenoid sinus. Posteriorly, there is a transition between the lateral walls of the sphenoid sinus with the solid cancellous clival bone. The sphenopetrosal synchondrosis represents another weak point that is often fractured, and this fibrocartilaginous junction between the greater wing of the sphenoid bone

Table 5
Markowitz classification of orbital fractures

Classification	Fracture Pattern
Type I	There is a single fracture fragment at the attachment site of the ligament, which is intact (**Fig. 10**)
Type II	Type II describes a comminuted fracture with the ligament attached to a single osseous fragment
Type III	type III is the most severe whereby the comminuted fracture involves the ligament attachment site with an avulsed tendon

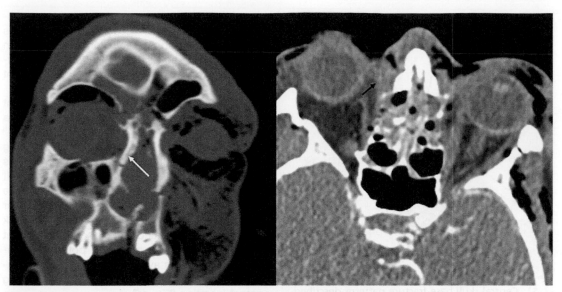

Fig. 10. Axial CT imaging on a bone and soft tissue window setting in a patient involved in an RTA. Significant naso-fronto-ethmoidal fractures with a Manson type 1 fracture with displacement of a large bone fragment with the attachment of the medial canthal tendon (*white arrow*). There is soft tissue stranding and hematoma at this site (*black arrow*).

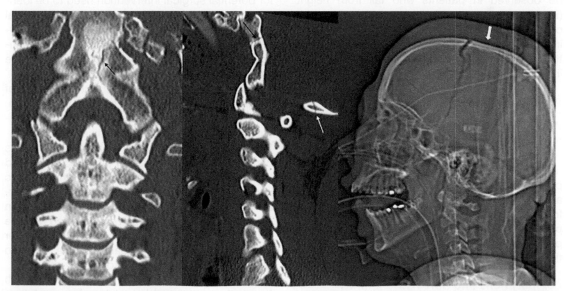

Fig. 11. Coronal and sagittal CT images and scout radiograph from a patient who fell from height. There is a vertically orientated fracture (*thick white arrow*) involving the calvarium with extension into the clivus (*thin black arrows*) and occipital bone (*thin white arrow*).

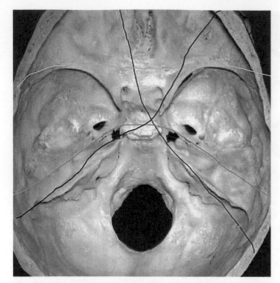

Fig. 12. Central skull base fracture patterns described by West and colleagues.[23] Yellow line, anterior transverse fracture pattern; blue line, posterior transverse fracture pattern; black line, lateral frontal diagonal fracture pattern, red line, mastoid diagonal fracture pattern.

and petrous temporal bone has a close relationship with the carotid canal. The stronger spheno-temporal buttress and petrous temporal bone can dissipate force to these sites of weakness, which is related to the fracture patterns described later.

Special consideration is given to axial loading forces and subsequent fracture pattern that can be observed in patients who fall from height (**Fig. 11**). The central skull base fractures can be orientated in a longitudinal plane, and clival involvement is a poor prognostic indicator given the risks of brainstem and vertebrobasilar arterial injury.[24]

Proposed Classification Systems

With severe lateral or frontal impact trauma, central skull base involvement may occur in the setting of additional anterior and posterior skull base fractures. West and colleagues[11] described 4 main patterns of central skull base involvement into anterior transverse, posterior transverse, lateral frontal diagonal, and mastoid diagonal fracture patterns (**Fig. 12**). The 2 diagonal patterns in particular are associated with increased complication rates and poorer outcomes (**Table 6**).

Complications and Soft Tissue Injuries

The soft tissue injuries and complications of central skull base fractures can be subdivided into vascular injuries, CSF leaks, and cranial nerve injuries. The spectrum of vascular injuries includes vascular transection, occlusion, incarceration within fracture fragments, dissection and aneurysm, pseudoaneursym, and arteriovenous shunt formation[24–26] (**Fig. 15**).

Vascular injury incidence in the setting of blunt trauma varies depending on the screening criteria applied to facilitate further vascular imaging.[26] Different criteria have been proposed, including the widely recognized Denver and Memphis criteria that have been modified[12,25] (**Table 7**). It is important to identify these injuries given the high risk of subsequent cerebrovascular ischemia/infarction and thus ameliorating this risk with appropriate anticoagulation or antiplatelet therapy.[25] In addition, given the potential endovascular treatments available, certain vascular injuries may be amenable to treatment with coiling or stent insertion (**Fig. 16**).

Although less frequent when compared with ASB fractures, CSF leaks can also occur in the setting of central skull base trauma secondary to disruption of the sphenoid sinuses. Penetrating trauma and sphenoid roof fractures are associated with higher risk of CSF leaks.[27]

Traumatic injury of the visual apparatus and optic nerves can occur secondary to a variety of different mechanisms including neuronal stretching, edema, and impairment of vascular supply.[28] Traumatic optic neuropathy (TON) is an uncommon cause of visual loss following blunt or penetrating head trauma with a reported incidence of 0.7% to 2.5%.[29] In an acute setting, candidates for potential surgical intervention need to be identified, and this requires assessment of orbital apex/canal fractures and their degree of comminution and displacement as well as soft tissue injuries, including any potentially compressive intraorbital hematoma (**Fig. 17**).

Indirect TON is caused by the transmission of forces to the optic nerve from a distant site, without any overt damage to the surrounding tissue structures.[29] The deformative stress transmitted the skull from blunt trauma is concentrated in the region of the optic canal, and thus the intracanalicular segment of the optic nerve is susceptible to this form of injury. Follow-up MR imaging in the setting of suspected can demonstrate altered signal change and volume loss within the affected optic nerve, and newer diffusion tensor imaging can also be used to assess potential traumatic axonal disruption.[30]

Cranial nerve deficits can be identified in both the acute setting and in a delayed presentation, the latter presumably related to worsening edema that is associated with a better prognosis. In

Table 6
Patterns of central skull base fracture

Fracture Pattern	Complications
Lateral frontal diagonal pattern Lateral impact to the lateral orbital and lateral maxillary wall propagates to the lateral and posterior walls of the sphenoid and often with extension to the contralateral skull base (Fig. 13)	This pattern is associated with cranial nerve injuries (typically the oculomotor, abducens, and facial nerves) and hearing loss
Mastoid diagonal pattern The fracture complex typically involves the occipital bone and occipitomastoid suture with anteromedial extension to involve the jugular foramen, petroclival fissure, and sphenoid body with potential subsequent lateral extension to the contralateral orbit and anterior skull base (Fig. 14)	This pattern is associated with cranial nerve injuries (typically the glossopharyngeal, vagus, and accessory nerves if there is jugular foramen involvement, whereas the extension of the central skull base is associated with abducens nerve palsy)
Anterior transverse pattern The fracture complex extends from the squamous temporal bone along the sphenotemporal buttress to intersect the transition between the ethmoid and sphenoid sinus in a coronal plane within the anterior sphenoid at the base of the anterior clinoid process The fracture complex involves the anterior skull base, and the fracture can extend to the contralateral greater wing of sphenoid	This fracture pattern is associated with CSF leaks, traumatic optic neuropathy, and oculomotor nerve injury
Posterior transverse pattern The fracture extends across the ipsilateral temporal bone involving first the tympanic and then petrous components and then across the central skull base involving the posterior sphenoid body and clivus (Fig. 15)	This pattern is often associated with cranial nerve injuries, typically the trochlear, abducens, and facial nerve, and there is a high risk of hearing impairment. The temporal bone involvement can also be associated with CSF otorrhea that will be discussed in the context of posterior skull base fractures

Data from West O, Mirvis S, Shanmuganathan K. Transsphenoid basilar skull fracture: CT patterns. *Radiology.* 1993 Aug;188:329-38.

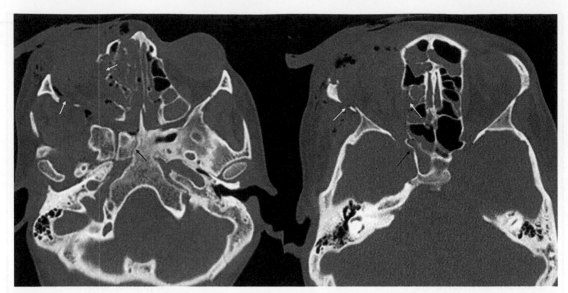

Fig. 13. Axial CT images in a patient involved in an RTA with lateral orbital and maxillary impact with right lateral/medial orbital wall fractures (*thin white arrows*) with central skull base extension (*thin black arrows*). This lateral frontal diagonal pattern is associated with increased complication rates, particularly cranial nerve palsies.

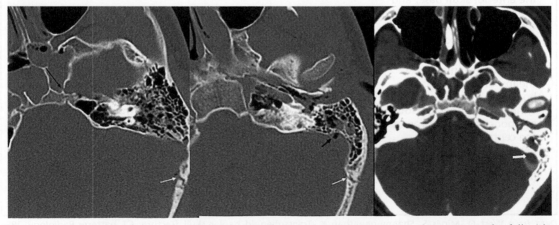

Fig. 14. Axial CT images of the posterior skull base and an axial CT venogram image in a patient who fell with a direct blow to the occiput. With the mastoid diagonal pattern, the fracture complex involves the occipital bone and occipitomastoid suture (*thin white arrow*) with anteromedial extension to involve the jugular foramen, petroclival fissure, and sphenoid (*thin black arrow*). Given the disruption of the sigmoid plate and small locule of pneumocephalus (*thick black arrow*) the CT venogram confirmed a small extradural hematoma (*thick white arrow*) but no venous thrombosis.

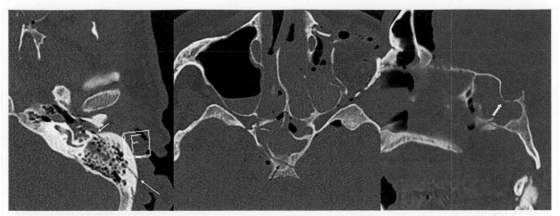

Fig. 15. Axial and sagittal CT in a patient involved in an RTA. In the posterior transverse pattern, the fracture extends across the ipsilateral temporal bone (thin *white arrows*) and central skull base involving the posterior sphenoid body and clivus (thin *black arrows*). There is disruption of the sella turcica (thick *white arrow*).

addition to cranial nerve palsies disruption of the postganglionic oculosympathetic pathway can also occur both as a direct result of the trauma or secondary to vascular injury of the internal carotid artery.[31,32]

Pituitary injury and dysfunction as a result of trauma can be observed in the presence or absence of central skull base fractures traversing the sella turcica. The incidence of posttraumatic panhypopituitarism is likely underestimated.[33] Pituitary dysfunction after a traumatic brain injury is usually transient, although delayed presentations can occur. There are various proposed mechanisms for pituitary dysfunction including shearing forces disrupting the vascular supply, compression due to increased intracranial pressure, general hypovolemia, and stalk amputation/displacement.

POSTERIOR SKULL BASE TRAUMA
Trauma Mechanisms and Anatomic Considerations

Posterior skull base fractures involve the occipital bone, petrous segment of the temporal bone, and if severe, the clivus and basiocciput. Posterior skull base fractures typically occur secondary to direct occipital impact because the crumple zone effect of the sinonasal compartment confers a degree of protection with anterior impact trauma.[34] Lateral impact to the calvarium and skull base is associated with a transverse fracture pattern and is associated with higher risk of internal carotid artery injury. Involvement of the carotid canal confers a higher risk of vascular complications particularly if the fracture traverses the petrous segment of the carotid canal.[35] A longitudinal fracture pattern secondary to axial loading involving

the clivus is associated with the risk of brainstem, vertebrobasilar arterial system, and cranial nerve injury (typically abducens nerve injury given the location of Dorello canal).[33]

Proposed Classification Systems

There are recognized fracture pattern classification systems for temporal bone fractures as well as occipital condyle fractures; the latter is considered here because the posterior skull base is an integral part of the craniocervical junction.

Temporal bone fractures can be classified based on the orientation of the fracture relative to the long axis of the temporal bone and subdivided into longitudinal, transverse, or mixed patterns for simplicity.[36] Most longitudinal fractures are indeed oblique fractures extending across the petrotympanic fissure, whereas longitudinal fractures run within it, and these latter fractures are rare.[37] This classification was based on cadaveric studies, and the more recent classification subdivided fractures in otic capsule into violating or nonviolating.[38] The latter classification is more clinically orientated and is a better predictor of the complications encountered, which include facial nerve palsy, sensorineural hearing loss, vestibular dysfunction, and CSF leak (**Fig. 18**).

Identification of fractures involving the facial nerve canal are important because this may be difficult to assess in the critically injured patient and may highlight the potential need for surgical intervention and decompression if appropriate (**Fig. 19**). In the patients with polytrauma with other life-threatening injuries, operative intervention may be delayed, but this does not necessarily worsen their prognosis because surgery can still be of benefit up to 3 months following injury.[39] Facial

Table 7
Modified Memphis and Denver criteria to guide additional cerebral angiography in the setting of blunt craniocerebral trauma

Modified Memphis Criteria	Modified Denver Criteria
Base of skull fracture carotid canal involvement Base of skull fracture with petrous temporal bone involvement Cervical spine fracture Abnormal neurologic examination not explained by imaging findings Horner's syndrome Le Fort II or III fracture pattern Neck soft tissue injury	Signs and symptoms • Potential arterial hemorrhage from the neck, nose, or mouth • Cervical bruit in patients <50 y of age • Expanding neck hematoma • Focal neurologic deficit (transient ischemic attack, hemiparesis, vertebrobasilar symptoms, Horner syndrome) • Neurologic deficit not explained by imaging findings • Stroke CT or MRI High-energy trauma and additional risk factors including • Le Fort II or III displaced midface fracture • Mandibular fracture • Complex skull fracture • Base of skull fracture (sphenoid, petrous temporal, clivus, and occipital condyle fractures) • Scalp degloving • Cervical spine fracture, subluxation, or ligamentous injury • Severe traumatic brain injury with Glasgow Coma Scale <6 • Near hanging with hypoxic-ischemic brain injury • Clothesline type injury or seat belt abrasion with significant swelling, pain, or altered mental status • Traumatic brain injury with thoracic injuries including upper rib fractures, thoracic vascular injuries and cardiac rupture

Data from Miller P, Fabian T, Croce M et al. Prospective Screening for Blunt Cerebrovascular Injuries: Analysis of Diagnostic Modalities and Outcomes. Ann Surg. 2002;236(3):386-395 and Cothren C, Moore E, Biffl W et al. Anticoagulation Is the Gold Standard Therapy for Blunt Carotid Injuries to Reduce Stroke Rate. Arch Surg. 2004;139:7.

nerve palsy may be immediate or have a delayed presentation with injury most commonly localized to the perigeniculate region. Immediate complete paralysis typically warrants surgical exploration particularly when neural degeneration of 90% or more is noted on electroneurography.[39] Delayed paralysis or incomplete paresis is typically

managed medically with good prognosis in these cases. In the author's institution, CT imaging of the temporal bone is used to identify whether the facial nerve canal has been involved with the temporal bone fracture to guide the operating surgeon. Identification of bony spicules that may impinge the nerve is important to highlight,

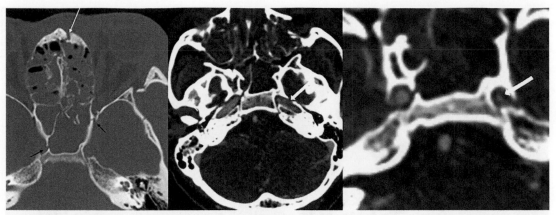

Fig. 16. Axial CT image of the skull base and axial CT angiogram images in a motorcyclist involved in an RTA. There are facial, orbital, and anterior skull base fractures (*thin white arrows*) extending to the central skull base (*thin black arrows*). The angiogram confirmed irregularity of the left internal carotid artery and luminal attenuation compatible with a nonocclusive arterial dissection (*thick white arrows*).

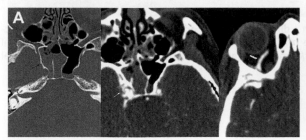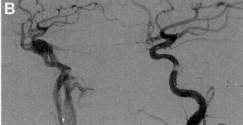

Fig. 17. (*A*) Axial CT image and selected axial images from a CT angiogram in a patient involved in an RTA. There is a fracture of the lateral wall of the sphenoid (*thin black arrow*) with a hemorrhagic effusion. Asymmetrical enhancement of the right cavernous sinus (*thin white arrow*) and early opacification of the right superior ophthalmic vein (*thick white arrow*) compatible with a direct caroticocavernous fistula. The patient underwent a diagnostic cerebral angiogram, Fig. 16B. (*B*) Lateral imaging from a cerebral angiogram with injections of the right common carotid artery performed before and after coil embolization of the direct caroticocavernous fistula. On the pretreatment angiogram there is abnormal early venous opacification that resolved following endovascular treatment with coil embolization to treat the traumatic fistulous connection.

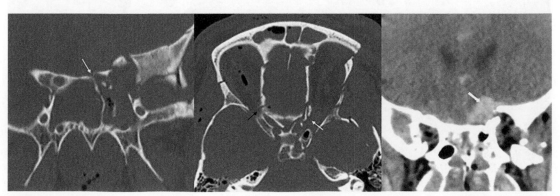

Fig. 18. Coronal and axial CT imaging in a patient who fell from height. There are facial, orbital, and skull base fractures with disruption of the left orbital apex and optic nerve canal (*thin white arrow*) and right optic nerve canal (*thin black arrow*); this resulted in a traumatic left optic neuropathy with loss of vision in the left eye. There was a significant extra-axial hemorrhage related to the anterior/central skull base (*thick white arrow*).

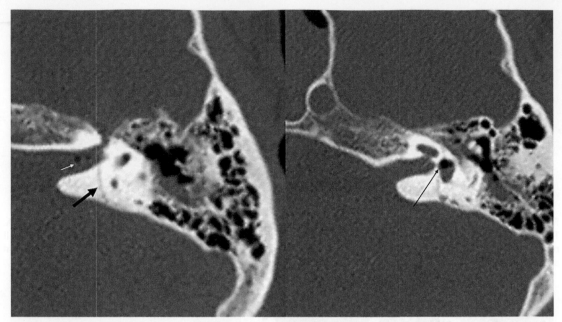

Fig. 19. Axial CT images in a patient assaulted with a direct blow to the occiput. There is an occipital bone fracture (not shown) extending to the temporal bone (*thick black arrow*) with an otic capsule violating temporal bone fracture. There is pneumolabyrinth (*thin black arrow*) and additional pneumocephalus within the internal auditory canal (*thin white arrow*).

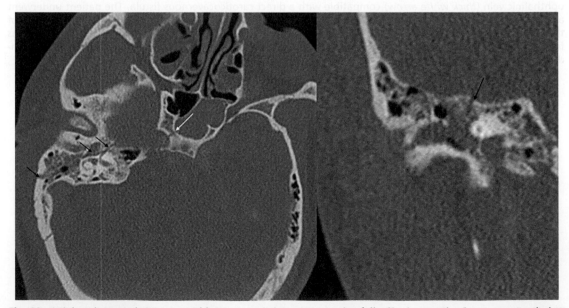

Fig. 20. Axial and coronal CT temporal bone images in a patient who fell off a horse. The fracture extended to involve the geniculate ganglion (*thin black arrows*) and proximal tympanic segment of the facial nerve canal that accounted for the patient's right-sided facial nerve palsy. The fracture complex extended to the central skull base (*thin white arrow*).

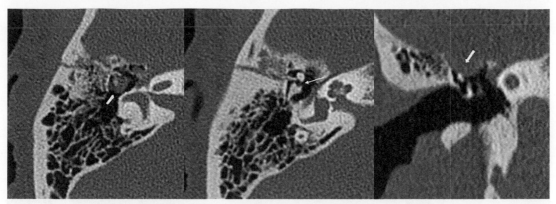

Fig. 21. Axial CT images and coronal image of a patient involved in an industrial accident with direct impact to the temporal bone. The temporal bone fracture resulted in ossicular chain disruption and malleoincudal dislocation (*thin white arrow*) with a fracture that extended through the tegmen tympani with a complicating meningoencephalocele (*thick white arrows*).

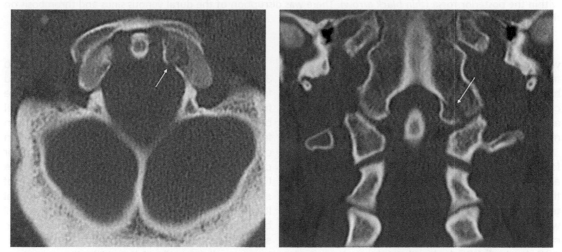

Fig. 22. Axial and coronal CT images of the craniocervical junction in a patient involved in a high-speed RTA. There is left occipital condyle fracture (*white arrows*) and alar ligament avulsion injury.

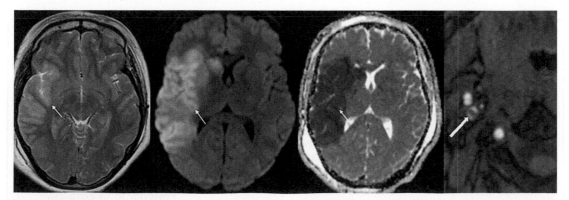

Fig. 23. MRI axial T2-weighted image, b1000 image, and ADC map and axial time-of-flight angiogram image. The patient developed left-sided weakness postinjury secondary to a right middle cerebral artery infarct (*thin white arrows*); this was secondary to the right-sided internal carotid artery traumatic dissection (*thick white arrow*).

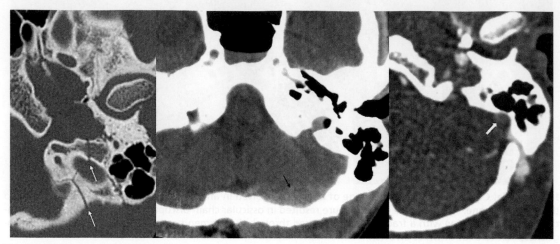

Fig. 24. Axial CT images with a CT venographic image in a patient assaulted with a baseball bat. There are fractures of the occipital bone extending to the jugular foramen (*thin white arrows*) with an extra-axial hematoma within the posterior fossa (*thin black arrow*). There was disruption of the dural venous sinus and thrombosis on the venogram (*thick white arrow*).

whereas intraneural hematoma or neural transection is difficult to predict. The presence of intact hearing and integrity of the rest of the otic capsule can also assist in guiding the intraoperative approach in terms of a middle cranial fossa transmastoid or translabyrinthine approach.

The tegmen tympani and tegmen mastoideum form part of the floor of the middle cranial fossa and separate the middle ear and mastoid from the intracranial compartment. Fractures of the tegmen can result in CSF leak that can present with otorrhea or postnasal discharge with CSF egress along the eustachian tube. As per the ASB fracture CSF leaks, there is an increased risk of meningitis and meningoencephalocele formation (**Fig. 20**).

Occipital condyle fractures can be classified into 3 main subtypes: type I representing an impacted fracture, type II representing a posterior skull base fracture extending into the condyle, and type III being the most unstable representing an avulsion facture involving the alar ligament.[40] Identification of these fractures prompts further evaluation for complicating vascular injuries (**Fig. 21**). The type I condylar fractures typically occur as a result of axial loading and are associated with potential lower cranial nerve palsies as they exit the skull base pass through a close osteoligamentous space in relationship to the condyle. Type II fractures result from direct impact to the calvarium, typically involving the occipital and temporal bones. Type III fractures can be observed in the

Table 8
Soft tissue complications in skull base trauma

Anterior Skull Base Trauma	Central Skull Base Trauma	Posterior Skull Base Trauma
CSF leak and intracranial sepsis	Vascular injuries affecting the internal carotid arteries	Vascular injuries: venous sinus thrombosis, petrous carotid canal disruption
Sinonasal compartment and impairment of frontal sinus drainage pathway	CSF leak	Temporal bone fractures with otic capsule violating and nonviolating patterns
Orbital blow-in and blow-out fractures, medial canthal tendon disruption	Traumatic optic neuropathy	CSF leaks due to temporal bone trauma
Olfactory pathway disruption	Cranial nerve palsies	Posterior fossa extra-axial hematomas
	Hypothalamic-pituitary axis dysfunction	Facial nerve palsy and other lower cranial nerve palsies

absence of other calvarial and cervical spine fractures and result from the combination of flexion, extension, and rotatory forces.

Complications and Soft Tissue Injuries

The intracranial and soft tissue injuries to consider with posterior skull base fractures are the presence of epidural hematoma, venous sinus thrombosis, and lower cranial nerve palsies with fracture involvement of the jugular foramen or hypoglossal canals. On the initial CT head imaging the differentiation between epidural hematoma and venous sinus thrombus can be difficult, and additional imaging with a CT venogram is required (Figs. 13, Fig. 22). The transverse, sigmoid, and upper internal jugular veins should be assessed for abnormal hyperdensity, and the presence of gas within the dural sinus is often a marker of venous sinus injury, although not necessarily thrombosis. Although infrequent, venous sinus thrombosis complicating posterior skull base fractures is a treatable cause of increased intracranial pressure and failure to identify is associated with adverse clinical outcomes.[41] Epidural hematomas are typically venous in origin and can result in significant mass effect on the posterior fossa structures that merits urgent neurosurgical intervention. Similarly, smaller hematomas with minimal mass effect at presentation should always be highlighted because these can potentially expand and result in rapid clinical deterioration.

Lower cranial nerve palsies can occur secondary to fracture disruption of the jugular foramen or the hypoglossal canal. In the setting of blunt trauma, lower cranial nerve palsies are uncommon and more frequently seen in the setting of penetrating neck trauma given the extracranial course of the lower cranial nerves (Figs. 23 and 24).

SUMMARY

Skull base traumatic fractures and soft tissue injuries are encountered in the setting of both penetrating and nonpenetrating trauma. Knowledge of both osseous skull base anatomy and relevant neurovascular structures is essential to provide accurate reports to the trauma team. Based on the pattern of skull base trauma, the radiologist can highlight potential complications that may ensue (Table 8).

REFERENCES

1. Lawrence T, Helmy A, Bouamra O, et al. Traumatic brain injury in England and Wales: prospective audit of epidemiology, complications and standardised mortality. BMJ Open 2016;6(11):e012197.

2. Hanrahan J, Matloob S, Paraskevopoulos D. Management of Skull Base Fractures in a UK Major Trauma Centre. J Neurol Surg B Skull Base 2018; 79(S 01):S1–188.

3. Baugnon KL, Hudgins PA. Skull Base Fractures and Their Complications. Neuroimaging Clin N Am 2014; 24(3):439–65.

4. Stephens JR, Holmes S, Bulters D, et al. The effect of direction of force to the craniofacial skeleton on the severity of brain injury in patients with a frontobasal fracture. Int J Oral Maxillofac Surg 2016; 45(7):872–7.

5. Solai C, C Domingues C, Nogueira L, et al. Clinical signs of basilar skull fracture and their predictive value in diagnosis of this injury. J Trauma Nurs 2018;25:301–6.

6. Faried A, Halim D, Widjaya I, et al. Correlation between the Skull Base Fracture and the Incidence of Intracranial Hemorrhage in Patients with Traumatic Brain Injury. Chin J Traumatol 2019;22:286–9.

7. Lin DT, Lin AC. Surgical Treatment of Traumatic Injuries of the Cranial Base. Otolaryngol Clin North Am 2013;46(5):749–57.

8. Kienstra MA, Loveren HV. Anterior skull base fractures. Facial Plast Surg 2005;21(03):180–6.

9. Borges A. Imaging of the central skull base. Neuroimaging Clin N Am 2009;19(3):441–68.

10. Connor SE, Tan G, Fernando R, et al. Computed tomography pseudofractures of the mid face and skull base. Clin Radiol 2005;60(12):1268–79.

11. West O, Mirvis S, Shanmuganathan K. Transsphenoid basilar skull fracture: CT patterns. Radiology 1993;188:329–38.

12. Miller P, Fabian T, Croce M, et al. Prospective screening for blunt cerebrovascular injuries: analysis of diagnostic modalities and outcomes. Ann Surg 2002;236(3):386–95.

13. Litschel R, Kühnel T, Weber R. Frontobasal Fractures. Facial Plast Surg 2015;31(04):332–44.

14. Garg RK, Afifi AM, Gassner J, et al. A novel classification of frontal bone fractures: The prognostic significance of vertical fracture trajectory and skull base extension. J Plast Reconstr Aesthet Surg 2015;68(5):645–53.

15. Piccirilli M, Anichini G, Cassoni A, et al. Anterior Cranial Fossa Traumas: Clinical Value, Surgical Indications, and Results—A Retrospective Study on a Series of 223 Patients. J Neurol Surg B Skull Base 2012;73(04):265–72.

16. Manson PN, Stanwix MG, Yaremchuk MJ, et al. Frontobasal Fractures: Anatomical Classification and Clinical Significance. Plast Reconstr Surg 2009; 124(6):2096–106.

17. Madhusudan G, Sharma RK, Khandelwal N, et al. Nomenclature of Frontobasal Trauma: A New Clinicoradiographic Classification. Plast Reconstr Surg 2006;117(7):2382–8.

18. Lee KF, Wagner LK, Lee YE, et al. The impact-absorbing effects of facial fractures in closed-head injuries. J Neurosurg 1987;66(4):542–7.

19. Sheth AA, Ngo V, Lam M. Traumatic cerebrospinal fluid oculorrhea managed with an external ventricular drain. J Surg Case Rep 2018;2018(8). https://doi.org/10.1093/jscr/rjy215.

20. Sarfraz M, Mustansir F, Khan N, et al. Acute Orbital Pseudomeningocele Due to Traumatic Fracture in an Infant. Neuro Ophthalmol 2019;44:339–43.

21. Nandapalan V, Watson ID, Swift AC. Beta-2-transferrin and cerebrospinal fluid rhinorrhoea. Clin Otolaryngol 1996;21(3):259–64.

22. Howell J, Costanzo RM, Reiter ER. Head trauma and olfactory function. World J Otorhinolaryngol Head Neck Surg 2018;4(1):39–45.

23. Markowitz BL, Manson PN, Sargent L, et al. Management of the medial canthal tendon in nasoethmoid orbital fractures: the importance of the central fragment in classification and treatment. Plast Reconstr Surg 1991;87(5):843–53.

24. Feiz-Erfan I, Horn EM, Theodore N, et al. Incidence and pattern of direct blunt neurovascular injury associated with trauma to the skull base. J Neurosurg 2007;107(2):364–9.

25. Cothren C, Moore E, Biffl W, et al. Anticoagulation Is the Gold Standard Therapy for Blunt Carotid Injuries to Reduce Stroke Rate. Arch Surg 2004;139:7.

26. Burlew CC, Biffl WL, Moore EE, et al. Blunt cerebrovascular injuries: Redefining screening criteria in the era of noninvasive diagnosis. J Trauma Acute Care Surg 2012;72(2):330–7.

27. Craig J, Goyal P. Patterns and Sequelae of Sphenoid Sinus Fractures. Am J Rhinology Allergy 2015;29: 211–4.

28. Yu-Wai-Man P. Traumatic optic neuropathy—Clinical features and management issues. Taiwan J Ophthalmol 2015;5(1):3–8.

29. Singman E, Daphalapurkar N, White H, et al. Indirect Traumatic Optic Neuropathy. Mil Med Res 2016;3:2.

30. Bodanapally U, Kathirkamanathan S, Elena Geraymovych E, et al. Diagnosis of Traumatic Optic Neuropathy: Application of Diffusion Tensor Magnetic Resonance Imaging. J Neuro Ophthalmol 2013;2:128–33.

31. Worthington JP, Snape L. Horner's syndrome secondary to a basilar skull fracture after maxillofacial trauma. J Oral Maxillofac Surg 1998;56(8): 996–1000.

32. Gilis-Januszewska A, Kluczyński L, Hubalewska-Dydejczyk A. Traumatic Brain Injuries Induced Pituitary Dysfunction: A Call for Algorithms. Endocr Connections 2020;9:112–23.

33. Winkler-Schwartz A, Correa JA, Marcoux J. Clival fractures in a Level I trauma center. J Neurosurg 2015;122(1):227–35.

34. Lee TS, Kellman R, Darling A. Crumple zone effect of nasal cavity and paranasal sinuses on posterior cranial fossa. Laryngoscope 2014;124(10):2241–6.

35. Resnick D, Subach B, Marion D. The Significance of Carotid Canal Involvement in Basilar Cranial Fracture. Neurosurgery 1997;40:1177–81.

36. Ishman SL, Friedland DR. Temporal bone fractures: traditional classification and clinical relevance: temporal bone fractures: traditional classification and clinical relevance. Laryngoscope 2004;114(10): 1734–41.

37. Ghorayeb B, Yeakley J. Temporal bone fractures: longitudinal or oblique? the case for oblique temporal bone fractures. Laryngoscope 1992;102:129–34.

38. Little SC, Kesser BW. radiographic classification of temporal bone fractures: clinical predictability using a new System. Arch Otolaryngol Neck Surg 2006; 132(12):1300.

39. Gordin E, Lee T, Ducic Y, et al. Facial nerve trauma: evaluation and considerations in management. Craniomaxillofac Trauma Reconstr 2015;8:1–13.

40. Anderson P, Montesano P. Morphology and treatment of occipital condyle fractures. Spine 1988; 13(7):731–6.

41. Zhao X, Rizzo A, Malek B, et al. Basilar skull fracture: a risk factor for transverse/sigmoid venous sinus obstruction. J Neurotrauma 2008;25:104–11.

Imaging of Developmental Skull Base Abnormalities

Ata Siddiqui, MBBS, MD, DNB, FRCR*, Steve E.J. Connor, MRCP, FRCR

KEYWORDS

- Skull base • Developmental skull base abnormalities • Skull base development • MRI • CT
- Neuroradiology

KEY POINTS

- The skull base largely develops from cartilaginous precursors (endochondral ossification) which are derived from the mesoderm and neural crest cells, the latter explaining the association of craniofacial anomalies with brain malformations.
- Common midline frontonasal lesions such as dermoids, cephaloceles and nasal 'gliomas' are related to anomalous regression of a transient dural diverticulum during early development.
- The ASB is largely unossified at birth and should not be confused with a defect on CT. MRI is advantageous in assessing intracranial extension/connections, especially in infants.
- Notochordal remnants and associated abnormalities include Thornwaldt cysts, fossa navicularis magna (FNM), persistent canalis basilaris medianus (PCBM), ecchordosis physaliphora (EP) & chordomas.
- The CSB is closely related to the developing pituitary (Rathke's pouch) and notochord, hence the association of anomalies.

INTRODUCTION

The skull base is a critical structure in the craniofacial region, supporting the developing brain and vital facial structures in addition to serving as a passageway for important structures entering and exiting the cranial cavity. Anatomically, it is subdivided into the anterior skull base (ASB), central skull base (CSB), and posterior skull base (PSB), forming the anterior, middle and posterior cranial fossae respectively. The endocranium refers to the inner aspect of the skull base, whereas the exocranium refers to the external aspect (Fig. 1). Key anatomic landmarks and constituents are described in Table 1. The posterolateral skull base, which incorporates much of the temporal bone, is beyond the scope of this article.

EMBRYOLOGY AND DEVELOPMENTAL ANATOMY

The skull base is phylogenetically one of the oldest parts of the skeletal framework, with ossification beginning early in fetal life. There are 110 ossification centers described in the fetal skull.[1] The skull base develops predominantly from cartilaginous precursors via a process of endochondral ossification. In contrast, the cranial vault and facial bones develop by intramembranous ossification.

The authors have nothing to disclose.
Department of Neuroradiology, King's College Hospital, Denmark Hill, London SE5 9RS, UK
* Corresponding author.
E-mail address: Ata.Siddiqui@nhs.net

Neuroimag Clin N Am 31 (2021) 621–647
https://doi.org/10.1016/j.nic.2021.06.004

neuroimaging.theclinics.com

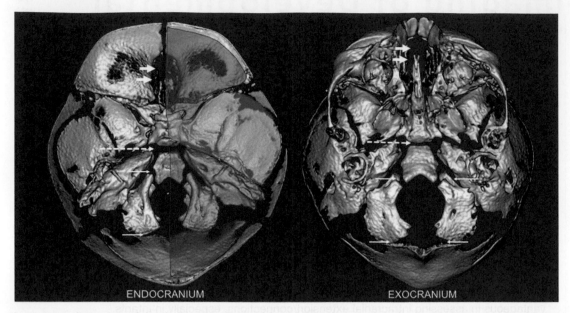

ENDOCRANIUM   EXOCRANIUM

Fig. 1. Normal anatomy of the skull base and cranial fossae at birth on a CT scan. The endocranium or the internal aspect of the skull base shows the anatomic structures forming the anterior (*blue*), central (*green*) and posterior (*orange*) skull base. Note the unossified bones (*arrows*), various unfused sutures and synchondroses such as the spheno-occipital synchondrosis (*long dashed arrows*) and the anterior and posterior interoccipital synchondroses (*short thin arrows*). The exocranium (external skull base), as seen from below, shows the anterior (facial), middle (jugular), and posterior (occipital) parts. Note the different unfused parts of the occipital bone (basal, 2 lateral and posterior parts).

The skull base derives from 2 components, the neural crest cells and the mesoderm. The ASB largely develops from neural crest cells, which lie rostral to the notochord, whereas the CSB and PSB develop largely from the para-axial mesoderm that surrounds the notochord. The developing brain and face share a neural crest origin with the ASB, which underlies the association of

Table 1
Parts and constituents of the skull

Skull Base Components	Interface	Bony Constituents
ASB	Separates the anterior cranial fossa from the orbits and sinonasal cavities	Orbital plates of frontal bone Ethmoid bone Lesser wings of the sphenoid
CSB	Separates the middle cranial fossa from the infratemporal fossa (masticator space) and sphenoid sinus	Body and greater wings of the sphenoid bone
PSB	Separates the posterior fossa from the cervical spine and subcranial deep neck spaces	Clivus (basisphenoid + basiocciput), dorsal petrous pyramid and the squamous part of the occipital bone
Posterolateral skull base	Separates the middle/posterior cranial fossa from the external, middle, and inner ear	Temporal bone (principally petromastoid)

Table 2	
The cartilaginous precursors of the skull base	
Final Bony Product	**Embryonic Precursors**
ASB	
Ethmoid	Trabecular and mesoethmoid cartilages (prechordal cartilage)
Frontal (orbital plate)	Forms by intramembranous ossification
CSB	
Sphenoid anterior body	Presphenoid (prechordal cartilage)
Sphenoid posterior body	Postsphenoid (hypophyseal/parachordal cartilage)
Sphenoid lesser wings and planum	Orbitosphenoid (lateral cartilage)
Sphenoid greater wings	Alisphenoid (lateral cartilage)
Sphenoid greater wings lateral	Forms by intramembranous ossification
Posterior and posterolateral skull base	
Petromastoid	Mesodermal condensations and parachordal cartilages
Basiocciput and clivus	Postsphenoid and basioccipital (parachordal cartilages/occipital somites 1, 2, and 4)
Occipital condyles	Basioccipital and exoccipital (parachordal cartilages/occipital somite 4)
Squamous occipital bone	Forms by intramembranous ossification

several craniofacial anomalies with telencephalic and diencephalic brain malformations such as holoprosencephalies.[2]

Chondrification (the development of cartilage from mesoderm) is closely related to the notochord, the rostral termination of which corresponds with the sella turcica. During the fifth and sixth weeks of development, the paraxial mesoderm and neural crest cells start condensing to form the chondrocranium.[3–5] The prechordal cartilage forms by condensations of neural crest cells rostral to the notochord and will form the ASB, whereas the parachordal cartilages formed by mesodermal condensations on either side of the notochord eventually form the bulk of the CSB and PSB. In the case of the PSB, there is formation of the basal plate by fusion of the parachordal cartilages with the occipital somites, with ossification beginning in the seventh week of life.[3,6] **Table 2** summarizes the cartilaginous derivatives of the various skull base components.

The pituitary gland is also developing at this time and in close relationship, starting at approximately 3 weeks of gestation, with the anterior pituitary being derived via the Rathke's pouch arising from the developing endoderm and stomodeum, and the posterior pituitary descending from the diencephalon. The endodermal attachment of the anterior pituitary subsequently regresses and becomes obliterated by progressive growth of the postsphenoid cartilages, which fuse in the midline. Failure of this fusion results

in a persistent craniopharyngeal canal. At the same time, posterolaterally, there is invagination of the otic placode with chondrification of the surrounding mesoderm, which surfaces with the parachordal cartilages to form the petromastoid bony structures surrounding the inner ear and the posterolateral skull base.[3]

Ossification follows chondrification, progressing from posterior to anterior.[7] Ossification starts in the occipital bone at 12 weeks of gestation and progresses anteriorly, to the postsphenoid (14 weeks of gestation), the presphenoid (17 weeks of gestation), and the ethmoid bones (**Figs. 2** and **3**). At around the same time, ossification is also seen laterally in the paired orbitosphenoid cartilages, which encase the developing optic nerves, and the alisphenoid cartilages, which encase the maxillary and mandibular nerves. Although there is variability in the timing of ossification, the pattern is well-defined and follows a clear sequence. The postnatal developmental anatomy is summarized in **Table 3** (see also **Figs. 4–7**) and key embryology points are summarized in **Box 1**.

Synchondroses and Foramina

Much of the cranial elongation of the skull base is dependent on the presence of synchondroses, which are cartilaginous junctions between the different ossification centers. The 3 main synchondroses from anterior to posterior are the spheno-ethmoid synchondrosis (fuses at 6–7 years

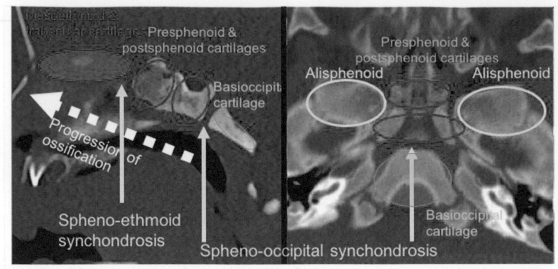

Fig. 2. Normal pattern and ossification centers of the developing skull base at birth on sagittal and axial CT scans. Similar to brain maturation, ossification progresses from posterior to anterior.

of age), the intersphenoid synchondrosis (fuses at birth) and the spheno-occipital synchondrosis (fuses 1–2 years earlier in girls, from superior to inferior, between 12 and 17 years of age).[11] The skull base foramina can be difficult to evaluate in infants owing to the variation in size, and asymmetry is a better marker of abnormality rather than absolute size.[12]

IMAGING TECHNIQUES AND PROTOCOLS

Ultrasound examination, CT scans, and MR imaging are the key imaging modalities and the relative advantages and pitfalls are summarized in **Table 4**. Although MR imaging is the mainstay, the choice of the appropriate imaging modality depends on the clinical indication and the different techniques are often complementary.

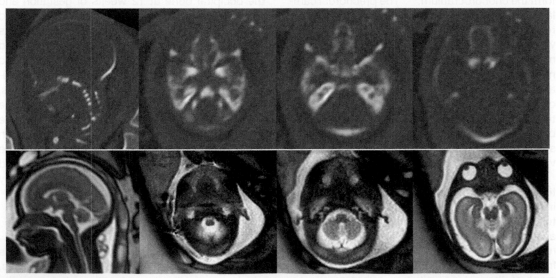

Fig. 3. Ossification in a 28-week-old fetus. (*Top*) Low-dose CT scan performed in view of the skeletal dysplasia preceded by an MR imaging (*bottom*). Note the posterior to anterior pattern of ossification with ossification of the basiocciput, postsphenoid, presphenoid, alisphenoid and orbitosphenoid, but no ossification of the ASB. The nonossified cartilaginous structures are less hypointense on MR imaging compared with the ossified structures.

Table 3
Key postnatal developmental anatomy

ASB	Almost completely unossified at birth
	Only orbital plates of the frontal bones ossified
	Median ASB ossifies from lateral to medial and posterior to anterior
	Earliest ASB bridging may be seen at 2 months of age
	About 50% ASB is ossified by around 6 months of age and 84% by 2 years of age[8]
	Fully ossified by about 4 years of age[9]
CSB	Largely ossified at birth
	Presphenoid and postsphenoid fuse to form sphenoid body
	Tuberculum sella delineates the junction between the presphenoid and postsphenoid
	Craniopharyngeal canal is obliterated by fusion of postsphenoid centers on both sides
	Paired lateral alisphenoid (forming greater wing of sphenoid) fuse with the sphenoid body in the first year
	Pneumatization begins at about 2–3 years in the presphenoid and extends posteriorly[10]
PSB	Consists of different parts at birth: basal, posterior squamous, and 2 lateral parts
	Lateral and squamous parts start to fuse from the second year
	Basal and lateral parts fuse between 3 and 7 years of age[10]

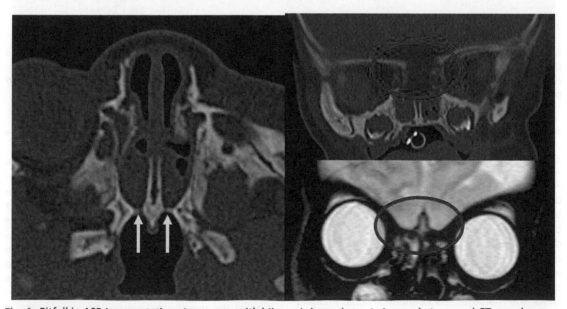

Fig. 4. Pitfall in ASB interpretation. A neonate with bilateral choanal atresia (*arrows*). A coronal CT scan shows an osseous deficiency of the median ASB. In combination with an opacified obstructed nasal cavity, this image could lead to an erroneous diagnosis of an encephalocele. The nasal opacification is due to pooling of secretions and MR imaging demonstrates an intact but unossified ASB (*blue circle*).

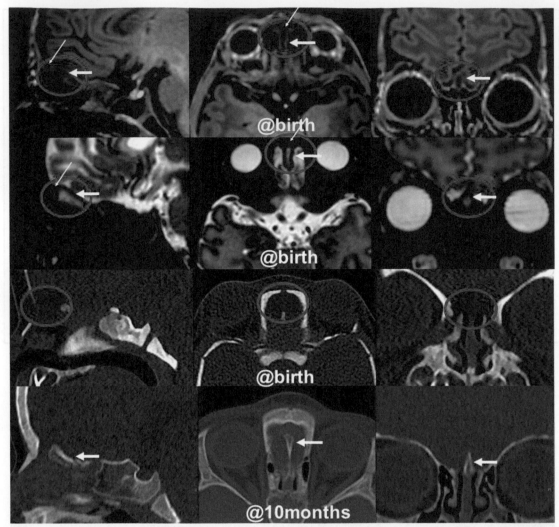

Fig. 5. Normal ASB development. (*Top*) T1W, (*second row*) T2W, and (*third row*) CT images in a term neonate shows the unossified ASB. Note the unossified crista galli (*thick arrow*) and the small foramen caecum more anteriorly (*thin arrow*) that falsely seems to be enlarged on bony CT windows. (*Bottom*) CT images at 10 months show progressive ossification of the ASB from posterior to anterior and lateral to medial.

ANTERIOR SKULL BASE DEVELOPMENTAL ABNORMALITIES
Midline Frontonasal Lesions

A midline and paramidline frontonasal lesion is an uncommon but specific clinical scenario encountered in the pediatric age group. The differential diagnosis of such lesions includes 3 key entities: dermoid/epidermoid, nasal glioma (neuroglial heterotopia), and cephalocele. Distinction of these entities and the demonstration of the presence or absence of a potential intracranial connection is vital for the management of these lesions. Imaging playing a key role in the diagnosis and mapping out any potential intracranial association. Other facial lesions such as hemangiomas may also

present with a frontonasal swelling; however, the clinicoradiologic features are usually diagnostic.

The developmental basis of these conditions is related to events around the closure of the anterior neuropore during early embryonic development.[13–16] A transient dural diverticulum extends extracranially through a gap called the fonticulus nasofrontalis at the junction of the developing frontal, nasal, and ethmoid bones. This traverses the midline prenasal space and reaches close to the skin. This diverticulum subsequently regresses with closure of foramen cecum and the bony margins of the nasofrontal suture. An abnormality of this normal process of regression can result in these 3 midline frontonasal lesions (**Table 5**):

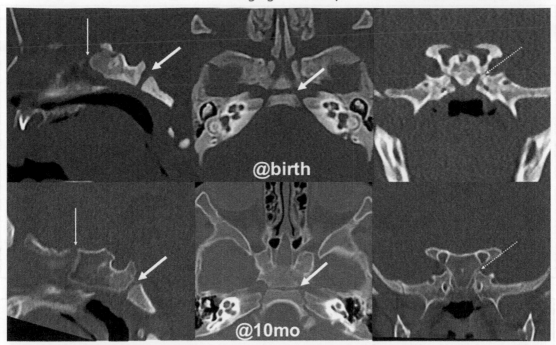

Fig. 6. Normal CSB development. Sagittal, axial, and coronal CT images at birth (*top*) and at 10 months of age (*bottom*) show a prominent spheno-occipital synchondroses (*thick arrow*) and the sphenoethmoid synchondrosis more anteriorly (*thin arrow*). The intersphenoid synchondrosis between the presphenoid and postsphenoid segments is obliterated. Coronal images show progressive fusion of the cartilaginous gap between the sphenoid body (postsphenoid) and greater wings (alisphenoid) (*dashed arrow*): the potential site of the lateral craniopharyngeal canal.

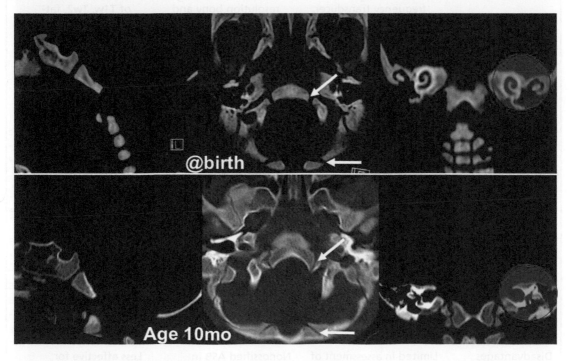

Fig. 7. Normal PSB development. Sagittal, axial, and coronal CT images in a term neonate at birth (*top*) and in a 10-month-old infant (*bottom*) show the unfused basal, lateral, and posterior squamous parts of the occipital bones and the petro-occipital fissures. Note the unossified tip of the dens and the anterior and posterior interoccipital synchondroses (*arrows*) which fuse at approximately 4 to 7 years of age. The middle ear clefts, ossicles, and inner ears have fully formed, but only the mastoid antrum is seen; the peripheral mastoid air cells are not pneumatized at this age.

Box 1
Key embryology pearls

Key embryology pearls

- The skull base predominantly develops from cartilaginous precursors (endochondral ossification) which are derived from the mesoderm and neural crest cells (the latter explaining the association of craniofacial anomalies with brain malformations)
- Chondrification starts very early at around 4 to 5 weeks of life
- Ossification starts in the occipital bones at approximately 12 weeks, progressing from posterior to anterior
- MR imaging is advantageous in assessing intracranial extension/connection, especially in infants
- ASB: largely unossified at birth (and should not be confused with a defect on a computed tomography [CT] scan)
- CSB: closely related to the developing pituitary (Rathke's pouch) and notochord, hence the association of anomalies
- PSB: development of the occipitocervical transition is key to understanding craniovertebral junction anomalies

---

Table 4
Summary of imaging techniques

	Ultrasound Examination	CT Scan	MR Imaging
Technique	High-resolution ultrasound examination with a standard high-frequency transducer. Doppler can be complementary Bedside test possible.	Multidetector, submillimeter slice thickness, typically 0.626 mm, with high resolution bony and soft tissue algorithms reconstructions. Modern PACS workstations allow quick 3D reformats from the isotropic volumetric data.	Multiplanar sequences, small field of view and high resolution/matrix. Combination of T1w, Tw2, fat-suppressed T2w/STIR, DWI and contrast enhanced T1w. Thin sagittal images most useful. DWI beneficial (with readout-segmented EPI techniques)
Ionizing radiation	No ionizing radiation.	Ionizing radiation.	No ionizing radiation.
Anesthesia or sedation	Usually does not require anesthesia or sedation.	Usually does not need anesthesia or sedation.	Usually a need for anesthesia or sedation, although 'feed and wrap' possible in young infants.
Advantages	Useful first-line test, particularly in the context of cystic calvarial or frontonasal lesions.	Most helpful to define bony anatomy.	Most useful modality in assessing developmental skull base lesions, especially with regards to intracranial connections Able to assess nonossified structures.
Disadvantages and pitfalls	Limited in assessment of deep facial or intracranial extent.	Nonossified ASB in young children could be confused with bony defects and less useful for assessing intracranial extension.	Less effective for assessing cortical bone.

Abbreviations: DWI, diffusion-weighted imaging; EPI, echo planar imaging; STIR, short T1 inversion recovery.

Table 5
Main developmental midline frontonasal lesions

Frontonasal Lesion	Pathophysiology	Imaging	Tips
Dermoid or epidermoid	Dural diverticulum reaches the nasal skin and pulls epidermal/dermal elements back during retraction	US examination - round to ovoid echogenic cystic avascular midline lesion. CT scan - low-density midline lesion MR imaging - dermoids may show fat or fluid signal whereas epidermoids show fluid signal with restricted diffusion Location: A nasoglabella or nasal dorsum/tip cyst, dermal sinus or fistula which may extend to the skull base at the foramen caecum anterior to the crista galli.	The normal foramen cecum can be of variable size (0–10 mm) with CT attenuation of fibrous tissue (higher than brain), and low to medium signal on MR imaging, although can be difficult to visualize when the crista galli is not ossified.[13] A bifid, dysplastic, or thickened crista galli is a useful clue to an intracranial dermoid. It is normally 1–8 mm thick with ossification progressing anteriorly.[13]
Nasal glioma and heterotopia	Dural diverticulum pinches off while regressing, leaving sequestrated neural, glial or meningeal tissues in the frontonasal region	CT scan - Soft tissue density. MR imaging - isointense on T1w/T2w and may enhance. Location: Usually paramidline extranasal where it is at the nasal bridge. Less frequently intranasal where it is medial to the middle turbinate.	A fibrovascular pedicle or stalk may be seen extending to the foramen caecum or skull base in 15%–20%, but typically no direct continuity with the subarachnoid space or brain. Differential from an encephalocele can sometimes be difficult owing to the small size of the dural/intracranial connection and limited resolution of imaging techniques.
Cephalocele	Dural diverticulum persists, resulting in an ongoing connection with the cranial cavity and subarachnoid space, with herniation of	CT scan - variable density depending on components. MR imaging - Variable signal depending on components. High resolution submillimeter 3D T2W MR imaging is	The foramen caecum is enlarged and crista galli is small in patients with nasoethmoid cephaloceles. May be associated with other craniofacial abnormalities (eg, (continued on next page)

Table 5
(continued)

Frontonasal Lesion	Pathophysiology	Imaging	Tips
	cerebrospinal fluid and/or brain	sometimes needed to delineate small intracranial connections (see Fig. 11) Location: Nasoethmoid type: widens the foramen cecum and extend caudally into the ethmoid/nasal soft tissues. Nasofrontal type (less common): extends anteriorly to the glabello-frontal region. Combination of these (rare). Lateral naso-orbital cephalocele (rare).[13]	hypoplasia of branchial arches or hemifacial macrosomia) or more extensive anomalies (eg, frontonasal dysplasia spectrum) (see Fig. 13)

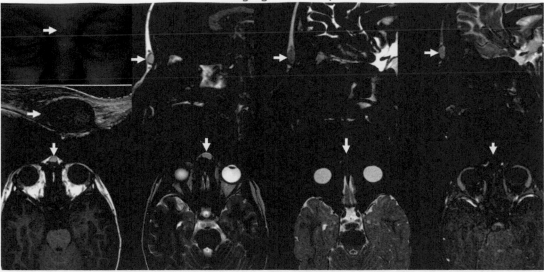

Fig. 8. Typical glabellar dermoid. A 2-year-old boy presented with a soft subcutaneous midline frontonasal swelling. (*Top*) A 3D MR imaging reconstruction, ultrasound image, and sagittal T1W and T2W images showing a well-defined rounded midline lesion at the glabella (*arrows*), demonstrating high T1 and T2 signal, without any vascularity on ultrasound imaging. No intracranial connection was demonstrated and the skull base was normal. (*Bottom*) Axial T1W, T2W, short T1 inversion recovery, and postcontrast T1W images demonstrate a fat signal lesion without contrast enhancement.

dermoid/epidermoid (**Figs. 8** and **9**), a nasal glioma or heterotopia (**Fig. 10**), and encephalocele (**Figs. 11** and **12**).

CENTRAL SKULL BASE DEVELOPMENTAL ABNORMALITIES
Persistent Hypophyseal Canal or Median Craniopharyngeal Canal

This developmental bony defect is related to Rathke's pouch, which is seen as a well-

corticated bony canal running in the midsagittal plane from the floor of the sella to the roof of the nasopharynx. It is seen anterior to the intersphenoid synchondrosis, as opposed to notochordal remnants, which are typically seen more posteriorly. The size of the canal can be variable and when larger than 1.5 mm it is typically referred to as the craniopharyngeal canal, rather than persistent hypophyseal canal. It is also important to describe its relationship with associated

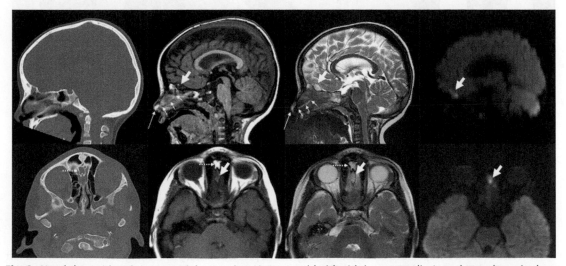

Fig. 9. Nasal dermoid with intracranial extension. A 4-year-old girl with known scoliosis and complex spinal segmentation anomalies presented with a nasal tip swelling. (*Top* and *bottom*) CT scan, T1W, T2W, and diffusion-weighted imaging in the sagittal and axial planes. A small fatty signal lesion at the nasal tip is seen (*thin long arrows*) with a thin track (short *arrows*) extending posterosuperiorly to the ASB. It terminates as a small extradural dermoid lesion which demonstrates diffusion restriction (*thick arrows*) just posterior to the thick dysplastic and posteriorly bifid crista galli (*dashed arrow*). Note craniocervical junction anomalies with fusion of C2 and C3, dysplastic C1 with nonfusion of the anterior and posterior arches, and moderate narrowing of the foramen magnum.

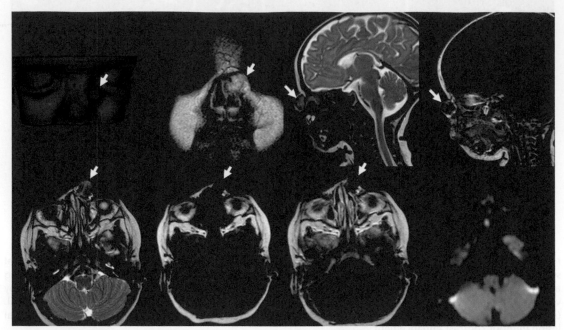

Fig. 10. Nasal glioma (glial heterotopia). A 1-year-old girl presented with a left paramidline nasal soft tissue swelling. (*Top*) A 3D virtual reality MR imaging reformat, coronal T2W, sagittal T2W, and postcontrast sagittal T1W images. (*Bottom*) Axial T2W, T1W, postcontrast T1W, and diffusion-weighted imaging. The images show a well-defined soft tissue lesion over the left nasal bridge (*arrows*) with a smaller deeper intranasal component but without any intracranial extension and a normal ASB.

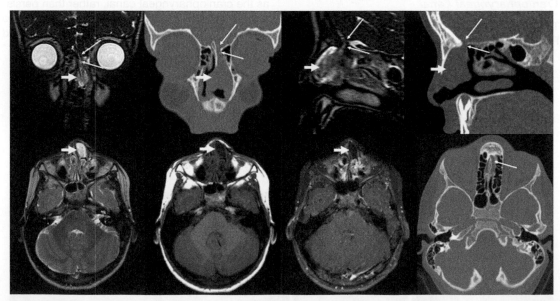

Fig. 11. Nasoethmoid encephalocele. A 5-year-old boy with a previous history of meningitis presented with a left nasal mass. (*Top*) Thin coronal T2W, coronal CT, sagittal T2W, and sagittal CT images. (*Bottom*) Axial T2W, T1W, postcontrast T1W, and CT images. A mixed signal left nasal cavity mass is seen (*thick arrow*) that extends to the skull base and is associated with a small defect of the left cribriform plate through which a very thin T2 high signal tract extended to the subarachnoid space with mild descent of the gyrus rectus and crowding of the olfactory fossa (*thin arrows*). Note the normal crista galli (compared with dysplastic/thickened crista galli often seen with intracranial dermoids).

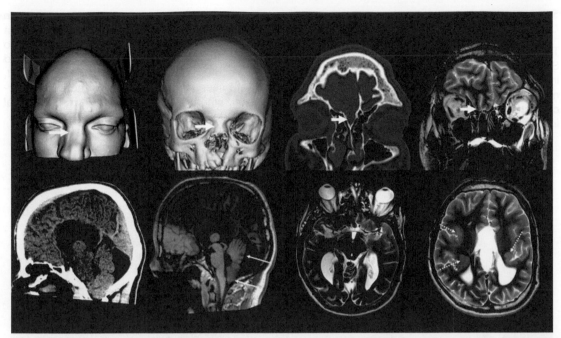

Fig. 12. Frontonasal dysplasia spectrum. A young male presented with a history of seizures, learning difficulties, developmental delay and facial dysmorphism. (*Top*) A 3D CT reformatted scan, coronal CT scan, and MR imaging show a broadened nasal bridge and hypertelorism, associated with a defect in the ASB and descent of the right frontal lobe (*arrows*). (*Bottom*) Sagittal CT scan and T1W and axial T2W MR imaging show agenesis of the corpus callosum, abnormal lateral ventricles, hypertelorism, bilateral cortical malformations (*long dashed arrows*) and a dysplastic cerebellum with low lying cerebellar tonsils (*long thin arrows*).

intracranial structures. Three types of craniopharyngeal canals have been described: incidental canals (type 1), canals with ectopic adenohypophysis (type 2), and canals containing cephaloceles (3A), tumors (3B), or both (3C).[17] Craniopharyngeal canals may be incidental findings or present with clinical features such as a postnasal space mass (**Fig. 13**).

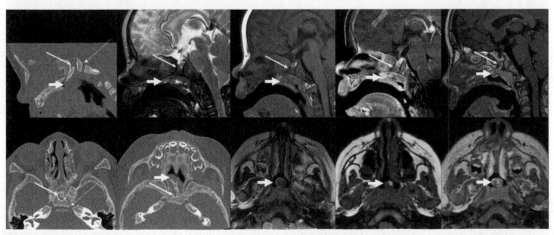

Fig. 13. Nasopharyngeal glioneuronal heterotopia a dilated craniopharyngeal canal. A 2-month-old boy presented with nasal obstruction. (*Top*) Sagittal CT scan and T2W, T1W, and postcontrast T1W images (far right image is a follow-up T1W image at 6 years of age). (*Bottom*) Axial CT scan and T2W, T1W, and postcontrast T1W images. (*Bottom*) Axial CT scan and T2W, T1W, and postcontrast T1W images. A polypoid mildly enhancing nasopharyngeal soft tissue mass (*thick short arrows*) is associated with a bony spur from the widened craniopharyngeal canal extending from the floor of the sella to the nasopharynx (*long thin arrows*). A biopsy showed glioneuronal heterotopia. The normal spheno-occipital synchondrosis (*dashed arrow*) is posterior to the craniopharyngeal canal. Low-lying cerebellar tonsils subsequently improved on images 6 years later (far right).

Sternberg's Canal (or Lateral Craniopharyngeal Canal)

This controversial entity was first described by Sternberg in 1888. It is proposed to be related to incomplete fusion of the greater wing of the sphenoid with the sphenoid body. Although this is consistently seen in children, it is rarely persistent in adults and may result in a cerebrospinal fluid leak or congenital sphenoid meningocele.[18] Given its embryologic basis, this congenital bony defect and associated cephaloceles should lie medial to the foramen rotundum. Most lateral sphenoid cephaloceles in adults are felt to be acquired, and are seen in the context of intracranial hypertension, where they are derived from osseodural defects developing lateral to V2[19] (Fig. 14).

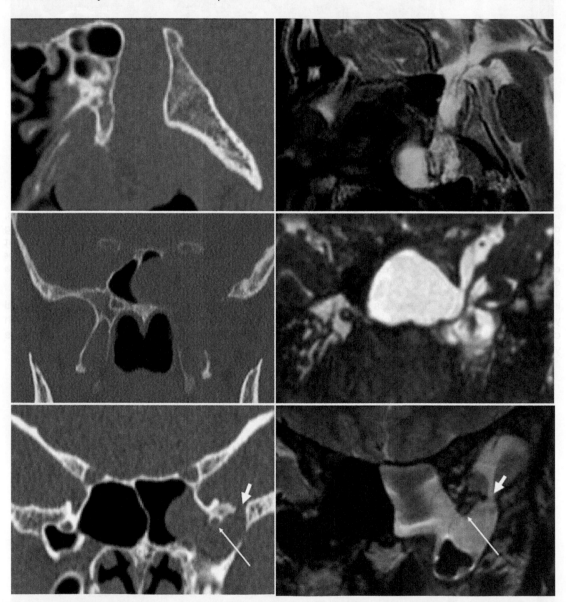

Fig. 14. Enlarged median and lateral craniopharyngeal canals with central skull cephaloceles. (*Top*) Median craniopharyngeal canal. Sagittal CT scan and T2W MR imaging in a young patient presenting with nasal obstruction. There is a large, well-corticated bony defect in the midline CSB that involves the floor of the pituitary fossa and with an associated large encephalocele. (*Middle*) Lateral craniopharyngeal canal. Coronal CT scan and T2W MR imaging demonstrate a large sphenoid cephalocele owing to a bony defect in the lateral sphenoid wall. This is medial to the foramen rotundum and presumed to be related to the lateral craniopharyngeal (Steinberg's) canal. (*Bottom*) Acquired sphenoid cephalocele. A middle-aged woman presenting with cerebrospinal fluid rhinorrhea showing a sphenoid encephalocele with an extensively pneumatized lateral recess and a defect of the sphenoid sinus (*small arrows*), lateral to the foramen rotundum (*long thin arrows*).

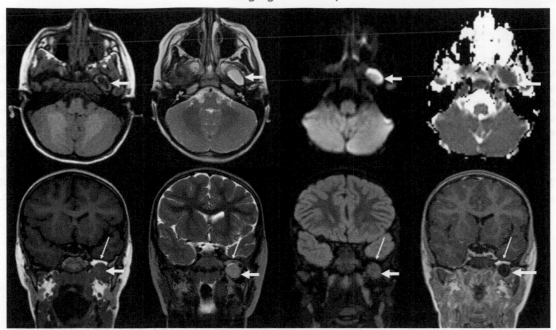

Fig. 15. CSB dermoid/epidermoid. A 5-year-old girl underwent MR imaging head for tremor and hypertonia. (*Top*) Axial T1W, T2W, diffusion-weighted imaging, and apparent diffusion coefficient maps show a well-defined rounded low T1 high T2 lesion centered in the region of the sphenoid body, showing diffusion restriction. (*Bottom*) Coronal T1W, T2W, fluid-attenuated inversion recovery, and postcontrast T1W images showing that the lesion is centered on the CSB and has 2 components: a cystic component inferiorly (*short arrows*) and a superior component with fat (*long thin arrows*). Also note the chemical shift artifact at the interface of the fat-fluid components on the coronal T2W image. There was no meningocele/cephalocele and no history of meningitis.

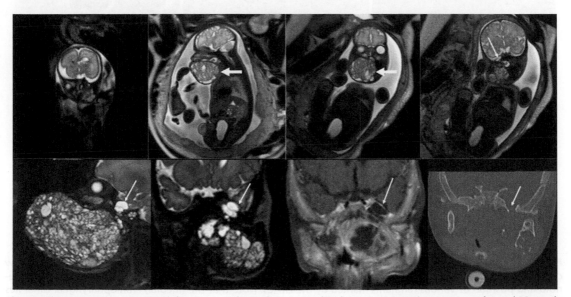

Fig. 16. Teratoma with intracranial extension through the CSB. (*Top*) Fetal MR imaging at 24 weeks and 32 weeks of gestation showing an enlarging complex solid–cystic mass in the face, extending to the oral cavity oropharynx and nasopharynx (*short thick arrows*). A small intracranial connection was suspected prenatally (*long thin arrows*). (*Bottom*) Sagittal T2W, coronal T2W, postcontrast T1W, and CT scan demonstrate the extent of the large orofacial mass filling the postnasal space and extending to the right side of the middle cranial fossa through a small bony skull base defect just lateral to the pterygoid plates (*long thin arrows*).

Dermoids, Epidermoids, and Teratomas

Dermoid and epidermoids can also be encountered in the CSB. The appearances are similar to lesions seen elsewhere, with fatty or cystic components in dermoids and diffusion restriction in epidermoids (**Figs. 15** and **16**).

Notochordal Remnants

The notochord, which lies between the ectoderm and endoderm, is the central axis around which the axial skeleton develops in vertebrates. It has an important role in the induction of the nervous system. It gradually regresses during development, but remnants are found in postnatal life (eg, the nucleus pulposus of the intervertebral discs). The cranial aspect of the notochord is intimately related to the developing central and PSB, terminating at the dorsum sella (**Fig. 17**). Anomalies of regression of the cranial end of the notochord result in postnatal developmental variants and pathologies such as the Thornwaldt (Tornwaldt) cyst, fossa navicularis magna,

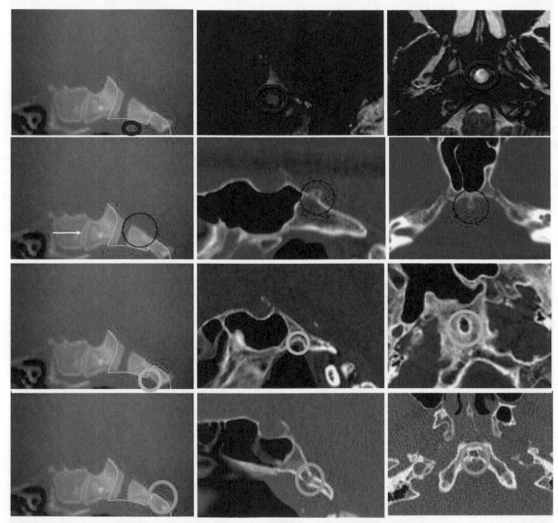

Fig. 17. Benign notochordal remnants. Normal comparative images. Left-sided image in each row with a *yellow curved line* showing the path taken by the cranial end of the notochord related to the basiocciput and basisphenoid and position of various remnants marked by the circles. Note that the (medial) craniopharyngeal canal lies anteriorly (*arrows*). The spheno-occipital synchondrosis is also seen. (*Top*) A Thornwaldt cyst (*purple*) typically directly abutting the prevertebral muscles in the midline of the nasopharynx. (*Second row*) Ecchordosis physaliphora (*red*) with a bony spur/excrescence along the posterior surface of in the upper/mid clivus. (*Third row*) Fossa navicularis (*blue*) as a small blind-ending pit grooving the anterior surface of the clivus in the roof of the nasopharynx. (*Bottom*) Persistent canalis basilaris medianus (*green*) seen as a well-demarcated bony canal in the midline of the lower clivus.

persistent canalis basilaris medianus, and ecchordosis physaliphora (**Table 6**).

Thornwaldt (Tornwaldt) Cyst

The notochord comes into close contact with the roof of the developing oral cavity and forms the nasopharyngeal bursa. Occlusion of the neck of this bursa and consequent obstruction results in the formation of the Thornwaldt cyst, a common incidental finding, typically seen in adults and rarely seen at the extremes of life. The autopsy prevalence has been reported to be around 4%, whereas the imaging incidence has been reported variably in up to 6%.[22]

Fossa Navicularis Magna

A fossa navicularis magna is a small, incidentally detected midline bony pit on the anterior aspect of the superior clivus, most likely owing to incomplete ossification at the site of adhesion between the pharyngeal bursa (endoderm) and the notochord.

Persistent Canalis Basilaris Medianus

As opposed to the notch-like defect seen with the fossa navicularis magna, the persistent canalis basilaris medianus is a small canal seen in the clivus, although numerous variants are described. They result from incomplete notochordal regression and are typically detected incidentally on imaging studies.

Ecchordosis Physaliphora

An ecchordosis physaliphora is a benign notochordal remnant first described on pathology in 1856 by Lusckha and in 1857 by Virchow. It was

Table 6
Notochordal remnants

Notochordal Remnant	Imaging Findings
Thornwaldt cyst	Small midline submucosal cyst ranging between 2 and 15 mm, located between longus colli and abutting the posterior nasopharyngeal wall CT density and MR imaging signal intensity are variable but commonly high on T2WI and iso to high on T1WI Should be differentiated from the more common mucosal retention cysts, which are generally of low T1 signal (reflecting their serous nature), typically paramidline and often multiple Rarely may enlarge or become infected
Fossa navicularis magna	Well-corticated midline bony notch in the anterior superior clivus, which may be filled with air or soft tissue. May coexist with a Thornwaldt cyst
Persistent canalis basilaris medianus	Small canal seen in the more inferior clivus as inferiorly as the basion May be complete or incomplete based on it's relationship to the basiocciput. Subtypes[20]: a. Superior, inferior and bifurcating subtypes in the complete type b. Long channel, superior and inferior recesses in the incomplete type
EP	Small cystic retroclival lesion in the prepontine cistern, often with an undulating margin and similar to cerebrospinal fluid signal intensity on MR imaging Difficult to detect on thicker sections – a clue is the lack of cerebrospinal fluid pulsation artifact (and therefore brighter T2 signal in the prepontine cistern) Subtypes: a. Classical EP with a typical cyst and dorsal clival excrescence (type A without and type B with some intraclival component) b. Incomplete EP when only a small T2 hypointense prominence of the clivus is seen without a cyst c. Variant EP when a small intraclival cyst is seen without a bony excrescence[21]

Abbreviation: EP, ecchordosis physaliphora.

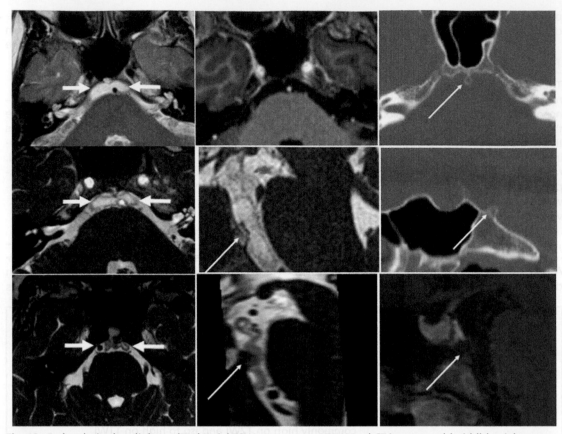

Fig. 18. Ecchordosis physaliphora. (*Top*) Axial T2W, postcontrast T1W, and CT images and (*middle*) axial constructive interference in steady state (CISS), sagittal CISS, and sagittal CT images in a young patient demonstrate a well defined thin walled nonenhancing prepontine cystic lesion isointense to cerebrospinal fluid (solid *arrows*) and better resolved on CISS imaging with small bony spur (*long thin arrows*). (*Bottom*) Axial and sagittal CISS and postcontrast sagittal T1W images in another patient with a retroclival prepontine cystic lesion with a clival bony spur (*thin long arrows*) and an additional cystic component within the clivus. Note the collapsed crenulated margins.

initially termed "ecchondrosis physaliphora" as it was believed to be related to cartilage, but it's notochordal origin was later recognized and it was renamed "ecchordosis physaliphora" by Rippert in 1894.[23] It is essentially a focus of gelatinous tissue which contains physalipherous cells with large vacuoles. It is found in approximately 2% of autopsies and is typically an incidental finding on imaging studies (**Fig. 18**). Complications such as hemorrhage or cerebrospinal fluid leak can occur, but are rare (**Fig. 19**).

Ecchordosis Physaliphora versus Chordoma

It is important to differentiate ecchordosis physaliphora from its malignant counterpart, chordoma. The key differentiating features of ecchordosis physaliphora include the lack of gadolinium contrast enhancement and a small bony excrescence or stalk, or an altered signal intensity seen with the adjacent clivus.[23] In contrast, chordoma typically present symptomatically as bulky T2 hyperintense soft tissue mass in the midline CSB with bony destruction (**Fig. 20**). Comparative findings are summarized in **Table 7**. Some controversy exists in the differentiation of giant ecchordosis physaliphora from the rarely encountered less aggressive extradural chordomas, particularly because there are overlapping histologic features, with physaliferous cells being present in both entities. Longitudinal studies are lacking and it remains uncertain whether ecchordosis physaliphora may be a precursor of chordoma. An intermediate form of benign notochordal cell tumor is also described in the context of a purely intraosseous lesion. When there are atypical imaging features or large lesions, then follow-up imaging is appropriate.

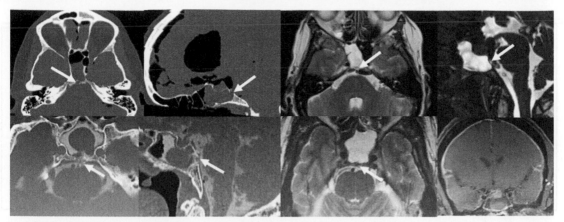

Fig. 19. Atypical ecchordosis physaliphora with a cerebrospinal fluid leak. Axial and sagittal CT scan and T2W MR imaging (*top*) in a patient presenting with acute alteration in consciousness. There is extensive pneumocephalus with a cystic lesion related to a defect in the dorsal clivus (*arrows*) as well as fluid opacification of the sphenoid sinus. The cerebrospinal fluid leak was repaired and histopathology of tissue confirmed ecchordosis physaliphora. (*Bottom*) Axial and sagittal CT cisternogram, axial T2W, and coronal postcontrast MR imaging in another patient presenting with meningitis shows a similar midline lytic lesion in the dorsal clivus (*arrows*) with a bony spur, associated cerebrospinal fluid leak (note the contrast leakage into the sphenoid sinus), and diffuse pachymeningeal enhancement related intracranial hypotension. (*Courtesy of* Dr Kuldeep Singh, India.)

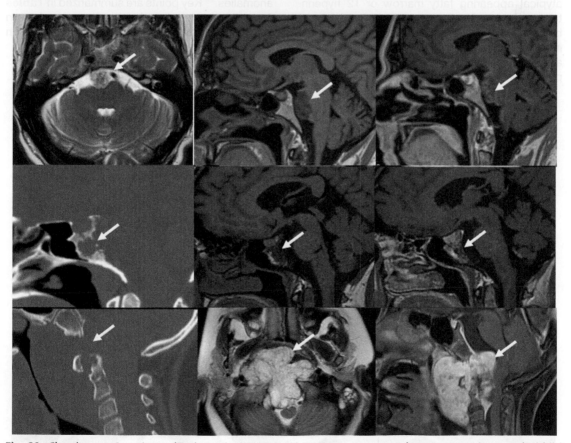

Fig. 20. Chordomas—3 patients. (*Top*) Axial T2W, sagittal T1W precontrast and postcontrast images. (*Middle*) Sagittal CT scan and T1W and postcontrast T1W images showing a purely extraosseous retroclival chordoma (*arrows*). (*Middle*) Sagittal CT scan and T1W precontrast and postcontrast images show a largely intraclival chordoma with irregular erosion of the clivus and contrast enhancement (*arrows*). (*Bottom*) Sagittal CT scan and T2W and postcontrast T1W images in another teenage patient presenting with nasal obstruction demonstrate a large intracranial and extracranial chordoma extending to the cervical spine and prevertebral space and occluding the nasopharynx.

Table 7
Ecchordosis physaliphora versus chordoma

Ecchordosis Physaliphora	Chordoma
Typically asymptomatic, incidental	Symptomatic
Cystic retroclival lesion	Solid/solid-cystic mass
No gadolinium enhancement	Gadolinium enhancement present
Bony stalk/excrescence	Bony destruction (although rarely purely extraosseous with a low risk of recurrence)
Lack of cellularity, pleomorphism, and mitoses No Ki-67, MIB-1 index	Cellularity, pleomorphism, and mitoses Ki-67 proliferation, MIB-1 index

Arrested Pneumatization of the Sphenoid Sinus

Arrested pneumatization of the sphenoid sinus is a commonly encountered variant, owing to failure of pneumatization of the sphenoid sinus with residual atypical appearing fatty marrow or T2 hyperintense microcystic change, typically involving the basisphenoid or pterygoid base (**Fig. 21**). It is important to recognize the imaging appearances and not confuse it with other lesions or aggressive pathologies.

POSTERIOR SKULL BASE AND CRANIOVERTEBRAL JUNCTION
Anatomy and Developmental Considerations

The development of the occipitocervical transition is key to understanding craniocervical junction anomalies.[24] Key points are summarized in **Tables 8** and **9** (see the embryology section, elsewhere in this article). Anatomic landmarks are shown in **Fig. 22**.

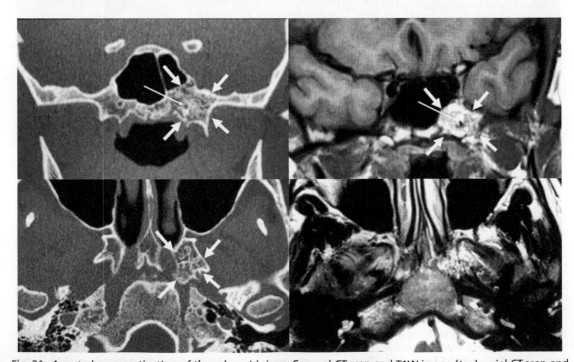

Fig. 21. Arrested pneumatization of the sphenoid sinus. Coronal CT scan and T1W image (*top*); axial CT scan and T2W image (*bottom*). Incidental finding of a sclerotic appearance to the left sphenoid body in a young man scan showing geographic area of sclerosis with fatty signal on MR imaging (*thick short arrows*). Note the lack of mass effect and preservation of the Vidian canal as it passes through this (*long thin arrow*).

Table 8
PSB and craniovertebral junction developmental pearls

PSB Boundaries	PSB formed by clivus (anteriorly), occipital squama (posteriorly), occipital condyles (inferolaterally) and petromastoid (superolaterally)
Foramen magnum	Almost fully ossified at birth May have persistent ossicle of Kerckring posteriorly
Occipitocervical transition	Skeletal and neural components develop in tandem, inducing each other reciprocally but also developing independently (explaining the finding of selective hypoplasia) Para-axial mesoderm condenses adjacent to developing neural tube in the fourth week of life to form bilateral segmented somites Four occipital somites (OS1–OS4) followed by seven cervical somites (CS1–CS7) OS1 and OS2 → basiocciput, OS3 → posterior supraocciput OS4 → basion anteriorly, occipital condyles laterally, tip of dens inferiorly Gap between OS3 and OS4 → hypoglossal canal Central mesenchymal cores (sclerotomes) eventually form the bony structures[24] Growth defect resulting in hypoplasia of occipital somite derivatives (mainly OS4, which is also called as proatlas is associated with a Chiari 1 malformation)[24]

Table 9
Key PSB and craniovertebral junction anatomic landmarks

Anatomic Landmarks	Location/Normative Value
Basion	Anterior margin of foramen magnum
Opisthion	Posterior margin of foramen magnum
Chamberlain's line	Hard palate to opisthion
McRae's line	Basion to opisthion
Clival line	Dorsum sella to basion, forms the Wackenheim's line when extended inferiorly tangentially to the posterior dens
Incisural line	Dorsum sella to vein of Galen–straight sinus junction (crossing midportion of midbrain)
Tentorial line	Along the straight sinus from the vein of Galen to the internal occipital protuberance
Basal angle (radiographic)	Angle between the line from the nasion to the center of the sella and from the sella to the basion (normally 125°–143°)
Basal angle (modified for MR imaging)[25]	Angle between the line along the anterior cranial fossa and the clival line (normally 114° ± 5° in children and 117° ± 6° in adults)
Posterior fossa pentagon	Formed by the McRae, clival, incisural, tentorial, and supraoccipital lines (typically regular in children)
pB-C2	Distance between posterior margin of dens and line drawn from basion to posterior margin of C2 inferior endplate to define posterior tilt of dens (normally ≤4 mm)

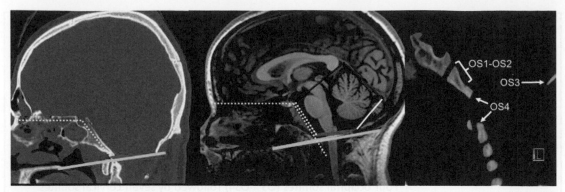

Fig. 22. Normal anatomic landmarks at the CCJ and development. See Table 9 for a description. *Dotted lines* show the basal angle between the ASB and the clival line, Chamberlain line (*yellow*), McRae line (*blue*), McGregor line (*green*), incisural line (*brown*), tentorial line (*purple*), supraocipital line (*white*), and the posterior fossa pentagon. The far right image shows derivatives of the occipital somites. Note the resegmentation of the fourth occipital somite OS4, which forms the basion as well as the tip of the dens.

Platybasia

Platybasia refers to an excessively obtuse basal angle resulting in a more horizontal orientation of

the clivus (**Fig. 23**). Although initially described on plain radiographs, it is now better assessed on cross-sectional imaging. The standard radiographic definition of the basal angle has now

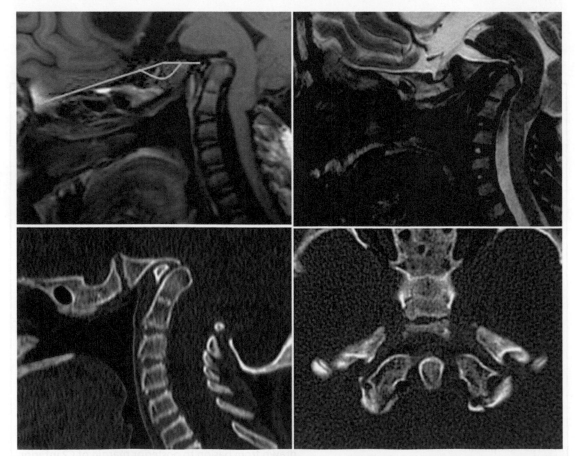

Fig. 23. Platybasia. MR imaging (*top*) and CT scans (*bottom*) showing severe horizontal orientation and shortening of the clivus with a significantly increased (obtuse) basal angle nearing 180° and cranial migration of the cervical spine impinging.

been refined and an easier to perform modified MR imaging technique has been proposed, which has a lower normative value[25] (see **Table 9**; see **Fig. 23**).

Basilar Invagination and Impression

Basilar invagination is a term generally reserved to describe a developmental anomaly whereby the tip of the dens projects above the plane of the foramen magnum, whereas basilar impression describes a similar upward displacement of the dens owing to acquired processes, often related to bone softening. It is also important to highlight venous variants, such as a persistent occipital sinus (which extends inferiorly along the occipital

bone in the midline/paramidline region) or the marginal sinus (at the margin of the foramen magnum), which present surgical risk during foramen magnum decompression.

Clival and Posterior Skull Base Hypoplasia and Clefts

PSB hypoplasia can occur in several conditions affecting endochondral bone growth, such as achondroplasia, with consequent shortening of the skull base and particularly the clivus. This may be associated with foramen magnum stenosis and neural compromise (**Fig. 24**). Clival clefts can also be seen in several conditions, such as CHARGE syndrome.

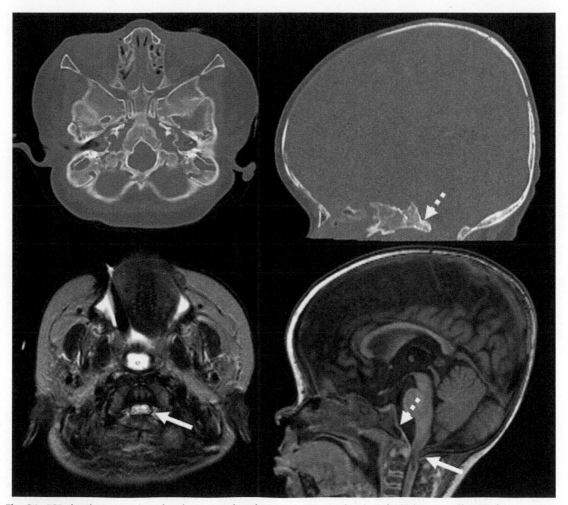

Fig. 24. PSB dysplasia in achondroplasia. Axial and sagittal CT scans (*top*) and MR imaging (*bottom*) in a patient with achondroplasia showing a large cranial vault and small skull base with a short clivus (*dashed arrows*). There is foramen magnum stenosis, resulting in compression of the upper spinal cord and myelopathic signal change (*solid arrow*). This is due to a mutation to the FGFR3 gene that affects bones forming by endochondral ossification, such as the skull base, but not the cranial vault, which forms by membranous ossification.

Chiari Malformations

Since the first description by Hans Chiari of "elongation of the tonsils and medial part of the inferior lobes of the cerebellum which go along the medulla into the cervical canal" in the late nineteenth century,[26] the literature abounds with numerous descriptions and proposed mechanisms for Chiari malformations. A full review of different types of Chiari malformations is beyond the scope of this article. The Chiari 2 malformation is a distinct entity and is seen in the context of a myelomeningocele, typically diagnosed antenatally or at birth. Discussion in this article is limited to certain aspects of the Chiari 1 malformation, which is increasingly being referred to as the Chiari 1 deformity (rather than malformation) and is not associated with a myelomeningocele (**Fig. 25**).

Pathophysiologically, a Chiari 1 malformation is believed to result from a disproportion or developmental mismatch of the container (posterior fossa) and contents (hindbrain).[24] The hindbrain and bony posterior fossa are metamerically associated and normally programmed to grow together, resulting in a normal position of the cerebellar tonsils superior to the foramen magnum and surrounded by cerebrospinal fluid. If there is a developmental mismatch in the rate of growth between the hindbrain and bony posterior fossa (more commonly owing to inadequate growth of the latter), the cerebellar tonsils may project inferiorly with crowding of the foramen magnum. This Chiari 1 malformation or deformity is typically defined as a tonsillar descent of 5 mm or more, although other factors such as the diameter of

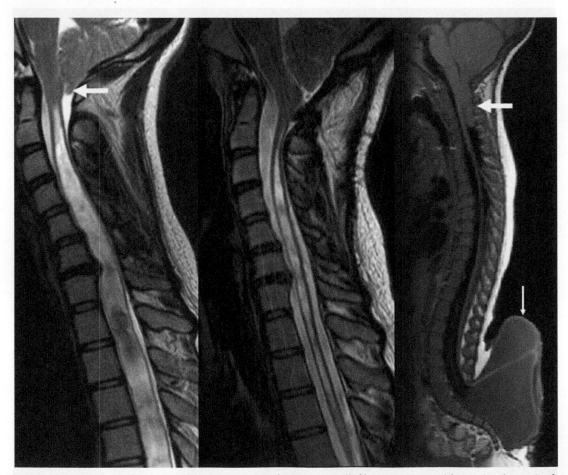

Fig. 25. Chiari 1 versus Chiari 2 malformation. Sagittal T2W image (*left*) in a patient with painless burns in the hands. The low lying, elongated, and peg-like cerebellar tonsils (*arrow*), elongation and descent of the cervicomedullary junction, and extensive spinal cord syrinx are compatible with a Chiari 1 malformation. (*Middle*) The same patient after foramen magnum decompression shows marked resolution of the syrinx. (*Right*) Sagittal T1W image in a neonate with a large lumbar myelomeningocele (*thin arrow*) shows striking descent and elongation of the cerebellar tonsils to the mid cervical canal (*thick arrow*) and marked crowding of a small sized posterior fossa, which is consistent with a Chiari 2 malformation.

the foramen magnum, shape of the tonsils (peg-like deformation), narrowing of the cerebrospinal fluid space, compression of neural structures, and syringomyelia are also relevant. Many patients are asymptomatic and the definition is anatomic rather than clinical. Syringomyelia is thought to be due to the Venturi effect, which is associated with high cerebrospinal fluid velocity across the narrowed foramen magnum. Although a midline sagittal section is the best imaging plane to evaluate the morphology, coronal imaging is also very useful to demonstrate shallowness of the posterior fossa. Additional hypoplasia of the upper cervical segments results in further bony narrowing and upward shift of the dens, which may therefore impinge on the medulla.

True versus False Chiari Malformation 1

Although a Chiari 1 malformation is typically developmental, it should be noted that tonsillar descent may also be acquired. Several classifications systems have been proposed to try and differentiate various causes or types of Chiari 1 malformations.[24,26–28] Most of the classification systems attempt at differentiating developmental variants of Chiari 1 malformations into those caused by a congenital or developmental defect of the container (skull base or cervical spine) from those owing to an increase in size of the contents (neural tissue overgrowth). Acquired processes resulting in tonsillar herniation include high or low intracranial pressure (**Fig. 26**). The most recent proposed classification (**Table 10**)

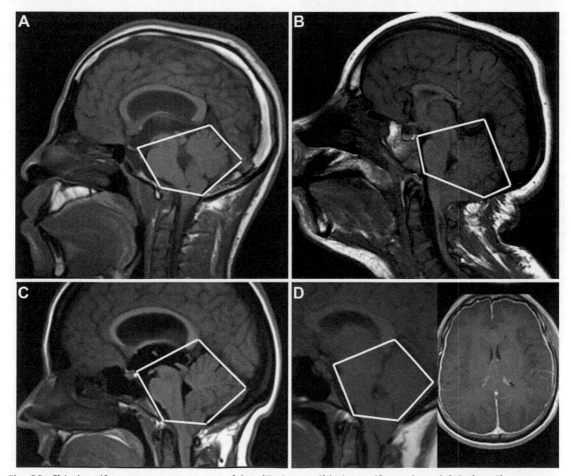

Fig. 26. Chiari malformations – true versus false. (*Top*) True Chiari 1 malformations. (*A*) Sathre Choetzen syndrome in a patient with platybasia, occipitalization of the atlas, atlantoaxial subluxation, Chiari 1 malformation, and medullary compression. (*B*) Rubinstein Taybi syndrome in a patient with abnormal dysplastic clivus, segmentation anomalies, callosal dysgenesis, Chiari 1 malformation, and syringomyelia. Note the abnormal posterior fossa polygons in these patients. (*Bottom*) False Chiari 1 malformations with a relatively regular posterior fossa pentagon. (*C*) Aqueductal stenosis with hydrocephalus, raised intracranial pressure and hindbrain herniation. (*D*) Intracranial hypotension in a patient with a spinal cerebrospinal fluid leak showing marked brain slumping, crowding at the tentorial hiatus, distortion of the brainstem, and hindbrain herniation (note also the dural enhancement in the same patient).

Table 10
Proposed etiologic classification of the tonsillar herniation spectrum/Chiari 1 malformation

True Chiari 1 malformation	a. Structural anomalies of the skull base and/or abnormal cervical segmentation b. Congenital overgrowth syndrome (eg, Beckwith-Wiedemann, Sotos, osteopetrosis, etc) c. Overcrowding caused by a congenitally small skull and/or posterior fossa (eg, craniosynostosis)
False Chiari 1 malformation	a. Excessive tissue in the posterior fossa or entire skull b. Craniospinal pressure imbalance c. Spinal malformation

Adapted from Fiaschi P, Morana G, Anania P, Rossi A, Consales A, Piatelli G, Cama A, Pavanello M. Tonsillar herniation spectrum: more than just Chiari I. Update and controversies on classification and management. Neurosurg Rev. 2020 Dec;43(6):1473-1492.

attempts at simplifying and separating Chiari 1 malformations into 2 broad groups, namely, true Chiari 1 malformations, which typically require occipitocervical decompression or fixation, and false Chiari 1 malformations, which typically involve the management of the contributing condition in the first instance.

SUMMARY

Using illustrative cases and tables, this article discusses some of the developmental anatomy and related abnormalities of the anterior, central and posterior skull base. An understanding of the embryology and varied imaging appearances of the wide spectrum of developmental skull base pathologies is critical in formulating a relevant differential diagnosis and guiding appropriate clinical management.

REFERENCES

1. Ricciardelli EJ. Embryology and anatomy of the cranial base. Clin Plast Surg 1995;22(3):361–72.

2. Hoyte DA. The cranial base in normal and abnormal skull growth. Neurosurg Clin N Am 1991;2(3): 515–37.

3. LoPresti MA, Sellin JN, DeMonte F. Developmental considerations in pediatric skull base surgery. J Neurol Surg B Skull Base 2018;79(1):3–12.

4. Noden DM. Cell movements and control of patterned tissue assembly during craniofacial development. J Craniofac Genet Dev Biol 1991;11(04): 192–213.

5. Bosma JF. Development of the Basicranium. In: Conference publication: symposium on the development of the basicranium. Bethesda, MD: National Institute of Health; 1975.

6. Gruber DP, Brockmeyer D. Pediatric skull base surgery. 1. Embryology and developmental anatomy. Pediatr Neurosurg 2003;38(01):2–8.

7. Nemzek WR, Brodie HA, Hecht ST, et al. CT, and plain film imaging of the developing skull base in fetal specimens. AJNR Am J Neuroradiol 2000; 21(9):1699–706.

8. Belden CJ, Mancuso AA, Kotzur IM. The developing anterior skull base: CT appearance from birth to 2 years of age. AJNR Am J Neuroradiol 1997;18(5): 811–8.

9. Hughes DC, Kaduthodil MJ, Connolly DJ, et al. Dimensions and ossification of the normal anterior cranial fossa in children. AJNR Am J Neuroradiol 2010; 31(7):1268–72.

10. Stranding S. Gray's anatomy-the anatomical basis of clinical practice. 39th edition. Elsevier; 2005. p. 463–80.

11. Krishan K, Kanchan T. Evaluation of spheno-occipital synchondrosis: a review of literature and considerations from forensic anthropologic point of view. J Forensic Dent Sci 2013;5:72–6.

12. Sepahdari AR, Mong S. Skull base CT: normative values for size and symmetry of the facial nerve canal, foramen ovale, pterygoid canal, and foramen rotundum. Surg Radiol Anat 2013;35(1):19–24.

13. Barkovich AJ, Vandermarck P, Edwards MS, et al. Congenital nasal masses: CT and MR imaging features in 16 cases. AJNR Am J Neuroradiol 1991; 12(1):105–16.

14. Lowe LH, Booth TN, Joglar JM, et al. Midface anomalies in children. Radiographics 2000;20(4):907–22.

15. Hedlund G. Congenital frontonasal masses: developmental anatomy, malformations, and MR imaging. Pediatr Radiol 2006;36(7):647–62.

16. Som PM, Curtin HD. Head & neck imaging, vol. 1. St. Louis, MO: Mosby Elsevier; 2003.

17. Abele TA, Salzman KL, Harnsberger HR, et al. Craniopharyngeal canal and its spectrum of pathology. AJNR Am J Neuroradiol 2014;35(4):772–7.

18. Schick B, Brors D, Prescher A. Sternberg's canal–cause of congenital sphenoidal meningocele. Eur Arch Otorhinolaryngol 2000;257(8):430–2.

19. Barañano CF, Curé J, Palmer JN, et al. Sternberg's canal: fact or fiction? Am J Rhinol Allergy 2009; 23(2):167–71.

20. Currarino G. Canalis basilaris medianus and related defects of the basiocciput. AJNR Am J Neuroradiol 1988;9(1):208–11.

21. Chihara C, Korogi Y, Kakeda S, et al. Ecchordosis physaliphora and its variants: proposed new classification based on high-resolution fast MR imaging employing steady-state acquisition. Eur Radiol 2013;23(10):2854–60.

22. Sekiya K, Watanabe M, Nadgir RN, et al. Nasopharyngeal cystic lesions: Tornwaldt and mucous retention cysts of the nasopharynx: findings on MR imaging. J Comput Assist Tomogr 2014;38(1):9–13.

23. Mehnert F, Beschorner R, Küker W, et al. Retroclival ecchordosis physaliphora: MR imaging and review of the literature. AJNR Am J Neuroradiol 2004; 25(10):1851–5.

24. Raybaud C, Jallo GI. Chiari 1 deformity in children: etiopathogenesis and radiologic diagnosis. Handb Clin Neurol 2018;155:25–48.

25. Koenigsberg RA, Vakil N, Hong TA, et al. Evaluation of platybasia with MR imaging. AJNR Am J Neuroradiol 2005;26(1):89–92.

26. Fiaschi P, Morana G, Anania P, et al. Tonsillar herniation spectrum: more than just Chiari I. Update and controversies on classification and management. Neurosurg Rev 2020;43(6):1473–92.

27. Buell TJ, Heiss JD, Oldfield EH. Pathogenesis and cerebrospinal fluid hydrodynamics of the Chiari I Malformation. Neurosurg Clin N Am 2015;26(4): 495–9.

28. Poretti A, Ashmawy R, Garzon-Muvdi T, et al. Chiari type 1 deformity in children: pathogenetic, clinical, neuroimaging, and management aspects. Neuropediatrics 2016;47(5):293–307.

Skull Base Neurointerventional Techniques

Zachary M. Wilseck, MD[a],*, Leanne Lin, MD, MPHS[a],
Joseph J. Gemmete, MD, FSIR, FCIRSE[b], Aditya S. Pandey, MD[c],
Ashok Srinivasan, MD[d], Neeraj Chaudhary, MD, MRCS, FRCR, FEBNI[e]

KEYWORDS

- Neurointervention • Skull base biopsy • Tumor ablation • Dural arteriovenous fistulas
- Venous sinus stenosis • Epistaxis and sinonasal bleeding

KEY POINTS

- Noninvasive cross-sectional imaging (computed tomography [CT], magnetic resonance [MR] imaging, and MR/CT angiography) plays a pivotal role in the diagnosis of patients with disorders of the deep face and skull lesions.
- The endovascular or percutaneous treatment of skull base tumors requires a thorough understanding of vascular anastomoses and anatomic variants.
- Dural arteriovenous fistulae increase the risk of venous hypertension and intraparenchymal hemorrhage. The preferred treatment method is an endovascular approach with either arterial, venous, or combination embolization.
- Venous sinus stenosis and jugular bulb abnormalities can lead to debilitating symptoms. Venous sinus stenting is a treatment option for patients with intracranial hypertension related to a dural venous sinus stenosis.
- Endovascular treatment of epistaxis has a high success rate and should be considered following the failure of conservative management.

INTRODUCTION

Neurointerventional radiology (NIR) plays a pivotal role in the diagnosis and treatment of deep face and skull base lesions. Endovascular and percutaneous access to these regions has dramatically improved, allowing improved histopathologic diagnosis of disorders, and therapies. This article discusses both vascular and nonvascular disorders of the deep face and skull base and the role of NIR in the diagnosis and treatment of vascular and nonvascular disorders of the skull base.

Imaging Protocols

Imaging modalities and techniques are described in **Table 1**.

SKULL BASE BIOPSY
Introduction

Superficial masses can be palpated and safely biopsied in a clinician's office without the need of image guidance. Biopsies of lesions involving the skull base and surrounding soft tissues typically require computed tomography (CT)

[a] Department of Radiology, University of Michigan, 1500 E. Medical Center Dr, B1D330, Ann Arbor, MI 48109, USA; [b] Department of Radiology, University of Michigan, 1500 E. Medical Center Dr, B1D328, Ann Arbor, MI 48109, USA; [c] Department of Neurosurgery, University of Michigan, 1500 E. Medical Center Dr, #5338 Attn: Dr. Pandey, Ann Arbor, MI 48109, USA; [d] Department of Radiology, University of Michigan, 1500 E. Medical Center Dr, B2A209D, Ann Arbor, MI 48109, USA; [e] Department of Radiology, University of Michigan, 1500 E. Medical Center Dr, B1D330A, Ann Arbor, MI 48109, USA
* Corresponding author.
E-mail address: zwilseck@med.umich.edu
Twitter: @ZWilseckMD (Z.M.W.); @LinYuanci (L.L.); @AshokSrini15 (A.S.)

Neuroimag Clin N Am 31 (2021) 649–664
https://doi.org/10.1016/j.nic.2021.06.007
1052-5149/21/

Table 1
Imaging protocols

Modality	Technique and Contrast
Computed tomography angiography	Helical scanning from the aortic arch to the cranial vertex following the intravenous administration of 80 mL of nonionic iodinated contrast, with imaging trigger of contrast density within the aortic arch. Section thickness of 0.625 mm. Multiplanar reformats are created in the coronal and sagittal planes. 3D reconstructions and MIP reformats are also created
Computed tomography venography	Helical scanning using 0.625-mm collimation following the intravenous administration of 100 mL of nonionic iodinated contrast and a 45-s delay with creation of 2-mm thickness sagittal and coronal reconstructions. 3D reconstructions and MIP reformats are also created
MRA	CE MRA includes 3-plane localizer, axial TOF (MOTSA), CE MRA, and axial TOF (MOTSA). Axial sequences are obtained at 4-mm thickness with 1.5-mm slice gap. COW protocol covers from the corpus callosum cranially to the distal cervical vertebral arteries caudally. Imaging is performed following the intravenous administration of 20 mL of gadolinium-based contrast at 2 mL/s
MRV	CE MRV includes a 3-plane localizer and CE 3D FFE MRV sequences. The scan includes whole-head coverage and slice thickness of 2 mm. The bolus tracker is set in the sagittal plane within the superior sagittal sinus. Imaging is performed following the intravenous administration of 20 mL of gadolinium-based contrast at 2 mL/s

Abbreviations: 3D, three-dimensional; CE, contrast enhanced; COW, circle of Willis; FFE, fast field echo; MIP, maximum intensity projection; MOTSA, multiple overlapping thin slab acquisition; MRA, magnetic resonance angiography, MRV, magnetic resonance venography; TOF, time of flight.

guidance given the anatomic complexity of these areas. Many procedures can be performed with local analgesia using 2% lidocaine and conscious sedation using a combination of midazolam and fentanyl citrate. For lesions requiring a transoral approach, general anesthesia is preferred. A coaxial technique, use of blunt trocars, and careful approach planning decrease the risk of vascular and nerve injury during biopsy. Based on lesion position, head position modification can facilitate access. In skull base lesions, neck hyperextension can make transbuccal or transmaxillary approach more accessible.[1] Complications can include bleeding, vasovagal reactions, and injury to vascular and nervous structures.

Imaging Findings/Pathology

Skull base lesions may be intrinsic to the skull base or arise from adjacent intracranial and extracranial soft tissues. Primary lesions of the suprahyoid

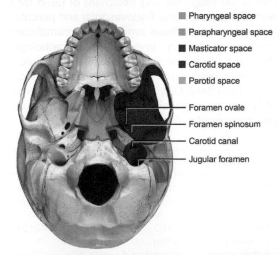

- Pharyngeal space
- Parapharyngeal space
- Masticator space
- Carotid space
- Parotid space

- Foramen ovale
- Foramen spinosum
- Carotid canal
- Jugular foramen

Fig. 1. View from below with color-coded skull base and suprahyoid neck spaces and the major osseous foramen.

neck spaces (**Fig. 1**) may extend directly to the skull base or via neurovascular channels.

Indication for Biopsy

Biopsies of the skull base are typically performed for lesions where pathognomonic imaging characteristics are not present and in cases where the patient may have multiple coexisting disorders. Fine-needle aspiration (FNA) is useful but highly dependent on the skill of the head and neck cytologist. A core biopsy obtains a high-quality specimen with reduced sampling error and allows for a spectrum of histochemical and immunohistochemical stains, further increasing chances of a tissue diagnosis.

Biopsy Technique

Typically 3-mm to 5-mm axial CT images are obtained for lesion localization and access planning. A coaxial technique involves the placement of an introducer needle, usually 18 or 19 gauge, through which a needle of 20 to 22 gauge can be placed for aspiration or core sampling.

Multiple biopsy approaches are available and can be used depending on the location of the lesion (**Table 2**). For example, the subzygomatic approach can allow access to lesions located in

the masticator space, parapharyngeal space, pharyngeal mucosal space, retropharyngeal space, pterygopalatine fossa, foramen ovale (**Fig. 2**A and B), and jugular foramen (**Fig. 3**A–C). The paramaxillary approach can allow access to the retropharyngeal space, prevertebral space, carotid space, skull base, and C1 and C2 lesions.

Pearls, pitfalls, variants

- CT, with its high spatial and contrast resolution, is the imaging modality of choice for biopsies of deep-seated face and skull base lesions.
- In cases where vascular anatomy is difficult to distinguish, the initial localizer CT images can be obtained following intravenous contrast administration.
- Many deep neck and skull base lesions can be biopsied via multiple approaches and the ideal approach is dictated by lesion location, extent, and adjacent neurovascular structures.

What referring physicians need to know

- Image-guided biopsies of the skull base can be performed in a safe and effective manner.
- Procedures can be performed with local analgesia and conscious sedation on an outpatient basis.
- Typically, procedures are performed with the use of CT guidance, but, depending on lesion, location, and operator experience, they can also be performed under fluoroscopic guidance.

Table 2
Barrow classification system of carotid cavernous fistulae

Type	Fistulous Vessels	Characteristics
A	Carotid artery to cavernous sinus	Direct, high flow, the most common
B	Dural ICA branches to cavernous sinus: • Meningohypophyseal trunk • Inferolateral trunk	Indirect, low flow
C	ECA branches to cavernous sinus: • Internal maxillary • Middle meningeal • Ascending pharyngeal	Indirect, low flow
D	Both ICA and ECA branches to cavernous sinus	Indirect, the most common of the low flow fistulas

Abbreviations: ECA, external carotid artery; ICA, internal carotid artery.

Summary

There are many available approaches to skull base biopsies. The lesion location, lesion extent, and the adjacent anatomic structures help guide access. Many lesions can be biopsied with local analgesia and conscious sedation. Familiarity with head and neck anatomy and the use of a small-caliber needle are important to decrease the risk of neurovascular injury.

ENDOVASCULAR AND PERCUTANEOUS SKULL BASE TUMOR EMBOLIZATION
Introduction

Preoperative embolization of vascular tumors of the skull base can decrease the difficulty of surgery, reduce perioperative blood loss, and is cost-

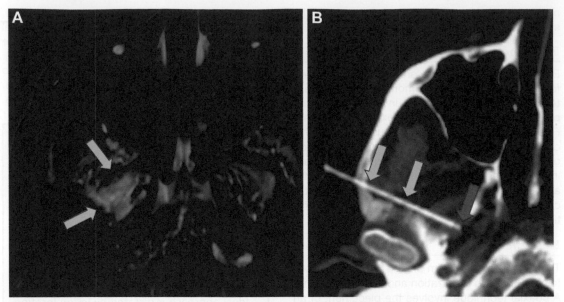

Fig. 2. An 83-year-old man with history of poorly differentiated cutaneous squamous cell carcinoma. Biopsy of right V3 nerve showed poorly differentiated carcinoma involving the soft tissue around the nerve. (*A*) Axial T1 fat-suppressed (FS) postcontrast MR imaging showing abnormal enhancing soft tissue within the right masticator space and foramen ovale. (*B*) Intraoperative CT during right subzygomatic approach. An introducer needle (*yellow arrows*) and an FNA needle (*blue arrow*) are located in abnormal skull base soft tissue.

effective.[2] The most commonly embolized tumors include meningiomas, glomus tumors, juvenile angiofibromas, and metastases. Preoperative embolization can also be performed for other hypervascular lesions such as endolymphatic sac tumor (**Fig. 4**A–E) and metastases. In addition to preoperative embolization, palliative ablation of head and neck carcinomas can be performed using percutaneous image-guided ablation techniques.

Imaging Findings/Pathology

Dedicated skull base imaging guides treatment planning. Accurate description of involved spaces, evaluation of important adjacent neurovascular structures, and imaging diagnosis can decrease anesthesia time and radiation exposure for the patients and operators during treatment.

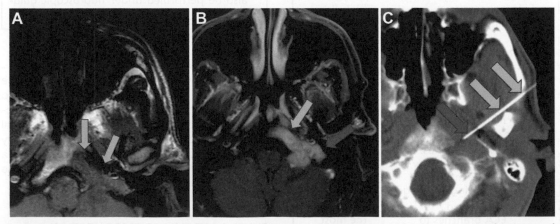

Fig. 3. A 62-year-old man with remote history of tongue SCCa who presented with progressive dysphagia, cough, and dysphonia. Biopsy-proven SCCa of the left jugular foramen and skull base. (*A*) Axial T1 FS precontrast MR imaging and (*B*) axial T1 FS postcontrast showing marrow replacing enhancing soft tissue involving the left aspect of the clivus, hypoglossal canal, and jugular foramen (*yellow arrows*). (*C*) Intraoperative CT during left subzygomatic approach with an introducer needle (*yellow arrow*) and an FNA needle (*blue arrow*) within the abnormal skull base soft tissue.

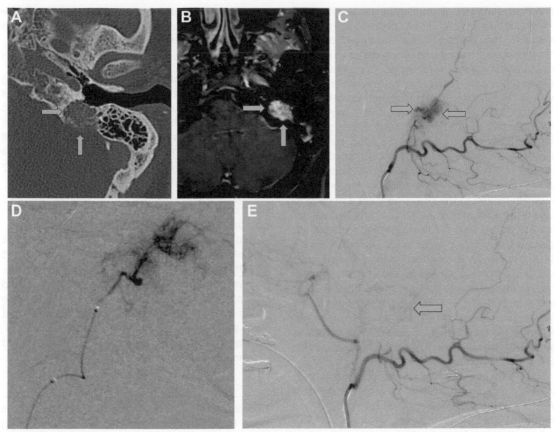

Fig. 4. A 64-year-old man with gradually progressive left-sided hearing loss. (*A*) Axial CT of the left temporal bone structures showing a destructive lytic lesion within the expected location of the vestibular aqueduct. (*B*) Axial T1 FS postcontrast MR imaging showing an avidly enhancing mass within the left temporal bone suggestive of an endolymphatic sac tumor, which was biopsy proved. (*C*) Lateral digital subtraction angiography (DSA) following left occipital artery injection showing hypertrophied transmastoid and jugular branches and tumoral blush within the location of the temporal bone mass. (*D*) High-magnification lateral DSA following selective injection of a hypertrophied transmastoid branch tumoral feeder arising from the left occipital artery. (*E*) Following particle and coil embolization of transmastoid tumoral feeders, left occipital artery injection shows no residual tumoral filling. Note minimal persistent tumoral blush via petrous branch of left middle meningeal artery (*arrow*).

Indications for Treatment

Preoperative embolization can decrease intraoperative blood loss through the control of surgically inaccessible arterial feeders, increase the chance of complete surgical resection, decrease operative procedure time, relieve intractable pain, decrease expected tumor recurrence, allow better visualization of the surgical field, and decrease overall surgical morbidity. Complications occur in less than 2% of patients and can be related to nontarget embolization, which can result in blindness or neurologic deficits.[3,4]

Treatment

Endovascular

The goal of preoperative embolization is to selectively occlude the vascular supply of the tumor at the precapillary level. Embolic materials most commonly used include polyvinyl alcohol (PVA), Embospheres (Merit Medical, South Jordan, UT), liquid embolic agents (*n*-butyl cyanoacrylate [*n*-BCA] glue [Trufill, Cerenovus, Miami, FL], ethylvinyl alcohol [EVOH] copolymer [Onyx, Medtronic, Irvine, CA]), gelatin sponge (Gelfoam; Pfizer, New York, NY), and coils. Embolization 24 to 72 hours before surgical resection allows maximal thrombosis of the occluded vessels.[5] Distal embolization at the capillary level is needed so arterial collateralization does not occur. Typically 100-μm to 300-μm Embospheres can be used to allow for distal penetration and devascularization. Larger particles (150–500 μm) can be used, but result in a lesser degree of tumor penetration but can decrease the risk of tissue necrosis and cranial nerve injury. If vigorous arteriovenous shunting is identified during angiography, larger particle size should be used (>500 μm) to prevent unimpeded flow into the venous system and embolization into the lungs.[2] The arterial field is dynamic and liberal use of digital subtraction angiography is required because anastomoses may emerge and open as the embolization procedure progresses.

Carotid artery sacrifice is sometimes required in the treatment of skull base tumors. Although most parents can tolerate permanent carotid occlusion, parent vessel occlusion (PVO) without balloon test occlusion (BTO) has an ischemic complication rate as high as 26%, with 12% of patients experiencing mortality related to the infarct.[6] BTO is a method to assess the efficiency of the intracranial collateral circulation and help determine whether a patient will tolerate PVO. The 2 most useful variables during BTO are the intraprocedural clinical examination and venous phase assessment on the angiogram. Venous phase assessment is based on the assumption that patients who have symmetry within the venous phase during BTO have enough intracranial collateral circulation to tolerate PVO. Venous phase asymmetry of more than 0.5 seconds correlates with a high ischemic risk for PVO.

A BTO including 4-vessel angiography is performed followed by inflation of a nondetachable balloon within the internal carotid artery (ICA) in question above the carotid bifurcation. The balloon is left inflated for 30 minutes and neurologic status is evaluated every 5 minutes. Some operators also access the opposite femoral artery and perform angiography of the contralateral ICA and 1 vertebral artery while the balloon is inflated.

In addition, a pharmacologic hypotensive challenge can provide additional information about whether a patient's intracranial collateral circulation can tolerate PVO. During the BTO, the patient's mean arterial blood pressure is decreased 30% below baseline and is maintained at this level for 15 to 20 minutes while neurologic evaluation continues.

Percutaneous

Tumors of the skull base frequently involve branches of the ICA and/or the vertebral arteries. Embolization of these vessels can be performed by experienced operators, but these procedures carry more risk of stroke and related complications. A variety of hypervascular tumors of the skull base, head, and neck can respond favorably to devascularization via direct percutaneous puncture, including hypervascular metastases, schwannomas, rhabdomyosarcomas, and paragangliomas.[7] Direct intratumoral injection provides easier access to the vascular tumor bed, and is not limited by vessel tortuosity or size, vasospasm, or atherosclerotic disease.[4] Options for direct embolic injection include n-BCA, EVOH, or absolute alcohol.

Cryotherapy

Cryoablation involves rapid freezing and thawing of tissue leading to intracellular ice formation, cell apoptosis, desiccation, and cellular ischemic injury during thawing.[8,9] Cryoablative techniques have several advantages compared with thermal ablation. The primary advantage is the ability to visualize the ice ball and treated lesion directly and in real time using sonography, CT, or MR.[9,10] Additional advantages include the absence of surgical scar, reduced recovery time, and less pain compared with heat-based techniques.[8,9]

Because of the protective effects of the heat sink phenomenon, cryoablation can be performed directly adjacent to head and neck vasculature. Severe complications such as stroke or carotid blowout are less likely than with other ablative techniques.[11] Other ablative techniques that have been used in the head and neck include microwave ablation, radiofrequency ablation, and irreversible electroporation.

Summary

Endovascular or percutaneous treatment of skull base tumors requires a thorough understanding of vascular anastomoses and anatomic variants. A variety of interventional techniques are available and are chosen based on the lesion being treated, the location, and the goal of treatment. Preoperative embolization can lead to reduced blood loss, operating time, and cost.

DURAL ARTERIOVENOUS FISTULAS
Introduction

Dural arteriovenous fistulas (dAVFs) are pathologic or congenital shunts between dural arteries and

---

Pearls, pitfalls, variants

- Tumors that most frequently require embolization in the head and neck include meningiomas, paragangliomas, and juvenile angiofibromas.

- Intracranial and extracranial arterial anastomoses are dynamic and high-quality digital subtraction angiography should be performed before and during embolization of skull base lesions.

- Nontarget embolization can result in complications, including cranial neuropathies, blindness, and cerebrovascular accident, and injury to skin, mucosa, tongue, larynx, and orbit.

dural venous sinuses, meningeal veins, or cortical veins typically supplied by pachymeningeal arteries.[12] dAVFs represent 10% to 15% of intracranial arteriovenous malformations, are typically acquired, and most involve the transverse, sigmoid, and cavernous sinuses.[2]

Carotid cavernous fistulas (CCFs) are the result of abnormal connections between the carotid artery and the cavernous sinus (**Fig. 5**A–E). CCFs can be either direct or indirect and can be the result of trauma or develop spontaneously. The Barrow classification system of CCFs is the most widely recognized.[13]

Symptoms and prognosis are variable and depend on the dAVF location, direction of venous flow, and size of involved territory. dAVFs can result in headaches, visual disturbances, tinnitus, focal neurologic deficits, subarachnoid hemorrhage, intraparenchymal hemorrhage, coma, or death.[12]

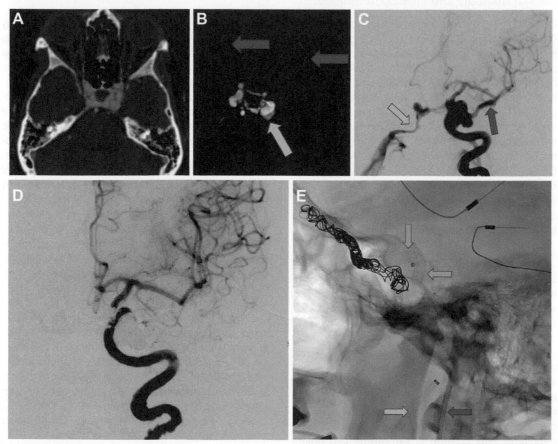

Fig. 5. A 62-year-old woman with history of migraine, worsening headache, left-sided pulsatile tinnitus, and new left cranial nerve VI palsy. (*A*) Axial CT angiography (CTA) shows abnormal early filling of the bilateral cavernous sinuses suggestive of a CCF. (*B*) Oblique time-of-flight (TOF) MR angiography (MRA) image showing flow-related enhancement within the cavernous sinus (*yellow arrow*) as well as dilated bilateral superior ophthalmic veins (*blue arrows*). (*C*) Anteroposterior (AP) DSA in the midarterial phase showing abnormal opacification of the cavernous sinus, intercavernous sinuses, contralateral inferior petrosal sinus (*yellow arrow*), and ipsilateral superior ophthalmic vein (*blue arrow*). (*D*) AP DSA following left ICA injection after ipsilateral flow-diverting stent placement and bilateral superior ophthalmic vein coil embolization shows no further early venous opacification. (*E*) Lateral single shot showing the left ICA flow-diverting stent (*green arrows*), superior ophthalmic vein coils. Catheter within the left ICA (*yellow arrow*) and left internal jugular vein (*blue arrow*).

Ophthalmologic manifestations of dAVFs near the cavernous sinus include the red-eye and white-eye shunts. Fistula near the dural sinuses can result in a papilledema shunt.[14] The fistulous drainage in a red-eye shunt is primarily into the orbit, leading to decreased visual acuity, increased intraocular pressures, and ocular venous congestion. The fistulous drainage in a white-eye shunt is primarily posteriorly into the petrosal or pterygoid venous sinuses, and typically does not present with orbital venous congestion but can develop reduced visual acuity and ophthalmoplegia caused by vascular steal from the optic nerve and vasa vasorum of the ocular motor cranial nerves. The papilledema shunt results from arterialization of the sagittal, transverse, or sigmoid sinuses and leads to increased venous and intracranial pressures (ICPs).

Normal Anatomy and Imaging Techniques

Initial imaging evaluation for dAVF should include CT angiography (CTA) and MR imaging. MR imaging has been suggested as the best first-line diagnostic modality for evaluation of dAVF, has a higher sensitivity in the detection of dAVF, and has been shown to be useful for clinical follow-up.[2] MR imaging can show findings including vascular enhancement, dilated and tortuous vessels, early and asymmetric venous enhancement, and signs of venous hypertension.[1] Noncontrast CT is limited to diagnosing secondary signs of dAVF, including intracranial hemorrhage and edema from venous hypertension. Conventional cerebral angiography remains the gold standard for the detection and classification of dAVF.[14,15]

Imaging Findings/Pathology

DAVF classification is based on the arterial connection to the dural venous sinus and/or cortical veins and the blood flow direction within the venous system. Cognard and colleagues[16] defined 5 types of dAVF (Fig. 6A–E) (fistulas with perimedullary venous drainage are not discussed here). The risk of venous hypertension and hemorrhage increases in the setting of a direct fistula to cortical veins or retrograde flow within the venous system. Although classification is helpful for risk stratification, dAVFs can be dynamic and classification may change over time. Any change in symptoms can reflect changes in venous drainage patterns and should prompt further diagnostic work-up.

Indications for Treatment

Given lesion complexity, treatment of dAVF requires a multidisciplinary treatment approach. Patients with angiographic high-grade lesions,

neurologic deficits, increased intraocular pressures, or papilledema typically require immediate treatment.[2] Low-grade lesions with severe debilitating symptoms are also candidates for endovascular repair.

Treatment

Although endovascular treatment has become the mainstay of therapy for dAVF, in the absence of neurologic symptoms, increased intracranial or intraocular pressures, or high-risk angiographic signs, the lesion can be closely followed with clinical examination and MR imaging. Although rare, dAVFs can spontaneously regress. The carotid-jugular compression protocol has been shown to be an effective noninvasive therapy but should be avoided in patients with atherosclerotic disease of the carotid bifurcation.[17]

Endovascular

Endovascular treatment of dAVFs is typically accomplished via a transarterial and/or transvenous approach.[12] Direct puncture of the cavernous sinus can be performed from an intraorbital approach in patients with CCF. The goal of treatment is the complete elimination of the arteriovenous shunt. Incomplete occlusion can lead to collateralization and a persistent risk of hemorrhage. Various embolic agents have been used, including platinum microcoils, EVOH (Onyx, Medtronic, Irvine, CA), and n-BCA (Trufill, Cerenovus, Miami, FL). The path of endovascular approach is typically determined by the type of fistula; for example, a Cognard type I can be treated via a transarterial approach and embolization of the arterial feeder (Fig. 7A–D). Liquid embolic use is common and has been successful in the treatment of dAVF.[18] Because of its cohesive properties, EVOH migration within the venous system can be better controlled than other liquid embolic materials.

Severe complications can occur following embolization, including the development of extensive thrombosis of the draining veins. This thrombosis can lead to increased risk of venous infarct and intraparenchymal hemorrhage. Risk of thrombosis can be decreased by treating patients with intravenous heparin and maintaining an activated clotting time twice the normal value for 48 hours postoperatively.

Surgery

Endovascular embolization may not always be feasible or completely treat the lesion. In complex dAVF, multistage endovascular embolization of arterial feeders may be required before surgical resection. In fistulas that show sinus drainage and/or reflux into cortical veins (Cognard types I

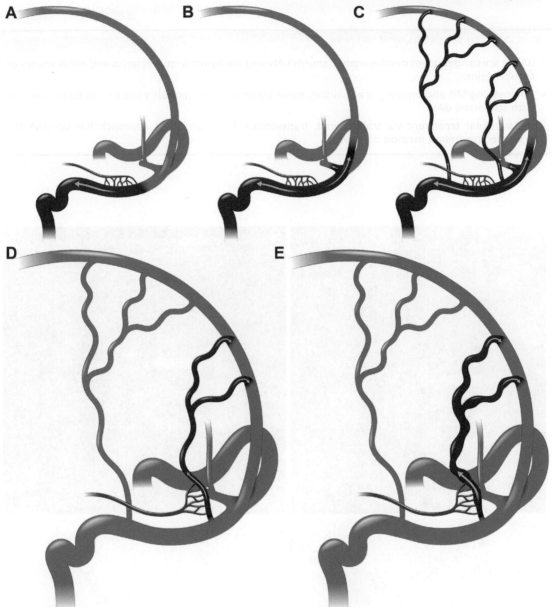

Fig. 6. Cognard classification of dAVF. (*A*) Cognard type I. (*B*) Cognard type IIa. (*C*) Cognard type IIb. (*D*) Cognard type III. (*E*) Cognard type IV.

and II), excision of the fistulous sinus segment is a definitive option. Treatment of fistulae with direct cortical venous drainage (Cognard types III and IV) may require interruption of the draining vein where it exits the dural wall of the sinus.[19]

Radiosurgery

Stereotactic radiosurgery (SRS) can be an effective in simple fistulas; however, complex fistulas with multiple arterial feeders and significant cortical venous reflux cannot be treated in a timely manner with SRS. Given the time from treatment to potential fistula closure, there is a continued risk of hemorrhage or rebleeding. SRS is typically used

as an adjunct to endovascular embolization in complex lesions or when there is high risk of nontarget embolization.[18]

Pearls, pitfalls, variants

- When present, dAVFs are typically located at the junction of the transverse and sigmoid sinuses.

- Most dAVFs present in adulthood and account for 10% to 15% of all cerebral vascular malformations.

- Dilated pial/leptomeningeal vessels in the subarachnoid space can be an important clue in the identification of dAVF.

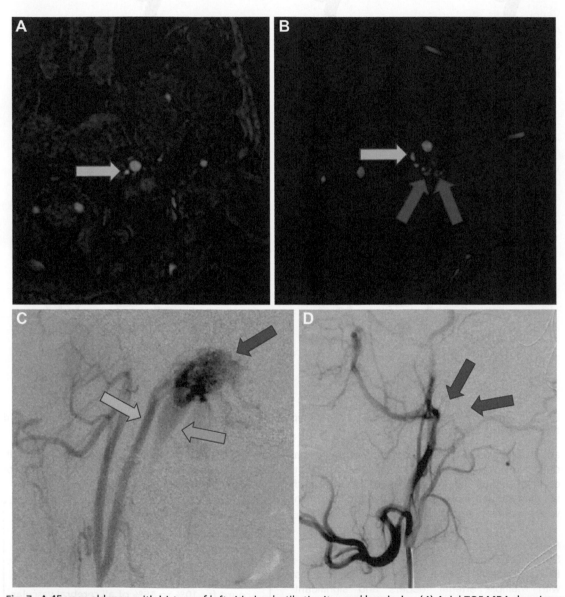

Fig. 7. A 45-year-old man with history of left-sided pulsatile tinnitus and headache. (*A*) Axial TOF MRA showing a hypertrophied left ascending pharyngeal artery lying medial to the left ICA. (*B*) Axial TOF MRA showing hypertrophied ascending pharyngeal branches (*yellow arrow*) with evidence of early flow-related enhancement within the left internal jugular vein (*blue arrows*). (*C*) Lateral DSA following left ascending pharyngeal artery (*yellow arrow*) injection showing a dAVF (*blue arrow*) and early antegrade filling of the left internal jugular vein (*green arrow*) (Cognard type I). (*D*) Late arterial phase lateral DSA via left external carotid artery (ECA) injection following coil embolization showing no residual filling of previously visualized dAVF.

Summary

dAVFs are abnormal connections between pachymeningeal arteries and dural sinuses or cortical veins. A dAVF can cause venous hypertension and potentially intraparenchymal hemorrhage. A multidisciplinary approach is recommended in diagnosing and treating these complex lesions. Various treatment options are available, but the preferred method is an endovascular approach.

VENOUS SINUS STENTING
Introduction

Venous sinus stenting can be used in the treatment of idiopathic intracranial hypertension (IIH) secondary to dural venous sinus stenosis, and vascular anatomic causes of pulsatile tinnitus, including venous diverticula, venous aneurysm, or jugular bulb dehiscence.

Imaging Findings/Pathology

Initial noninvasive imaging of the dural venous sinuses can include CT venography (CTV) or MR venography (MRV). Venous sinus stenosis most commonly occurs at the junction of the transverse and sigmoid sinuses (**Fig. 8**).

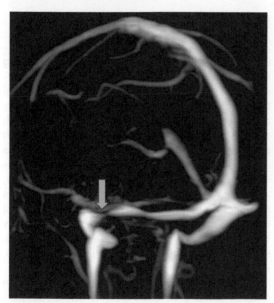

Fig. 8. Oblique three-dimensional MRV showing a focal stenosis (*arrow*) at the junction of the left transverse and sigmoid sinuses.

IIH, also known as pseudotumor cerebri, is a disorder characterized by increased ICP without radiographic evidence of dilated ventricles or mass lesion and normal CSF content. Patients with IIH commonly have significant bilateral transverse sinus stenoses and outflow obstruction.[20]

Diagnostic criteria are listed in **Box 1**. Venous sinus stenosis can be secondary to focal intrinsic narrowing (eg, fenestrations, arachnoid granulations, septations, organized chronic thrombus) or extrinsic compression.

Box 1
Criteria for diagnosis of pseudotumor cerebri

Required for diagnosis of pseudotumor cerebri syndrome

1. Papilledema

2. Normal neurologic exemption except for cranial nerve abnormalities

3. Neuroimaging: normal brain parenchyma without hydrocephalus, mass, structural lesion, or meningeal enhancement

4. Normal cerebrospinal fluid (CSF) composition

5. Increased lumbar puncture opening pressure (≥250 mm H_2O CSF in adults and ≥280 mm CSF in children)

Diagnosis of pseudotumor cerebri syndrome without papilledema

In the absence of papilledema, pseudotumor cerebri can be diagnosed if (2) to (5) from above are satisfied, and in addition the patient has unilateral or bilateral abducens nerve (cranial nerve VI) palsy.

In the absence of papilledema and abducens nerve palsy, a diagnosis of pseudotumor cerebri can be suggested but not made if (2) to (5) from above are satisfied, and in addition at least 3 of the following neuroimaging criteria are satisfied:

1. Empty sella

2. Flatting of the posterior aspect of the globe

3. Distension of the perioptic subarachnoid space with or without a tortuous optic nerve

---

Jugular bulb anomalies include high-riding jugular bulb, jugular bulb diverticula, jugular bulb dehiscence, and spontaneous venous aneurysm and occur in 10% to 15% of patients. Jugular bulb anomalies can lead to erosion into the adjacent structures (vestibular aqueduct, facial nerve canal, and posterior semicircular canal) and can result in pulsatile tinnitus.[10]

Indication for Treatment

In the setting of IIH, medical management is typically the first-line treatment and includes weight loss programs, a low-salt diet, and potentially the initiation of a carbonic anhydrase inhibitor. Serial lumbar punctures can be used to decrease ICP. When lifestyle changes and medical therapy fail to prevent vision loss or when the disease onset is fulminant, surgical or endovascular treatment options should be considered.

Treatment

Endovascular

Venous sinus stenting has gained increased acceptance as a treatment option for IIH in the setting of venous sinus stenosis and has been proved to decrease ICP and improve symptoms.[21] MRV and CTV show anatomic stenosis in up to 93% of patients with IIH.[22] Dural venous sinus stenosis can also be measured endovascularly, using intravascular ultrasonography or by measuring pressure gradients across the stenosis.[23] For many operators, the indications for endovascular treatment include symptomatic IIH unresponsive to conservative treatment with evidence of transverse sinus stenosis and a pressure gradient greater than 8 mm Hg documented on a catheter venogram (Fig. 9A–C).[22,24,25]

Rarely, venous stenting and stent-assisted coiling have also been used in the setting of venous diverticulum or aneurysm and jugular bulb dehiscence with successful amelioration of clinically significant pulsatile tinnitus (Fig. 10A,B).[10]

Surgery

In the setting of IIH, the two most commonly used surgical treatments are CSF diversion (ventriculoperitoneal and lumboperitoneal shunting) and optic nerve sheath fenestration (ONSF). ONSF may be chosen if the patient has visual loss but mild or no symptoms associated with increased ICP. CSF diversion is preferable in patients with visual loss, papilledema, and significant symptoms of increased ICP.

Abbreviations

MIP (maximum intensity projection)

TOF (time of flight)

MOTSA (multiple overlapping thin slab acquisition)

Pearls, pitfalls, variants

- Venous sinus stenosis is a significant and treatable vascular cause of pulsatile tinnitus and increased ICP.

- Venous sinus stenosis can be secondary to intrinsic causes (fenestrations, prominent arachnoid granulations, septations, organized chronic thrombus) or extrinsic compression.

- Jugular bulb abnormalities include a high-riding jugular bulb, venous diverticulum/aneurysm, and jugular bulb dehiscence.

What referring physicians need to know

- Consultation with a neuro-ophthalmologist and formal visual field testing are essential to guide management decisions in IIH.

- The main goals of treatment of IIH are symptom alleviation and visual preservation.

- Noninvasive evaluation of intracranial venous abnormalities can include CTV or MRV.

Summary

Venous sinus stenosis and jugular bulb abnormalities can lead to debilitating symptoms. Noninvasive evaluation of the dural venous sinuses includes CTV or MRV. Venous sinus stenosis can be evaluated endovascularly, including venous sinus stenosis gradient measurements. Venous sinus stenting has gained increased acceptance as a treatment option for patients with IIH and significant dural venous sinus stenosis. Venous sinus stenting has also proved effective in the treatment of venous diverticulum and jugular bulb dehiscence.

EPISTAXIS AND SINONASAL BLEEDING
Introduction

Epistaxis is a common clinical problem affecting more than 60% of the normal population. Episodes of bleeding can be caused by mucosal trauma from chronic excoriation, mucosal fragility and dryness, and inflammatory conditions such as viral rhinitis. Epistaxis can be associated with anticoagulation, vascular abnormalities such as aneurysm, or neoplasm. Other factors that increase the risk of epistaxis include coagulopathy, arteriosclerosis, or inherited conditions such as hereditary hemorrhagic telangiectasia. Most epistaxis can be controlled conservatively. Only 6% of patients with epistaxis require medical or surgical attention and, although uncommon, epistaxis can be life threatening.[26]

Up to 90% of cases of epistaxis arise from the anterior septal area (Little area), which is vascularized by the Kiesselbach plexus (Fig. 11). Typically, these cases can be managed with direct pressure, chemical cautery or electrocautery, application of topical hemostatic or vasoconstriction agents, or packing. Approximately 10% of cases originate from posteriorly and receive vascular supply from branches of the sphenopalatine artery. The success of conservative management in posterior nasal cavity bleeding lies between 48% and 83%.[29] The optimal surgical option in posterior

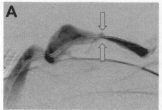
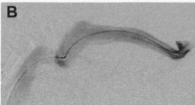
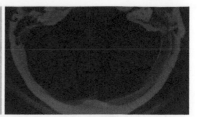

Fig. 9. (*A*) Lateral DSA via injection of the left transverse sinus shows focal stenosis (*arrows*) at the transverse sigmoid sinus junction. (*B*) Lateral DSA via injection of the left transverse sinus following stent deployment showing resolution of the previous stenosis and patency of indwelling stent. (*C*) Maximum intensity projection DynaCT showing a left transverse sigmoid sinus stent.

nasal bleeding remains unclear; however, endoscopic sphenopalatine artery ligation (ESPAL) is an effective treatment option to control refractory epistaxis with low morbidity.[27]

Endovascular embolization of the internal maxillary artery using Gelfoam (Pfizer, New York, NY) for intractable epistaxis was first reported in 1974.[28] Endovascular embolization is an effective alternative to surgery, has few complications, and has success rates from 71% to 100%.[26]

Imaging Findings/Pathology

The termination of the internal maxillary artery as it enters the sphenopalatine foramen is the sphenopalatine artery (SPA). The SPA is the major arterial supply to the nasal cavity and has been known as

the artery of epistaxis. The SPA supplies the Kiesselbach plexus, which is a vascular region composed of 4 arterial anastomoses: the anterior ethmoidal artery, sphenopalatine artery, greater palatine artery, and superior labial artery.

Indications for Treatment

The treatment of epistaxis depends on the location of the source of bleeding, either anterior or posterior. The treatment of anterior epistaxis should be done in a stepwise fashion using attempts at tamponade via nasal packing, cautery, thrombogenic foams, and gels.[29] The treatment of epistaxis arising from a posterior source can also include nasal packing, cautery, and in some cases ESPAL.

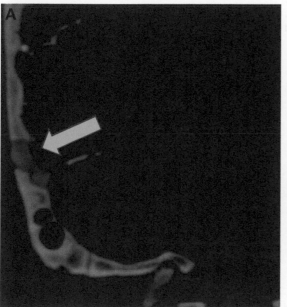
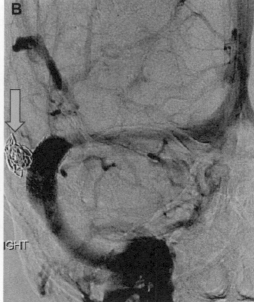

Fig. 10. A 36-year-old man with pulsatile right-sided tinnitus. (*A*) Coronal DynaCT following left ICA injection shows a venous diverticulum arising from the superolateral margin of the right transverse and sigmoid sinus junction (*yellow arrow*). (*B*) AP DSA in the venous phase following right ICA injection shows no further filling of the venous diverticulum, which has been coiled (*arrow*) with a stent in the adjacent venous sinus.

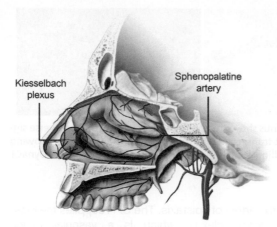

Kiesselbach plexus

Sphenopalatine artery

Fig. 11. Kiesselbach plexus.

In the setting of intractable epistaxis, endovascular embolization can also be considered.

Treatment

General anesthesia is typically used to decrease the risk of aspiration, but the procedure can be performed under conscious sedation for patients at high risk for anesthesia. Selective angiography of the bilateral ICAs and external carotid arteries (ECAs) is first performed to identify the location of bleeding.

The angiogram should be evaluated for evidence of contrast extravasation, tumor blush, vascular malformation, or pseudoaneurysm. Identification of vascular variants and anastomoses is critical before embolization. The most dangerous vascular anastomoses in the head and neck involve communications of the ICA and/or the vertebral artery with the first-order and second-order branches of the ECA. These connections are dynamic and visualization can change during the embolization procedure. The operator must keep these connections and their dynamic state in mind during any embolization procedure to avoid potentially catastrophic complications.

Embolization should only be performed with a stable microcatheter position within the internal maxillary artery distal to the origins of the middle meningeal artery, accessory meningeal, and deep temporal arteries, ideally just proximal to the branches supplying the nasal mucosa. Typical technique includes injection of a mixture of contrast material and particles sized 150 to 500 μm (**Fig. 12**A–C). The use of smaller particles should be avoided to decrease risk of nontarget embolization or tissue necrosis. Liquid embolic material such as n-BCA glue can also be used and Gelfoam pledgets can be placed in the vessel lumen after particulate embolization. Permanent occlusion should be avoided to not preclude vessel access if future bleeding occurs.

Complications of the procedure are similar to other neurointerventional procedures, including groin hematoma or vascular injury. Other complications can include facial numbness or pain, mucosal necrosis, and sinusitis. Stroke or blindness can also occur, but the incidence is very low.[30,31]

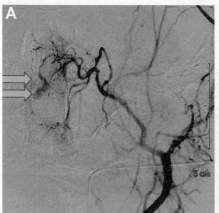
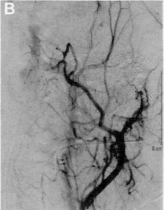
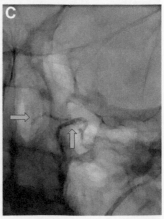

Fig. 12. An 80-year-old man with recurrent left-sided epistaxis previously treated with right-sided SPA ligation. (A) Lateral DSA following left ECA injection showing irregularity of the posterior septal branches of the distal SPA with active extravasation of contrast (arrows). (B) Lateral ECA angiogram following glue embolization shows no further filling of distal mucosal branches and no further contrast extravasation. (C) Nonsubtracted AP image showing the appearance of a glue cast within the distal left SPA (arrows).

Pearls, Pitfalls, Variants

- Kiesselbach plexus is a rich arterial anastomotic area where greater than 90% of epistaxis occurs.
- The anastomotic connections between the ICA and ECA are dynamic and must be considered during any embolization procedure.
- Permanent occlusion of the SPA with vascular plugs or coils should be avoided so access is not precluded if future bleeding occurs.

What Referring Physicians Need to Know

- Conservative management with thorough examination and surgical packing is typically the first step in management of epistaxis.
- CTA can be performed in cases where alternative causes of epistaxis are a consideration.
- Endovascular embolization for epistaxis is a safe and highly effective treatment option.

Summary

Epistaxis is a common clinical problem. Although many episodes of epistaxis can be managed conservatively, uncontrollable epistaxis can be a life-threatening condition. The management of uncontrollable epistaxis requires a collaborative effort between otorhinolaryngologists and neurointerventionalists. Endovascular embolization for epistaxis is a safe and effective method of treatment.

SUMMARY

Image-guided biopsy can allow safe, efficient, and accurate tissue sampling. NIR plays an important role in the treatment of many skull base disorders given the anatomic complexities and limited surgical windows. NIR plays an important role in the treatment of vascular tumors, arteriovenous fistulae/malformations, dural sinus stenosis, and epistaxis.

DISCLOSURE

The authors have nothing to disclose.

REFERENCES

1. Connor SE, Chaudhary N. CT-guided percutaneous core biopsy of deep face and skull-base lesions. Clin Radiol 2008;63(9):986–94.

2. Morris P. Interventional and endovascular therapy of the nervous system: a Practical guide. New York: Springer; 2013.

3. Abud DG, Mounayer C, Benndorf G, et al. Intratumoral injection of cyanoacrylate glue in head and neck paragangliomas. AJNR Am J Neuroradiol 2004;25(9):1457–62.

4. Quadros RS, Gallas S, Delcourt C, et al. Preoperative embolization of a cervicodorsal paraganglioma by direct percutaneous injection of onyx and endovascular delivery of particles. AJNR Am J Neuroradiol 2006;27(9):1907–9.

5. Dean BL, Flom RA, Wallace RC, et al. Efficacy of endovascular treatment of meningiomas: evaluation with matched samples. AJNR Am J Neuroradiol 1994;15(9):1675–80.

6. Elias AE, Chaudhary N, Pandey AS, et al. Intracranial endovascular balloon test occlusion: indications, methods, and predictive value. Neuroimaging Clin N Am 2013;23(4):695–702.

7. Casasco A, Herbreteau D, Houdart E, et al. Devascularization of craniofacial tumors by percutaneous tumor puncture. AJNR Am J Neuroradiol 1994; 15(7):1233–9.

8. Gandhi D, Gemmete JJ, Ansari SA, et al. Interventional neuroradiology of the head and neck. AJNR Am J Neuroradiol 2008;29(10):1806–15.

9. Erinjeri JP, Clark TW. Cryoablation: mechanism of action and devices. J Vasc Interv Radiol 2010;21(8 Suppl):S187–91.

10. Shastri RK, Chaudhary N, Pandey AS, et al. Venous diverticula causing pulsatile tinnitus treated with coil embolization and stent placement with resolution of symptoms: report of two cases and review of the literature. Otol Neurotol 2017;38(9):e302–7.

11. Guenette JP, Tuncali K, Himes N, et al. Percutaneous image-guided cryoablation of head and neck tumors for local control, preservation of functional status, and pain relief. AJR Am J Roentgenol 2017; 208(2):453–8.

12. Gandhi D, Chen J, Pearl M, et al. Intracranial dural arteriovenous fistulas: classification, imaging findings, and treatment. AJNR Am J Neuroradiol 2012; 33(6):1007–13.

13. Barrow DL, Spector RH, Braun IF, et al. Classification and treatment of spontaneous carotid-cavernous sinus fistulas. J Neurosurg 1985;62(2):248–56.

14. Chaudhary N, Griauzde J, Gemmete JJ, et al. Issues in the diagnosis and management of the papilledema shunt. J Neuroophthalmol 2014;34(3):259–63.

15. Gökçe E, Pınarbaşılı T, Acu B, et al. Torcular Herophili classification and evaluation of dural venous sinus variations using digital subtraction angiography and magnetic resonance venographies. Surg Radiol Anat 2014;36(6):527–36.

16. Cognard C, Gobin YP, Pierot L, et al. Cerebral dural arteriovenous fistulas: clinical and angiographic

correlation with a revised classification of venous drainage. Radiology 1995;194(3):671–80.

17. Kai Y, Morioka M, Yano S, et al. External manual carotid compression is effective in patients with cavernous sinus dural arteriovenous fistulae. Interv Neuroradiol 2007;13(Suppl 1):115–22.

18. Cognard C, Januel AC, Silva NA, et al. Endovascular treatment of intracranial dural arteriovenous fistulas with cortical venous drainage: new management using Onyx. AJNR Am J Neuroradiol 2008;29(2): 235–41.

19. Collice M, D'Aliberti G, Arena O, et al. Surgical treatment of intracranial dural arteriovenous fistulae: role of venous drainage. Neurosurgery 2000;47(1): 56–67.

20. Dinkin M, Patsalides A. Venous sinus stenting in idiopathic intracranial hypertension: results of a prospective trial. J Neuroophthalmol 2017;37:8.

21. Patsalides A, Oliveira C, Wilcox J, et al. Venous sinus stenting lowers the intracranial pressure in patients with idiopathic intracranial hypertension. J Neurointerven Surg 2019;11:3.

22. Levitt MR, Hlubek RJ, Moon K, et al. Incidence and predictors of dural venous sinus pressure gradient in idiopathic intracranial hypertension and non-idiopathic intracranial hypertension headache patients: results from 164 cerebral venograms. J Neurosurg 2017;126(2):347–53.

23. Liu R, Sun R, Huang F, et al. Endovascular treatment of cerebral venous sinus stenosis based on hemodynamic assessment using pressure wire. World Neurosurg 2020;136:2.

24. Cappuzzo JM, Hess RM, Morrison JF, et al. Transverse venous stenting for the treatment of idiopathic intracranial hypertension, or pseudotumor cerebri. Neurosurg Focus 2018;45(1):E11.

25. Koovor JM, Lopez GV, Riley K, et al. Transverse venous sinus stenting for idiopathic intracranial hypertension: safety and feasibility. Neuroradiol J 2018;31(5):513–7.

26. Andersen PJ, Kjeldsen AD, Nepper-Rasmussen J. Selective embolization in the treatment of intractable epistaxis. Acta Otolaryngol 2005;125(3):293–7.

27. Schaitkin B, Strauss M, Houck JR. Epistaxis: medical versus surgical therapy: a comparison of efficacy, complications, and economic considerations. Laryngoscope 1987;97(12):1392–6.

28. Sokoloff J, Wickbom I, McDonald D, et al. Therapeutic percutaneous embolization in intractable epistaxis. Radiology 1974;111(2):285–7.

29. Pollice PA, Yoder MG. Epistaxis: a retrospective review of hospitalized patients. Otolaryngol Head Neck Surg 1997;117(1):49–53.

30. Strutz J, Schumacher M. Uncontrollable epistaxis. Angiographic localization and embolization. Arch Otolaryngol Head Neck Surg 1990;116(6):697–9.

31. Terada T, Kinoshita Y, Yokote H, et al. Preoperative embolization of meningiomas fed by ophthalmic branch arteries. Surg Neurol 1996;45(2):161–6.

New and Advanced Magnetic Resonance Imaging Diagnostic Imaging Techniques in the Evaluation of Cranial Nerves and the Skull Base

Philip Touska, MBBS, FRCR[a],*, Steve E.J. Connor, MRCP, FRCR[a,b,c]

KEYWORDS

- Skull base • Cranial nerves • Magnetic resonance imaging • Diffusion-weighted imaging (DWI)
- Diffusion tensor imaging (DTI) • MR neurography
- Dynamic contrast enhancement (DCE) MR imaging

KEY POINTS

- Developments in three-dimensional T2-weighted and postgadolinium T1-weighted sequences have improved the imaging of cranial nerves in their cisternal and foraminal portions.
- Diffusion tensor tractography can be used to delineate cranial nerves not visible on conventional sequences, such as those displaced by tumors, and diffusion tensor imaging can be used to derive functional metrics.
- A variety of magnetic resonance (MR) neurography techniques have been developed that use vascular and fat suppression techniques (such as diffusion weighting, motion-sensitized driven equilibrium and selective water excitation) to facilitate visualization of the extracranial portions of the cranial nerves.
- Diffusion-weighted imaging and dynamic contrast-enhanced MR imaging have been evaluated for their contribution to differential diagnosis, prognostication, and posttreatment follow-up of skull base lesions.

INTRODUCTION

Magnetic resonance (MR) imaging evaluation of the skull base and its traversing cranial nerves is one of the most technically challenging areas of head and neck imaging. It requires strategies that not only mitigate deleterious artifacts such as magnetic susceptibility created by air-bone interfaces but also provide excellent spatial and contrast resolution. Over the last 2 decades, considerable efforts have been made to address these challenges, aided by the widespread adoption of high field MR imaging systems, improvements in coil design, parallel imaging, three-dimensional (3D) techniques, and more efficient k-space sampling strategies. As a result, an increasing number of advanced techniques for cranial nerve and skull base imaging are

[a] Department of Radiology, Guy's and St. Thomas' NHS Foundation Trust, London, UK; [b] Department of Neuroradiology, Kings College Hospital NHS Trust, Denmark Hill, London SE5 9RS, UK; [c] School of Biomedical Engineering & Imaging Sciences Rayne Institute, 4th Floor, Lambeth Wing Street, Thomas' Hospital Westminster Bridge Road, London SE1 7EH, UK
* Corresponding author. Department of Radiology, Guy's Hospital, 2nd Floor Tower Wing, Great Maze Pond, London SE1 9RT, UK.
E-mail address: p.touska@nhs.net

Neuroimag Clin N Am 31 (2021) 665–684
https://doi.org/10.1016/j.nic.2021.06.006
1052-5149/21/© 2021 Elsevier Inc. All rights reserved.

beginning to enter clinical practice and are the focus of this article.

CRANIAL NERVE IMAGING

Cranial nerves may be conceptually divided into segments (nuclear, fascicular, cisternal, intradural, foraminal, and extraforaminal).[1,2] Sequences and MR imaging protocols are typically tailored to the cranial nerve segments being examined, as a result of the significant differences in anatomic microenvironments encountered along the courses of the nerves.

Nuclear and Fascicular Segments

The parenchyma of the brainstem is typically evaluated using a combination of conventional turbo spin-echo (TSE), fluid-attenuated inversion recovery (FLAIR), and diffusion-weighted imaging (DWI) sequences.[3] Gradient echo sequences that acquire multiple echoes during a single repetition time (TR) increase both the signal to noise ratio (SNR) and contrast to noise ratio (CNR). Therefore, sequences such as multiecho data image combination (MERGE) (GE Healthcare), multiecho data image combination (Siemens), and multiecho fast field gradient echo (mFFE) (Philips) can aid imaging of brainstem nuclei and the paths of the fascicular segments of the cranial nerves.[4,5]

Cisternal Segment

Cisternographic sequences

The abundance of cerebrospinal fluid (CSF) surrounding the cisternal portions of cranial nerves enables excellent delineation on heavily T2-weighted (cisternographic) sequences. Two principal approaches may be used, using either fast gradient echo or fast spin-echo (FSE) techniques (Box 1).

Diffusion tensor imaging and diffusion tensor tractography

Although cisternographic sequences are extremely useful for routine imaging protocols, they provide limited depiction of cranial nerves when they are effaced by large tumors. Diffusion tensor imaging (DTI) offers a means of addressing these limitations and can also provide functional information.

Principles and metrics The diffusion of water molecules within highly organized tissues, such as the cranial nerves, is anisotropic, with the orientation of maximal diffusion (diffusion tensor) occurring parallel to the axes of neuronal bundles.[10,11] Data obtained using DTI can not only be used to provide qualitative directionally encoded color

---

Box 1
Cisternographic techniques

FSE

- Involve variations of balanced steady-state free precession and provide high SNR.
- Although banding artifacts secondary to field inhomogeneities and magnetic susceptibility can be problematic, these are reduced by frequency phase alterations, such as in constructive interference into steady state (Siemens) or fast imaging using steady-state acquisition with phase cycling (GE).[6]

Fast gradient echo

- Three-dimensional FSE techniques typically use short non–spatially selective radiofrequency pulses (significantly shortening echo spacing) and variable flip angles for the refocusing radiofrequency pulses.[7]
- Examples include sampling perfection with application-optimized contrasts by using different flip angle evolutions (SPACE [**sampling perfection** with application optimized contrasts using different flip angle evolutions]) (Siemens), CUBE (GE) and volume isotropic turbo spin-echo acquisition (Philips).
- These sequences are resistant to susceptibility, flow, and chemical shift artifacts with low levels of blurring; furthermore, differing contrast properties are provided by altering the effective echo time and flip angle.[8,9]

---

maps but also yield quantitative metrics. Among the most commonly encountered metrics are fractional anisotropy (FA), which is a measure of the orientation dependence of diffusion, and mean diffusivity (MD), which is a measure of overall diffusion.[11] Reductions in MD and FA are thought to correlate with abnormalities such as axonal loss, impaired myelination, and abnormal fiber organization.[11]

Diffusion tensor tractography (DTT) is an extension of DTI whereby algorithms are used to infer connections between voxels based on diffusion vectors, and can be used to produce 3D images of neuronal structures.[11]

Practicalities In order to obtain 3D DTT images that can be used for clinical applications, several steps need to be undertaken, which has been termed the tractography pipeline.[12] Examples of the principal steps involved, based on the authors' institutional experience, are summarized in **Table 1**.

Table 1
Steps involved in diffusion tensor tractography

	Example Parameters	Comments
Step 1: Acquisition	Field strength: 3 T	DTT can be undertaken at 1.5 T but angular resolution is limited
	Sequence: RESOLVE (with acceleration techniques such as multislice excitation, if available)	Although ss-EPI is rapid and widely available sequence, it suffers from off-resonance effects along the phase-encoding direction
		These can be addressed by readout-segmented EPI, although at the expense of longer acquisition times.[13] More recently, sequences using >1 b value (multishell) and multislice excitation (multiband) techniques in combination with probabilistic tractography have proved superior to single-shell techniques, owing to reduced partial volume effects and improved visualization of fibers with high angular curvature[14]
	Number of gradient directions: 64	A minimum of 32 directions has been proposed for cranial nerve DTT, with acquisition of >50 directions, known as high angular resolution diffusion imaging, improving discrimination of multiple fiber orientations within the same voxel[12,15]
	Voxel size: 1.5–2 mm (isotropic)	Smaller voxel sizes are limited by low SNR, increased scanning times, or reduced field of view
Step 2: Distortion Correction	Geometric distortion correction	Additional phase-encoding acquisitions of opposite polarities (anteroposterior and posteroanterior) allow the degree of susceptibility-induced off-resonance field effects to be estimated and corrected[16]
	Eddy current distortion correction	Rapid gradient switching leads to off-resonance distortion caused by eddy current formation within the machine bore; software correction is performed retrospectively[16]
Step 3: ROI	Primary sequence for anatomic coregistration and ROI placement: 3D T2 CISS/SPACE	Tracts are typically propagated by manually defining a seed point ROI with or without additional ROI used as "include" or "exclude" regions. For cranial nerves, ROI may be placed at cranial nerve REZ, brainstem nuclei, or in multiple locations along the expected

(continued on next page)

Table 1
(continued)

	Example Parameters	Comments
		anatomic courses of nerves (eg, REZ and foramen for the CN VII–VIII complex)[12,17]
Step 4: Fiber tracking	Algorithm: probabilistic fiber tracking using constrained spherical deconvolution	Probabilistic techniques that account for multiple fiber orientations in a single voxel have been shown to provide superior fiber tracking compared with standard deterministic techniques (which only propagate fiber tracts in line with the dominant vectors of adjacent voxels) when applied to cranial nerve DTT[18,19]
	Software package: MRtrix 3.0[20]	Various DTT software packages are available and can be chosen depending on the type of algorithm used (eg, deterministic DTT using 3DSlicer www.slicer.org/)
	Additional variables: number of seeds and streamlines, FA threshold, step size, curvature threshold, and fiber length	There are various parameters to fiber tracking that may be specified and will alter the number of true and spurious streamlines generated; in the authors' experience, optimal thresholds, for FA and curvature in particular, can differ between patients

Abbreviations: CISS, constructive interference into steady state; CN VII–VIII, facial and vestibulocochlear cranial nerve complex; FA, fractional anisotropy; RESOLVE, readout segmentation of long variable echo trains (Siemens); REZ, root-entry zone; ROI, regions of interest; ss-EPI, single-shot echoplanar imaging

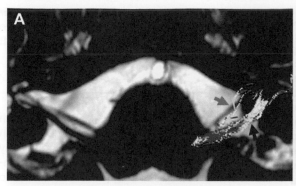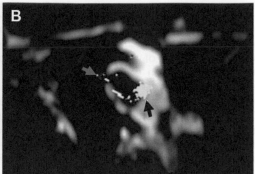

Fig. 1. Example of DTT in vestibular schwannoma. DTT data coregistered with a 3D constructive interference into steady state (CISS) sequence in a patient with a small left-sided vestibular schwannoma centered on the porus acusticus. Tractography streamlines generated using MRtrix 3.0 and a probabilistic algorithm (CSD). (*A*) Coregistered axial image shows streamlines extending anteriorly along the line of the facial nerve (*gray arrow*) and posteriorly in the line of the vestibulocochlear nerve (*black arrow*) around the left-sided schwannoma. (*B*) Coregistered oblique sagittal sequence through the left internal auditory meatus shows displaced bundles of streamlines, which cluster anterosuperior to (*gray arrow*) and posterolateral to (*black arrow*) the left-sided vestibular schwannoma (in the approximate trajectories of the facial and vestibulocochlear nerves, respectively).

Applications

Trigeminal nerve DTI of the trigeminal nerve has been predominantly directed toward the evaluation of trigeminal neuralgia (TN). There is agreement among most studies that a reduction in FA at the root-entry zone (REZ) is associated with the symptomatic side and it is suggested that this correlates with pathologic microstructural change within the nerve.[21,22] Approximately 80% of studies included in a recent systematic review found lower REZ FA levels in patients with TN secondary to neurovascular compression; furthermore, patients with lower FA values tended to show a positive response to decompressive therapy.[10] However, lower FA values can be seen in other causes of TN, including multiple sclerosis, and precise correlation between quantitative DTI metrics and histopathology remains to be elucidated.[23]

Facial and vestibulocochlear nerves Almost all studies pertaining to cranial nerve tractography address the facial-vestibulocochlear nerve complex in the context of posterior fossa tumors (**Fig. 1**), because of the debilitating consequences of inadvertent facial nerve injury during extirpation (preservation of facial nerve function is possible in only 70%–80% of vestibular schwannomas [VSs] larger than 3 cm).[24] Although a priori visualization of the facial component of the facial-vestibulocochlear nerve complex is usually impossible using conventional anatomic MR imaging sequences, because of mass effect and anatomic distortion, tractography has proved to be a promising alternative. A systematic review of tractography for preoperative nerve localization in VS found an overall rate of concordance between tractographic and surgical findings

of 87.1%, with discordance in 7.6% and failure of tract generation of 3.4%.[25] However, a more recent review found the range of accuracy for cranial nerve fiber tractography to be highly variable (30%–100%).[10]

Limitations and future directions Real-world application of DTI and DTT for cranial nerve imaging depends on a multitude of factors (see **Table 1**). As a result, awareness of its limitations is required; for example, small-caliber structures, such as the abducens, trochlear, and lower cranial nerve rootlets, may be invisible because of partial volume effects caused by CSF pulsation.[12,26] Furthermore, reductions in voxel size and increases in the number of diffusion directions are limited by reductions in SNR, increased eddy current generation, and bulk motion (caused by scanning time). Variations can also be introduced by region of interest (ROI) placement (reliant on accurate coregistration and a priori knowledge of cranial nerve anatomy) and numerical thresholds (such as FA and curvature; see **Box 1**). FA thresholds can be varied in a systematic manner, but the process is time consuming.[27] It is therefore possible that whole-brainstem DTT techniques will prove useful in future as they obviate manual ROI placement.[28] An optimal tractography algorithm has also yet to be defined, and, although probabilistic techniques may be superior (see **Table 1**), advanced deterministic techniques have shown promise.[29] Although significant challenges remain, increased use of compressed-sensing techniques as well as artificial intelligence (AI)–driven automation are likely to facilitate the future integration of cranial nerve tractography clinical imaging workflows.[10,30]

Foraminal Segment

Imaging of neural structures passing through cranial foramina is often technically challenging owing to the juxtaposition of vascular and osseous structures. The detection of individual cranial nerves within foramina with a large venous compartment, such as the jugular foramen, cavernous sinus, or Dorellos canal, can be achieved through the visualization of nonenhancing nerves contrasted against the enhancing blood. So-called white blood 3D T1-weighted postgadolinium gradient echo techniques, such as volumetric interpolated brain examination magnetization-prepared rapid gradient echo (MP-RAGE), or contrast-enhanced steady-state imaging, such as constructive interference into steady state (CISS), have proved useful. Enhancing cranial nerve lesions may be better depicted by using high-resolution black-blood 3D spin-echo postcontrast sequences that use flow-suppression techniques, such as delay alternating with nutation for tailored excitation (DANTE), and improved motion-sensitized driven equilibrium (MSDE).[5]

The intratemporal facial nerve has a long and complex intraosseous segment and additional sequences may be used to enhance the contrast between the nerve and the bone. Recently, a noncontrast technique known on Siemens systems as pointwise encoding time reduction with radial acquisition (PETRA) has been developed. It uses a near-zero echo time (TE) of less than 1 millisecond to obtain signal from tissues with extremely short T2, such as cortical bone; furthermore, the ultrashort TE minimizes susceptibility artifacts.[31,32] It has been shown to enable visualization of the entire course of the intrapetrous facial nerve, which is not normally possible on conventional sequences (Fig. 2).[31] Similarly black bone MR imaging uses a proton density–weighted spoiled gradient echo volumetric sequence that is optimized for delineating the

bone–soft tissue interfaces by using a short TE/TR and low flip angle, and is optimized to minimize soft tissue contrast, thereby enhancing bone–soft tissue boundaries.[33]

Extraforaminal segment

Magnetic resonance neurography

The term MR neurography (MRN) has been applied to various sequences, including DTI (which is considered separately), but is more commonly ascribed to a group of sequences that use a combination of fat and flow suppression in order to selectively accentuate the signal from neural structures within the extracranial soft tissues.[34]

Techniques Three principal sequences have shown promise for MRN in the head and neck: 3D reversed fast imaging in steady-state free precession (3D PSIF), 3D double-echo steady state with water excitation (3D DESS WE), and 3D sampling perfection with application-optimized contrasts using different flip angle evolution short-tau inversion recovery (3D SPACE STIR) (Table 2).

Applications of magnetic resonance neurography

MRN uses strategies adapted from neuromuscular applications such as brachial plexus imaging, where neural injury results in endoneurial fluid and increased T2-weighted signal.[44] In the head and neck, MRN has been applied to the definition of normal neural anatomy (Fig. 3), cranial neuropathies, mandibular trauma, and parotid gland lesions (where the relationship with the facial nerve can only ordinarily be estimated using anatomic landmarks on standard sequences) (Table 3).

General limitations of magnetic resonance neurography

Application of MRN in the head and neck is challenging owing to a combination of vascular pulsation and susceptibility artifacts (found at dental and air-bone interfaces). In addition, with respect to the extracranial facial nerve, differentiation of nerve branches from nonfatty salivary gland parenchyma is typically limited using MRN; similarly, all MRN techniques struggle to reliably depict smaller facial nerve branches, which can be problematic when determining the relationship to anteriorly located parotid tumors.[40,41,45]

Diffusion tensor imaging and diffusion tensor tractography Although limited to a few small case series, DTI and DTT have been applied to the extracranial portions of certain cranial nerves. In particular, the mandibular nerves (using a readout-segmented echoplanar imaging [EPI] sequence)[13] and intraparotid facial nerves in

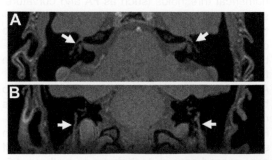

Fig. 2. PETRA ultrashort-TE sequence. Axial (*A*) and coronal (*B*) reconstructions from a PETRA sequence obtained through the temporal bones showing the intrapetrous course of the facial nerve (*white arrows*).

Table 2
Magnetic resonance neurography techniques

Sequence	How It Works	Benefits and Drawbacks
3D PSIF	Involves establishment of a coherent steady state (SSFP) with fat suppression (using selective water excitation) and a small diffusion moment (b = >20–50 sec/mm²)[35,36]	Aided by the use of a diffusion moment, 3D PSIF provides effective suppression of signal from adjacent vessels; furthermore, the selective water excitation provides reliable fat suppression and the sequence is relatively resistant to field inhomogeneities.[34,36–38] However, although this technique provides a good CNR, its SNR is limited because the echo formed by the pulse sequence is not derived from a spin echo but is formed by a weaker Hahn echo; furthermore, it is sensitive to motion artifacts and susceptibility effects[34,37,39]
3D DESS WE	Like 3D PSIF, this sequence is based on SSFP and achieves fat suppression by selective water excitation; however, in addition to the PSIF echo, a free induction decay gradient echo is also acquired[40,41]	Compared with 3D PSIF, it can produce a higher SNR because it involves the sampling of 2 echoes during each TR (from both free induction decay and a radiofrequency echo).[40] Furthermore, flip angle variation can aid discrimination between the facial nerve and T2-weighted hyperintense fluid-containing structures such as the parotid ducts.[40] However, the long scan time may lead to motion artifacts, and wrap artifacts can be problematic when attempting to image parts of the intraparotid facial nerve, which lie at the periphery of the field of view[40]
3D SPACE STIR	Based on an FSE pulse sequence and is highly versatile; STIR is used to provide fat suppression. Contrast enhancement may be applied to aid suppression of background signal from vessels, muscle, and salivary gland parenchyma, via a T2 relaxation shortening effect[42]	Although 3D SPACE STIR provides reliable and homogeneous fat suppression and is widely used in brachial plexus imaging, its use in cranial nerve imaging is challenging, particularly because of signal from intravascular flow. However, improvements to vascular suppression may be achieved using advanced techniques. In particular, a technique termed 3D CRANI has been developed with a pseudo–steady-state sweep in conjunction with an MSDE pulse to provide more uniform suppression of signal from fat, muscle, and blood. However, sparse sampling of k-space data (compressed sensing) is required to achieve clinically acceptable scanning times[43]

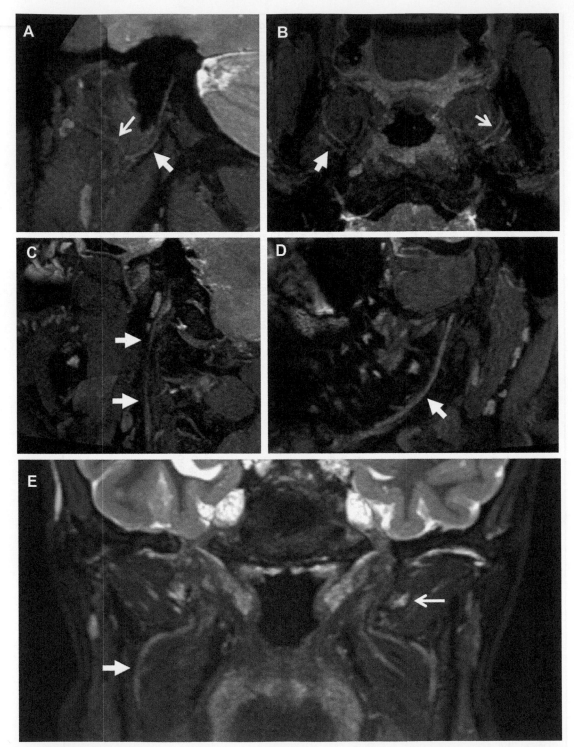

Fig. 3. Examples of anatomic visualization using MRN techniques. (*A–D*) Images obtained using a 3D DESS WE sequence. (*A*) Oblique sagittal reconstruction through the right parotid gland showing the main trunk (*solid arrow*) and temporofacial branch (*thin arrow*) of the intraparotid facial nerve. (*B*) Axial reconstruction at the level of the medial pterygoid muscles showing branching of the mandibular division of the trigeminal nerve, with the inferior alveolar (*solid arrow*) and lingual (*thin arrow*) nerves clearly shown. (*C*) Oblique sagittal reconstruction showing the right vagus nerve. (*D*) Oblique sagittal reconstruction through the right hemimandible showing the inferior alveolar nerve (*arrow*). (*E*) Image obtained from a 3D SPACE STIR sequence clearly showing the right inferior alveolar nerve (*solid arrow*), but artifact from flow within small venous structures is evident (*thin arrow*).

Table 3
Parameters and applications of magnetic resonance neurography techniques

Sequence	Parameters	Applications
3D PSIF	TR/TE: 9.3/4.2 ms FOV: 220 × 220 mm Flip angle: 35° Matrix size: 256 × 256 Spatial resolution: 0.6 mm isotropic Diffusion moment: 40 mT/m(*)msec Approximate acquisition time: 7 min IV contrast: none System: Siemens 3T Source: adapted from Chu et al.[45]	Anatomy: • The intracranial and larger extracranial portions of CN II–XII have been satisfactorily visualized in normal volunteers[37] • The intraparotid CN VII (main trunk and primary divisions) were well depicted in a small case series; delineation was further improved using microsurface coils (particularly for the secondary branches)[45] Cranial neuropathies: • Small case series of patients with clinically suspected neuropathies of the inferior alveolar and lingual nerves found moderate to excellent correlation between MRN and intraoperative findings, with neuromata and transections correctly identified in all cases[39] • Small case series of patients with migraine thought to be secondary to greater occipital neuropathy found significantly increased signal and diameter of the greater occipital nerves on the symptomatic sides[35] Parotid disorder: • The intraparotid CN VII and parotid duct were visualized in most a small case series of patients with parotid disease, including Sjögren syndrome and parotid neoplasia[38]
3D DESS WE	TR/TE: 11/4.21 ms FOV: 200 × 200 mm Flip angle: 30° Matrix size: 384 × 244 Effective slice thickness = 0.82 mm GRAPPA factor: 3 Approximate acquisition time: 4 min IV contrast: none System: Siemens 3T Source: adapted from Fujii et al.[41]	Anatomy: • The intraparotid CN VII has been depicted, showing the main trunks, cervicofacial divisions, and temporofacial divisions in 100%, 94.4%, and 55.6% of patients respectively[40] • Branches of the mandibular division of CN V were shown, including excellent depiction of the lingual and inferior alveolar nerves, although evaluation of the buccal and masseteric nerves was limited by susceptibility effects[46] Parotid neoplasms: • MRN was superior (in terms of accuracy, sensitivity, and negative predictive value) to indirect methods using standard sequences when localizing deep lobe of parotid gland tumors[41]

(continued on next page)

Table 3
(continued)

Sequence	Parameters	Applications
		Trauma: • MRN (in combination with 3D STIR and T1 fast field echo) provides a comprehensive assessment of mandibular trauma to assess for inferior alveolar nerve injury, beyond what can be achieved using radiography or computed tomography alone[47]
Black-blood 3D SPACE STIR (3D CRANI)	TR/TE: 2300/150 ms FOV: 200 × 200 × 100 mm Matrix size: 224 × 222 Acquired voxel size: 0.9 mm (isotropic) Compressed sense factor: 5 Black-blood pulse: MSDE Approximate acquisition time: 5 min IV contrast: none System: Philips 3T Source: Van der Cruyssen et al.[43]	Anatomy: • The 3D CRANI sequence showed good to excellent visualization of the extraforaminal trigeminal, greater occipital, and facial nerves in healthy volunteers[43] • A contrast-enhanced 3D SPACE STIR sequence was also able to show excellent selective cranial nerve delineation (including of the intraparotid facial nerve), while suppressing the background signal from vessels, muscle, and parotid parenchyma in healthy volunteers, albeit with a scan time of ~ 14 min[42]

Abbreviations: CN, cranial nerve; FOV, field of view; GRAPPA, generalized autocalibrating partially parallel acquisitions; IV, intravenous.

Table 4
Diffusion-weighted imaging techniques used at the skull base

Technique	Comments (Including Benefits and Drawbacks)
ss-EPI	• Commonest DWI technique • Benefits: rapid (insensitive to motion) and high SNR • Drawbacks: highly sensitive to susceptibility effects encountered at air-bone interfaces, which can cause geometric disrtion and signal dropout at the skull base (particularly problematic for cholesteatoma imaging leading to false-positive and false-negative results)[51,52]
Non-EPI ss-TSE	• Typically accelerated by a half-Fourier transform acquisition in order to shorten the echo train • Benefits: markedly improved resistance to susceptibility-related distortions; superior to ss-EPI for detection of cholesteatoma[52,53] • Drawbacks: lower resolution and SNR[51]
ms-EPI	• Multiple echo trains; often further improved using techniques that reduce sensitivity to motion as well as improving SNR and CNR via oversampling of the center of k-space, either through readout-segmented EPI (eg, RESOLVE on Siemens systems) or radial acquisitions (eg, PROPELLER on GE systems or BLADE on Siemens systems)[51,54,55] • Benefits: reduced susceptibility to artifacts while maintaining resolution; superior to ss-EPI for cholesteatoma detection[52,53] • Drawbacks: longer sequence (more prone to bulk motion artifacts)[51] • Note: ms-EPI (RESOLVE) has been compared with non-EPI (HASTE ss-TSE) in the detection of primary and postoperative cholesteatoma, finding similar positive predictive values for both techniques, but a slightly lower negative predictive value for ms-EPI[56]

Abbreviations: ms-EPI, multishot-EPI; PROPELLER, periodically rotated overlapping Parallel lines with enhanced reconstruction; ss-TSE, single-shot TSE.

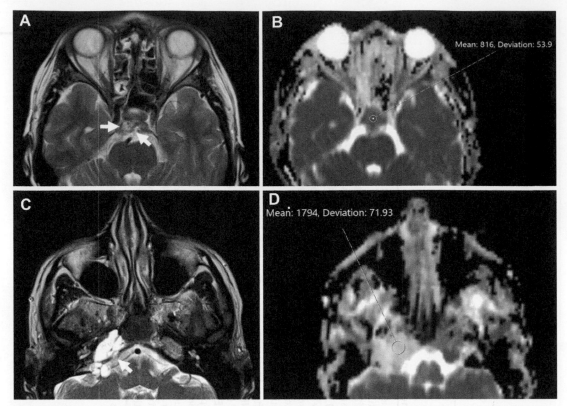

Fig. 4. Applications of DWI at the skull base. Axial T2 sequence (*A*) and ADC map (*B*) through the skull base in a patient with a chordoma (*white arrows*) with an ROI placed on the tumor on the ADC map. Axial T2 sequence (*C*) and ADC map (*D*) through the skull base in a patient with chondrosarcoma (*white arrow*) with an ROI placed on the tumor; note the considerably higher ADC values compared with the chordoma.

patients with parotid lesions (outperforming an anatomic balanced fast field echo technique).[48] Functional metrics applied to DTT of the extracranial facial nerves have shown promise (FA being reduced where there is contact with parotid tumors and average pathlength being increased in nerves affected by perineural tumor spread).[49]

SKULL BASE IMAGING
Diffusion-weighted Imaging

DWI is based on the relative freedom of movement of extracellular water within tissue, which is affected by microstructural differences at a voxel level.[11] Furthermore, diffusivity may be quantitively assessed by drawing an ROI on an apparent diffusion coefficient (ADC) map.[50] DWI techniques used at the skull base (along with their benefits and drawbacks) are considered in **Table 4**.

Clinical utility

DWI has a wide range of utilities at the skull base, not only for diagnosis but also for prognostication and posttreatment follow-up.[50] For example, it may aid differentiation between chordoma and chondrosarcoma as well as predict aggressiveness and dedifferentiation in chordoma

(**Fig. 4**).[57–59] Additional details and examples are provided in (**Table 5**).

Limitations

Aside from technical factors at the skull base (including susceptibility effects that can affect qualitative imaging), note that, although ADC values and cutoffs may be helpful, they are influenced by the MR imaging system, sequence parameters, and analysis methods, which limits their wider application.[69]

Perfusion and Permeability Imaging

Neoangiogenesis typically accompanies tumor development, which leads to alterations in vascular dynamics that can be detected and interrogated using a variety of dynamic MR imaging techniques, enabling the derivation of diagnostic or prognostic biomarkers.[70,71]

Techniques

Two techniques have proved useful in head and neck and skull base imaging: dynamic contrast-enhanced (DCE) MR imaging and arterial spin labeling (ASL).

Table 5
Clinical utility of diffusion-weighted imaging

Diagnosis and Differential Diagnosis	**Benign calvarial lesions**
	• Lesions such as hemangiomas and fibrous dysplasia tend to have high ADC values or lesion/white matter ADC ratios, but others, such as intradiploic dermoid and epidermoid cysts, can show variable diffusivity, and Langerhans cell histiocytosis typically shows restricted diffusion[50]
	Cholesteatoma
	• Non-EPI DWI accurately detects residual and recurrent cholesteatoma following canal wall down mastoidectomy, aided by T1-weighted sequences to increase specificity[60,61]
	Chordoma and chondrosarcoma
	• Although conventional MRI sequences can be limited, a significantly higher ADC value has been observed in chondrosarcomas compared with chordomas, with Welzel et al.[57] proposing a cutoff value of $1.585 \times 10^{(-3)}$ mm^2/s.[57,58]
	• Although ADC values do not aid differentiation between classic and chondroid chordoma subtypes, they are helpful in differentiating these from aggressive dedifferentiated forms (characterized by lower ADC values)[59,62]
	NOE and skull base osteomyelitis
	• Lower ADC values have been found in patients with NOE where skull base osteomyelitis had developed[63]
	• Higher ADC values are seen in skull base osteomyelitis compared with tumors that can invade the skull base (such as lymphoma or nasopharyngeal carcinoma); however, ADC values in skull base osteomyelitis are not significantly different from skull base metastases[64]
	Lymphoma and nasopharyngeal carcinoma
	• Lower ADC values (0.51–0.59×10–3 mm^2/s) are observed in skull base lymphoma compared with nasopharyngeal carcinoma
Prognostication	**Skull base invasion**
	• Lower ADC values are observed in the portions of head and neck tumors involving the skull base found to have dural and osseous invasion[65]
	Meningioma
	• Lower ADC values and ADC ratios have been found in skull base meningiomas that show early progression or recurrence[66]

	VS • Midrange ADC values correlated with lower postoperative House-Brackmann score, but ADC values have not been found to correlate with treatment response or progression in VSs treated with Gamma Knife radiosurgery[67,68]
Posttreatment Evaluation	**Chordoma** • ADC values have also been shown to be helpful in detecting and delineating residual chordoma following treatment; furthermore, lower ADC values (proposed cutoff ADC value of $1.494 \times 10 -3 \times mm^2/s$) have been associated with tumor progression[59,62]

Abbreviation: NOE, necrotising otitis externa.

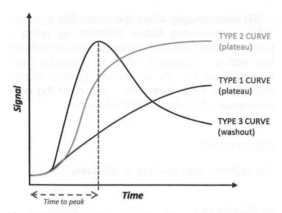

Fig. 5. Time-signal curves. Graphic examples of the 3 principal types of time-signal curve, which can be used to qualitatively assess DCE MR imaging data.

Dynamic contrast-enhanced magnetic resonance imaging

This technique makes use of rapid two-dimensional or 3D T1-weighted sequences (eg, FSE, fast imaging with steady-state free precession (FISP), variable flip angle spoiled gradient recalled echo, and turbo fast field echo) to initially perform T1 tissue mapping and then to follow a Gd-based contrast bolus within a defined volume of tissue over time.[70–72] Imaging at a high temporal resolution (2–4 seconds) provides a dataset that can be postprocessed to yield a variety of qualitative, semiquantitative, and quantitative metrics.[70]

Qualitative and semiquantitative Data from tissue enhancement can be displayed in the form of time-signal curves, with refinements performed by user-defined ROI placement on tumor or normal tissue.

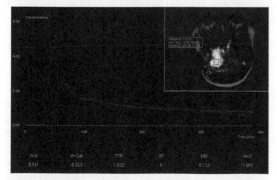

Fig. 6. Qualitative assessment of DCE MR imaging in skull base PGL. Example of a time-signal curve and semiquantitative parameters obtained using DCE MR imaging in a patient with a residual right-sided skull base paraganglioma with intracranial extension (axial image with ROI placed on the enhancing tumor is inset at the top right of the image).

Time-signal curves may be viewed qualitatively and given a type according to shape and washout characteristics (**Fig. 5**).[73] From these curves, further semiquantitative metrics can be obtained. These metrics include wash-in and washout velocities, peak enhancement, time to maximum enhancement, and area under the curve.[71]

Quantitative

Derivation of quantitative metrics from DCE MR imaging data requires more complex postprocessing and typically relies on the Tofts model (or variations thereof), which assumes the presence of 2 compartments: a vascular space and an extravascular extracellular space (ESS).[74] Using ROIs placed on a large vessel within the volume as well as within the target lesion, alterations in Gd-related signal change can be used to compute aspects of intralesional perfusion and permeability. Metrics such as the volume transfer constant between the vascular space and ESS (K^{trans}), the flux rate constant between ESS and the vascular space (K_{ep}), as well as the fractional volumes Gd in the ESS (V_e) or plasma (V_p) are among the most frequently encountered.[70,74]

Arterial spin labeling

ASL is a technique capable of measuring perfusion and is based on measuring Gd-related dephasing on T2 or T2*-weighted sequences.[71] ASL offers the significant advantage of not requiring an exogenous contrast medium; instead, it involves the application of continuous, pulsed, or pseudocontinuous radiofrequency inversion pulses to magnetically label water within a volume of blood below the area of interest; the signal from the labeled blood can then be measured as it passes through the target area.[71,72]

Clinical applications

Diagnosis and differential diagnosis Paragangliomas (PGLs) and nerve sheath tumors may be encountered at similar locations (eg, jugular foramen) and, although they can often be distinguished on conventional sequences, differentiation may be challenging. In such scenarios, qualitative and semiquantitative DCE MR imaging metrics may be helpful, because PGLs yield a significantly shorter time to maximum enhancement as well as a higher peak enhancement compared with schwannomas.[76] Furthermore, a type 3 time-intensity curve (characterized by a rapid increase in enhancement followed by significant washout) is seen in PGL (**Fig. 6**).[77] With respect to quantitative metrics, PGLs typically show low K^{trans}, K_{ep}, V_p, and V_e because of vascular shunting.[76]

Pseudocontinuous ASL can be helpful in differentiating nonhypervascular tumors (such as meningiomas from schwannomas) from hypervascular tumors (such as PGL from meningiomas or metastases) by measuring and comparing the total blood flow, which can be normalized to healthy cerebellar parenchyma.[75] The technique has also been found to be helpful in detecting skull base metastases owing to increased conspicuity.[78]

Prognostication Quantitative DCE MR imaging parameters have garnered significant interest in the setting of head and neck cancer where lower K^{trans} levels have been associated with reduced permeability and hypoxia, which can impair the effectiveness of chemoradiotherapy, leading to unfavorable outcomes.[70,71] Use at the skull base has been limited, but it has been used to aid preoperative characterization of meningiomas, with some correlation between increased V_e and K^{trans} parameters and the time to progression as well as a lower V_p and higher Ki-67 scores.[79] Similarly, ASL has been found to aid prediction of higher-grade meningiomas, which are characterized by lower hyperperfusion metrics.[80] In addition, features of hyperperfusion on ASL can be used to confirm the presence of a hypervascular VS, which, although rarely encountered, represents a neurosurgical challenge.[81]

Multiparametric Imaging

Multiparametric imaging uses techniques such as convolutional neural networks, artificial intelligence, and texture analysis to identify radiomic signatures from MR imaging data that might reflect otherwise imperceptible microstructural changes.[82] Although it remains operator dependent and has yet to find a defined role in skull base imaging, it has been used to help differentiate chordoma from chondrosarcoma (with the latter showing features of greater tissue complexity)[83] as well as to identify meningiomas likely to undergo progression or recurrence.[82]

Magnetic Resonance Spectroscopy and Elastography

MR spectroscopy is capable of noninvasive detection of a range of metabolites (such as myoinositol, choline creatine, lactate, and amino acids such as alanine).[84] It is typically used to interrogate brain tissue, but has been used in a case series of cerebellopontine angle (CPA) cistern masses, finding that a myoinositol peak was common to schwannomas, whereas a delayed alanine peak occurred in most meningiomas.[85]

MR elastography offers the possibility of noninvasively assessing tissue stiffness by using a phase contrast MR imaging sequence in combination with a mechanical driver to generate sheer waves. Thus far, the technique remains experimental, but it has been used to predict the ease of removal of pituitary and CPA tumors.[86,87]

DISCLOSURE

The authors have nothing to disclose.

REFERENCES

1. Blitz AM, Aygun N, Herzka DA, et al. High Resolution Three-Dimensional MR Imaging of the Skull Base: Compartments, Boundaries, and Critical Structures. Radiol Clin North Am 2017;55(1):17–30.
2. Gandhi MR, Panizza B, Kennedy D. Detecting and defining the anatomic extent of large nerve perineural spread of malignancy: Comparing "targeted" MRI with the histologic findings following surgery. Head Neck 2011;33(4):469–75.
3. Kitajima M, Hirai T, Shigematsu Y, et al. Comparison of 3D FLAIR, 2D FLAIR, and 2D T2- weighted MR imaging of brain stem anatomy. AJNR Am J Neuroradiol 2012;33(5):922–7.
4. Martin N, Malfair D, Zhao Y, et al. Comparison of MERGE and Axial T2-Weighted Fast Spin-Echo Sequences for Detection of Multiple Sclerosis Lesions in the Cervical Spinal Cord. AJR Am J Roentgenol 2012;199(1):157–62.
5. Krainik A, Casselman JW. Imaging evaluation of patients with cranial nerve disorders. Springer; 2020. p. 143–61.
6. Touska P, Connor SEJ. Recent advances in MRI of the head and neck, skull base and cranial nerves: New and evolving sequences, analyses and clinical applications. Br J Radiol 2019;92(1104):20190513.
7. Mugler JP. Optimized three-dimensional fast-spin-echo MRI. J Magn Reson Imaging 2014;39(4):745–67.
8. Naganawa S, Koshikawa T, Fukatsu H, et al. MR Cisternography of the Cerebellopontine Angle: Comparison of Three-dimensional Fast Asymmetrical Spin-echo and Three-dimensional Constructive Interference in the Steady-state Sequences. AJNR Am J Neuroradiol 2001;22(6):1179–85.
9. Kojima S, Suzuki K, Hirata M, et al. Depicting the semicircular canals with inner-ear MRI: A comparison of the SPACE and TrueFISP sequences. J Magn Reson Imaging 2013;37(3):652–9.
10. Shapey J, Vos SB, Vercauteren T, et al. Clinical applications for diffusion MRI and tractography of cranial nerves within the posterior fossa: A systematic review. Front Neurosci 2019;13(Feb):23.

11. Winston GP. The physical and biological basis of quantitative parameters derived from diffusion MRI. Quant Imaging Med Surg 2012;2(4):254–65.

12. Jacquesson T, Frindel C, Kocevar G, et al. Overcoming Challenges of Cranial Nerve Tractography: A Targeted Review. Clin Neurosurg 2019;84(2): 313–25.

13. Manoliu A, Ho M, Piccirelli M, et al. Simultaneous multislice readout-segmented echo planar imaging for accelerated diffusion tensor imaging of the mandibular nerve: A feasibility study. J Magn Reson Imaging 2017;46(3):663–77.

14. Castellaro M, Moretto M, Baro V, et al. Multishell Diffusion MRI-Based Tractography of the Facial Nerve in Vestibular Schwannoma. AJNR Am J Neuroradiol 2020;41(8):1480–6.

15. Berman JI, Lanza MR, Blaskey L, et al. High angular resolution diffusion imaging probabilistic tractography of the auditory radiation. AJNR Am J Neuroradiol 2013;34(8):1573–8.

16. Andersson JLR, Sotiropoulos SN. An integrated approach to correction for off-resonance effects and subject movement in diffusion MR imaging. Neuroimage 2016;125:1063–78.

17. Yoshino M, Kin T, Ito A, et al. Combined use of diffusion tensor tractography and multifused contrast-enhanced FIESTA for predicting facial and cochlear nerve positions in relation to vestibular schwannoma. J Neurosurg 2015;123(6):1480–8.

18. Zolal A, Sobottka SB, Podlesek D, et al. Comparison of probabilistic and deterministic fiber tracking of cranial nerves. J Neurosurg 2017;127:613–21.

19. Behan B, Chen DQ, Sammartino F, et al. Comparison of Diffusion-Weighted MRI Reconstruction Methods for Visualization of Cranial Nerves in Posterior Fossa Surgery. Front Neurosci 2017;11:554.

20. Tournier JD, Smith R, Raffelt D, et al. MRtrix3: A fast, flexible and open software framework for medical image processing and visualisation. Neuroimage 2019;202:116137.

21. Lutz J, Linn J, Mehrkens JH, et al. Trigeminal neuralgia due to neurovascular compression: High-spatial- resolution diffusion-tensor imaging reveals microstructural neural changes. Radiology 2011; 258(2):524–30.

22. Alper J, Shrivastava RK, Balchandani P. Is There a Magnetic Resonance Imaging-Discernible Cause for Trigeminal Neuralgia? A Structured Review. World Neurosurg 2017;98:89–97.

23. Lummel N, Mehrkens JH, Linn J, et al. Diffusion tensor imaging of the trigeminal nerve in patients with trigeminal neuralgia due to multiple sclerosis. Neuroradiology 2015;57(3):259–67.

24. Betka J, Zvěřina E, Balogová Z, et al. Complications of microsurgery of vestibular schwannoma. Biomed Res Int 2014;2014:315952.

25. Savardekar AR, Patra DP, Thakur JD, et al. Preoperative diffusion tensor imaging-fiber tracking for facial nerve identification in vestibular schwannoma: A systematic review on its evolution and current status with a pooled data analysis of surgical concordance rates. Neurosurg Focus 2018;44(3):E5.

26. Jacquesson T, Cotton F, Attyé A, et al. Probabilistic Tractography to Predict the Position of Cranial Nerves Displaced by Skull Base Tumors: Value for Surgical Strategy Through a Case Series of 62 Patients. Clin Neurosurg 2019;85(1):E125–36.

27. Zhang Y, Mao Z, Wei P, et al. Preoperative Prediction of Location and Shape of Facial Nerve in Patients with Large Vestibular Schwannomas Using Diffusion Tensor Imaging–Based Fiber Tracking. World Neurosurg 2017;99:70–8. Available at: https://www.sciencedirect.com/science/article/pii/ S187887501631258X?via%3Dihub. Accessed May 2, 2018.

28. Jacquesson T, Yeh FC, Panesar S, et al. Full tractography for detecting the position of cranial nerves in preoperative planning for skull base surgery: Technical note. J Neurosurg 2020;132(5):1642–52.

29. Epprecht L, Kozin ED, Piccirelli M, et al. Super-resolution Diffusion Tensor Imaging for Delineating the Facial Nerve in Patients with Vestibular Schwannoma. J Neurol Surg B Skull Base 2019;80(6): 648–54.

30. Kuhnt D, Bauer MHA, Egger J, et al. Fiber tractography based on diffusion tensor imaging compared with high-angular-resolution diffusion imaging with compressed sensing: Initial experience. Neurosurgery 2013;72(SUPPL. 1). Available at: https://www. ncbi.nlm.nih.gov/pmc/articles/PMC3784319/. Accessed December 13, 2020.

31. Guenette JP, Seethamraju RT, Jayender J, et al. MR Imaging of the Facial Nerve through the Temporal Bone at 3T with a Noncontrast Ultrashort Echo Time Sequence. AJNR Am J Neuroradiol 2018; 39(10):1903–6.

32. Lu A, Gorny KR, Ho ML. Zero TE MRI for craniofacial bone imaging. AJNR Am J Neuroradiol 2019;40(9): 1562–6.

33. Connor SEJ, Borri M, Pai I, et al. 'Black Bone' magnetic resonance imaging as a novel technique to aid the pre-operative planning of posterior tympanotomy for cochlear implantation. Cochlear Implants Int 2020. https://doi.org/10.1080/14670100.2020. 1823126.

34. Chhabra A, Zhao L, Carrino JA, et al. MR Neurography: Advances. Radiol Res Pract 2013;2013:1–14.

35. Hwang L, Dessouky R, Xi Y, et al. MR neurography of greater occipital nerve neuropathy: Initial experience in patients with migraine. AJNR Am J Neuroradiol 2017;38(11):2203–9.

36. Chhabra A, Bajaj G, Wadhwa V, et al. MR neurographic evaluation of facial and neck pain: Normal

and abnormal craniospinal nerves below the skull base. Radiographics 2018;38(5):1498–513.

37. Zhang Z, Meng Q, Chen Y, et al. 3-T imaging of the cranial nerves using three-dimensional reversed FISP with diffusion-weighted MR sequence. J Magn Reson Imaging 2008;27(3):454–8.

38. Naganawa S, Ishihara S, Satake H, et al. Simultaneous three-dimensional visualization of the intraparotid facial nerve and parotid duct using a three-dimensional reversed FISP sequence with diffusion weighting. Magn Reson Med Sci 2010; 9(3):153–8.

39. Cox B, Zuniga JR, Panchal N, et al. Magnetic resonance neurography in the management of peripheral trigeminal neuropathy: experience in a tertiary care centre. Eur Radiol 2016;26(10):3392–400.

40. Qin Y, Zhang J, Li P, et al. 3D double-echo steady-state with water excitation MR imaging of the intraparotid facial nerve at 1.5T: A pilot study. AJNR Am J Neuroradiol 2011;32(7):1167–72.

41. Fujii H, Fujita A, Kanazawa H, et al. Localization of parotid gland tumors in relation to the intraparotid facial nerve on 3D double-echo steady-state with water excitation sequence. AJNR Am J Neuroradiol 2019;40(6):1037–42.

42. Wu W, Wu F, Liu D, et al. Visualization of the morphology and pathology of the peripheral branches of the cranial nerves using three-dimensional high-resolution high-contrast magnetic resonance neurography. Eur J Radiol 2020;132. https://doi.org/10.1016/j.ejrad.2020.109137.

43. Van der Cruyssen F, Croonenborghs T-M, Hermans R, et al. 3D Cranial Nerve Imaging, a Novel MR Neurography Technique Using Black-Blood STIR TSE with a Pseudo Steady-State Sweep and Motion-Sensitized Driven Equilibrium Pulse for the Visualization of the Extraforaminal Cranial Nerve Branches. AJNR Am J Neuroradiol 2020. https://doi.org/10.3174/ajnr.A6904.

44. Filler A. Magnetic resonance neurography and diffusion tensor imaging: Origins, history, and clinical impact of the first 50 000 cases with an assessment of efficacy and utility in a prospective 5000-patient study group. Neurosurgery 2009; 65(SUPPL. 4). https://doi.org/10.1227/01.NEU.0000351279.78110.00.

45. Chu J, Zhou Z, Hong G, et al. High-resolution MRI of the intraparotid facial nerve based on a microsurface coil and a 3d reversed fast imaging with steady-state precession DWI sequence at 3T. Am J Neuroradiol 2013;34(8):1643–8.

46. Fujii H, Fujita A, Yang A, et al. Visualization of the peripheral branches of the Mandibular division of the trigeminal nerve on 3D double-echo steady-state with water excitation sequence. AJNR Am J Neuroradiol 2015;36:1333–7.

47. Burian E, Sollmann N, Ritschl LM, et al. High resolution MRI for quantitative assessment of inferior alveolar nerve impairment in course of mandible fractures: an imaging feasibility study. Sci Rep 2020;10(1). https://doi.org/10.1038/s41598-020-68501-5.

48. Attyé A, Karkas A, Troprès I, et al. Parotid gland tumours: MR tractography to assess contact with the facial nerve. Eur Radiol 2016;26(7):2233–41.

49. Rouchy R-CC, Attyé A, Medici M, et al. Facial nerve tractography: A new tool for the detection of perineural spread in parotid cancers. Eur Radiol 2018; 28(9):3861–71.

50. Ginat DT, Mangla R, Yeaney G, et al. Diffusion-weighted imaging of skull lesions. J Neurol Surg B Skull Base 2014;75(3):204–13.

51. Schwartz KM, Lane JI, Neff BA, et al. Diffusion-weighted imaging for cholesteatoma evaluation. Ear Nose Throat J 2010;89(4):E14–9. Available at: https://pubmed.ncbi.nlm.nih.gov/20397131/. Accessed December 13, 2020.

52. Algin O, Aydın H, Ozmen E, et al. Detection of cholesteatoma: High-resolution DWI using RS-EPI and parallel imaging at 3 tesla. J Neuroradiol 2017; 44(6):388–94.

53. Li PMMC, Linos E, Gurgel RK, et al. Evaluating the utility of non-echo-planar diffusion-weighted imaging in the preoperative evaluation of cholesteatoma: A meta-analysis. Laryngoscope 2013;123(5):1247–50.

54. Porter DA, Heidemann RM. High Resolution Diffusion-Weighted Imaging Using Readout-Segmented Echo-Planar Imaging, Parallel Imaging and a Two-Dimensional Navigator-Based Reacquisition. Magn Reson Med 2009. https://doi.org/10.1002/mrm.22024.

55. Pipe JG, Farthing VG, Forbes KP. Multishot Diffusion-Weighted FSE Using PROPELLER MRI. Magn Reson Med 2002. https://doi.org/10.1002/mrm.10014.

56. Dudau C, Draper A, Gkagkanasiou M, et al. Cholesteatoma: multishot echo-planar *vs* non echo-planar diffusion-weighted MRI for the prediction of middle ear and mastoid cholesteatoma. BJR Open 2019; 1(1):20180015.

57. Welzel T, Meyerhof E, Uhl M, et al. Diagnostic accuracy of DW MR imaging in the differentiation of chordomas and chondrosarcomas of the skull base: A 3.0-T MRI study of 105 cases. Eur J Radiol 2018; 105:119–24.

58. Müller U, Kubik-Huch RA, Ares C, et al. Is there a role for conventional MRI and MR diffusion-weighted imaging for distinction of skull base chordoma and chondrosarcoma? Acta Radiol 2016; 57(2):225–32.

59. Sasaki T, Moritani T, Belay A, et al. Role of the apparent diffusion coefficient as a predictor of tumor

progression in patients with chordoma. Am J Neuroradiol 2018;39(7):1316–21.

60. Dremmen MHG, Hofman PAM, Hof JR, et al. The diagnostic accuracy of non-echo-planar diffusion-weighted imaging in the detection of residual and/or recurrent cholesteatoma of the temporal bone. Am J Neuroradiol 2012;33(3):439–44.

61. De Foer B, Vercruysse JP, Bernaerts A, et al. Detection of postoperative residual cholesteatoma with non-echo-planar diffusion-weighted magnetic resonance imaging. Otol Neurotol 2008;29(4):513–7.

62. Guler E, Ozgen B, Mut M, et al. The Added Value of Diffusion Magnetic Resonance Imaging in the Diagnosis and Posttreatment Evaluation of Skull Base Chordomas. J Neurol Surg B Skull Base 2017;78(3):256–65.

63. Abdel Razek AAK, Mahmoud W. Prediction of skull base osteomyelitis in necrotising otitis externa with diffusion-weighted imaging. J Laryngol Otol 2020;134(5):404–8.

64. Ozgen B, Oguz KK, Cila A. Diffusion MR imaging features of skull base osteomyelitis compared with skull base malignancy. Am J Neuroradiol 2011;32(1):179–84.

65. Ogawa T, Kojima I, Wakamori S, et al. Clinical utility of apparent diffusion coefficient and diffusion-weighted magnetic resonance imaging for resectability assessment of head and neck tumors with skull base invasion. Head Neck 2020;42(10):2896–904.

66. Ko CC, Lim SW, Chen TY, et al. Prediction of progression in skull base meningiomas: additional benefits of apparent diffusion coefficient value. J Neurooncol 2018;138(1):63–71.

67. Kunigelis KE, Hosokawa P, Arnone G, et al. The predictive value of preoperative apparent diffusion coefficient (ADC) for facial nerve outcomes after vestibular schwannoma resection: clinical study. Acta Neurochir (Wien) 2020;162(8):1995–2005.

68. Killeen DE, Perez CL, Chkheidze R, et al. Exploring the Association Between Apparent Diffusion Coefficient Values on Magnetic Resonance Imaging and the Response of Vestibular Schwannoma to Radiation. In: 30th Annual Meeting North American Skull Base Society. Vol 81. Georg Thieme Verlag KG; 2020:P228. San Antonio, February 7-9, 2020.

69. Moreau B, Iannessi A, Hoog C, et al. How reliable are ADC measurements? A phantom and clinical study of cervical lymph nodes. Eur Radiol 2018;28(8):3362–71.

70. Gaddikeri S, Gaddikeri RS, Tailor T, et al. Dynamic Contrast-Enhanced MR Imaging in Head and Neck Cancer: Techniques and Clinical Applications. AJNR Am J Neuroradiol 2015;37(4):1–8.

71. Kabadi SJ, Fatterpekar GM, Anzai Y, et al. Dynamic Contrast-Enhanced MR Imaging in Head and Neck Cancer. Magn Reson Imaging Clin N Am 2018;26(1):135–49.

72. Essig M, Shiroishi MS, Nguyen TB, et al. Perfusion MRI: The five most frequently asked technical questions. AJR Am J Roentgenol 2013;200(1):24–34. https://doi.org/10.2214/AJR.12.9543.

73. Choi YJ, Lee JH, Sung YS, et al. Value of dynamic contrast-enhanced MRI to detect local tumor recurrence in primary head and neck cancer patients. Med (United States) 2016;95(19). https://doi.org/10.1097/MD.0000000000003698.

74. Tofts PS, Brix G, Buckley DL, et al. Estimating kinetic parameters from dynamic contrast-enhanced T1-weighted MRI of a diffusable tracer: Standardized quantities and symbols. J Magn Reson Imaging 1999;10(3):223–32.

75. Geerts B, Leclercq D, Tezenas du Montcel S, et al. Characterization of Skull Base Lesions Using Pseudo-Continuous Arterial Spin Labeling. Clin Neuroradiol 2019;29(1):75–86.

76. Gaddikeri S, Hippe DS, Anzai Y. Dynamic Contrast-Enhanced MRI in the Evaluation of Carotid Space Paraganglioma versus Schwannoma. J Neuroimaging 2016;26(6):618–25.

77. Yuan Y, Shi H, Tao X. Head and neck paragangliomas: diffusion weighted and dynamic contrast enhanced magnetic resonance imaging characteristics. BMC Med Imaging 2016;16:12.

78. Ryu KH, Baek HJ, Cho SB, et al. Skull metastases detecting on arterial spin labeling perfusion Three case reports and review of literature. Med (United States). 2017;96(44). https://doi.org/10.1097/MD.0000000000008432.

79. Chidambaram S, Pannullo SC, Roytman M, et al. Dynamic contrast-enhanced magnetic resonance imaging perfusion characteristics in meningiomas treated with resection and adjuvant radiosurgery. Neurosurg Focus 2019;46(6):E10.

80. Qiao XJ, Kim HG, Wang DJJ, et al. Application of arterial spin labeling perfusion MRI to differentiate benign from malignant intracranial meningiomas. Eur J Radiol 2017;97:31–6.

81. Tanaka Y, Kohno M, Hashimoto T, et al. Arterial spin labeling imaging correlates with the angiographic and clinical vascularity of vestibular schwannomas. Neuroradiology 2020;62(4):463–71.

82. Zhang Y, Chen JH, Chen TY, et al. Radiomics approach for prediction of recurrence in skull base meningiomas. Neuroradiology 2019;61(12):1355–64.

83. Li L, Wang K, Ma X, et al. Radiomic analysis of multiparametric magnetic resonance imaging for differentiating skull base chordoma and chondrosarcoma. Eur J Radiol 2019;118:81–7.

84. Dickerson E, Srinivasan A. Advanced Imaging Techniques of the Skull Base. Radiol Clin North Am 2017;55(1):189–200.

85. Khaled M, Moghazy K, Elsaadany W, et al. Additional diagnostic role of MRI spectroscopy, diffusion and susceptibility imaging in differentiation of CPA masses: our experience with emphasis on schwannomas and meningiomas. Egypt J Radiol Nucl Med 2020;51(1):137.

86. Hughes J, ElSheikh M, Yin Z, et al. Magnetic Resonance Elastography in Vestibular Schwannoma. J Neurol Surg B Skull Base 2017;78(S 01):S1–156.

87. Huston J, Arani A, Hughes J, et al. Magnetic Resonance Elastography for Presurgical Assessment of Skull Base Lesions. J Neurol Surg B Skull Base 2015;76(S 01):A137.

1. Publication Title	2. Publication Number	3. Filing Date
NEUROIMAGING CLINICS OF NORTH AMERICA	010 – 548	9/18/2021

4. Issue Frequency	5. Number of Issues Published Annually	6. Annual Subscription Price
FEB, MAY, AUG, NOV	4	$397.00

7. Complete Mailing Address of Known Office of Publication (Not printer) (Street, city, county, state, and ZIP+4®)

ELSEVIER INC.
230 Park Avenue, Suite 800
New York, NY 10169

Contact Person
Malathi Samayan

Telephone (Include area code)
91-44-4299-4507

8. Complete Mailing Address of Headquarters or General Business Office of Publisher (Not printer)

ELSEVIER INC.
230 Park Avenue, Suite 800
New York, NY 10169

9. Full Names and Complete Mailing Addresses of Publisher, Editor, and Managing Editor (Do not leave blank)

Publisher (Name and complete mailing address)

Dolores Meloni, ELSEVIER INC.
1600 JOHN F KENNEDY BLVD. SUITE 1800
PHILADELPHIA, PA 19103-2899

Editor (Name and complete mailing address)

JOHN VASSALLO, ELSEVIER INC.
1600 JOHN F KENNEDY BLVD. SUITE 1800
PHILADELPHIA, PA 19103-2899

Managing Editor (Name and complete mailing address)

PATRICK MANLEY ELSEVIER INC.
1600 JOHN F KENNEDY BLVD. SUITE 1800
PHILADELPHIA, PA 19103-2899

10. Owner (Do not leave blank. If the publication is owned by a corporation, give the name and address of the corporation immediately followed by the names and addresses of all stockholders owning or holding 1 percent or more of the total amount of stock. If not owned by a corporation, give the names and addresses of the individual owners. If owned by a partnership or other unincorporated firm, give its name and address as well as those of each individual owner. If the publication is published by a nonprofit organization, give its name and address.)

Full Name	Complete Mailing Address
WHOLLY OWNED SUBSIDIARY OF REED/ELSEVIER, US HOLDINGS	1600 JOHN F KENNEDY BLVD. SUITE 1800 PHILADELPHIA, PA 19103-2899

11. Known Bondholders, Mortgagees, and Other Security Holders Owning or Holding 1 Percent or More of Total Amount of Bonds, Mortgages, or Other Securities. If none, check box ▸ ☐ None

Full Name	Complete Mailing Address
N/A	

12. Tax Status (For completion by nonprofit organizations authorized to mail at nonprofit rates) (Check one)
The purpose, function, and nonprofit status of this organization and the exempt status for federal income tax purposes:
☒ Has Not Changed During Preceding 12 Months
☐ Has Changed During Preceding 12 Months (Publisher must submit explanation of change with this statement)

PS Form 3526, July 2014 [Page 1 of 4 (see instructions page 4)] PSN: 7530-01-000-9931   PRIVACY NOTICE: See our privacy policy on www.usps.com.

13. Publication Title	14. Issue Date for Circulation Data Below
NEUROIMAGING CLINICS OF NORTH AMERICA	MAY 2021

15. Extent and Nature of Circulation			Average No. Copies Each Issue During Preceding 12 Months	No. Copies of Single Issue Published Nearest to Filing Date
a. Total Number of Copies (Net press run)			394	371
b. Paid Circulation (By Mail and Outside the Mail)	(1)	Mailed Outside-County Paid Subscriptions Stated on PS Form 3541 (Include paid distribution above nominal rate, advertiser's proof copies, and exchange copies)	293	276
	(2)	Mailed In-County Paid Subscriptions Stated on PS Form 3541 (Include paid distribution above nominal rate, advertiser's proof copies, and exchange copies)	0	0
	(3)	Paid Distribution Outside the Mails Including Sales Through Dealers and Carriers, Street Vendors, Counter Sales, and Other Paid Distribution Outside USPS®	63	49
	(4)	Paid Distribution by Other Classes of Mail Through the USPS (e.g., First-Class Mail®)	0	0
c. Total Paid Distribution [Sum of 15b (1), (2), (3), and (4)]		▸	356	325
d. Free or Nominal Rate Distribution (By Mail and Outside the Mail)	(1)	Free or Nominal Rate Outside-County Copies included on PS Form 3541	22	31
	(2)	Free or Nominal Rate In-County Copies Included on PS Form 3541	0	0
	(3)	Free or Nominal Rate Copies Mailed at Other Classes Through the USPS (e.g., First-Class Mail)	0	0
	(4)	Free or Nominal Rate Distribution Outside the Mail (Carriers or other means)	0	0
e. Total Free or Nominal Rate Distribution (Sum of 15d (1), (2), (3) and (4))		▸	22	31
f. Total Distribution (Sum of 15c and 15e)		▸	378	356
g. Copies not Distributed (See Instructions to Publishers #4 (page #3))		▸	16	15
h. Total (Sum of 15f and g)			394	371
i. Percent Paid (15c divided by 15f times 100)		▸	94.17%	91.29%

* If you are claiming electronic copies, go to line 16 on page 3. If you are not claiming electronic copies, skip to line 17 on page 3.

PS Form **3526**, July 2014 (Page 2 of 4)

16. Electronic Copy Circulation	Average No. Copies Each Issue During Preceding 12 Months	No. Copies of Single Issue Published Nearest to Filing Date
a. Paid Electronic Copies ▸		
b. Total Paid Print Copies (Line 15c) + Paid Electronic Copies (Line 16a) ▸		
c. Total Print Distribution (Line 15f) + Paid Electronic Copies (Line 16a) ▸		
d. Percent Paid (Both Print & Electronic Copies) (16b divided by 16c × 100) ▸		

☒ I certify that 50% of all my distributed copies (electronic and print) are paid above a nominal price.

17. Publication of Statement of Ownership

☒ If the publication is a general publication, publication of this statement is required. Will be printed
in the NOVEMBER 2021 issue of this publication.

☐ Publication not required.

18. Signature and Title of Editor, Publisher, Business Manager, or Owner

Malathi Samayan

Malathi Samayan - Distribution Controller

Date 9/18/2021

I certify that all information furnished on this form is true and complete. I understand that anyone who furnishes false or misleading information on this form or who omits material or information requested on the form may be subject to criminal sanctions (including fines and imprisonment) and/or civil sanctions (including civil penalties).

PS Form **3526**, July 2014 (Page 3 of 4)   PRIVACY NOTICE: See our privacy policy on www.usps.com.

Printed and bound by CPI Group (UK) Ltd, Croydon, CR0 4YY

03/10/2024

01040307-0004